Introduction to
Health Assessment

Introduction to
Health Assessment

Willa L. Fields, R.N., M.S.Ed.
Karen M. McGinn-Campbell, R.N., M.S.N.

Reston Publishing Company, Inc.
A Prentice-Hall Company
Reston, Virginia

Library of Congress Cataloging in Publication Data

Fields, Willa L.
  Introduction to health assessment.

  Includes bibliographical references and index.
  1. Nursing.   2. Medical history taking.
3. Physical diagnosis. I. McGinn-Campbell, Karen M.
II. Title. [DNLM: 1. Diagnosis—Nursing texts.
2. Nursing process. WY 100 I613]
RT48.F53 1983   616.07′5   82-9149
ISBN 0-8359-3191-9   AACR2

© 1983 by Reston Publishing Company, Inc.
A Prentice-Hall Company
Reston, Virginia 22090

10   9   8   7   6   5   4   3   2   1

Printed in the United States of America

We dedicate this book to our husbands,
Edward and Cameron,
and to our children,
Lisa and Alison
and
Erin, Eric, and Corinne

Contents

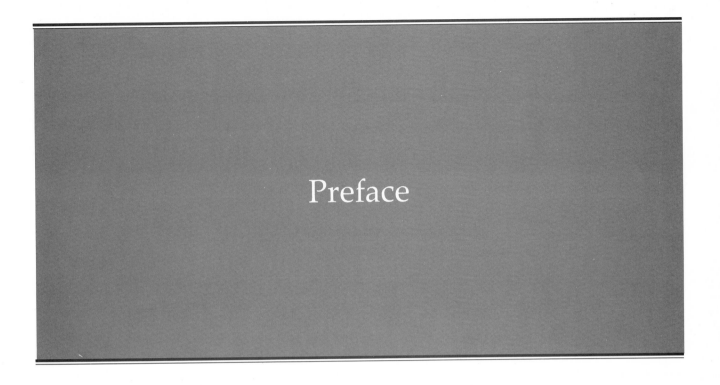

Preface

Health assessment techniques are the foundation of health care delivery. In all aspects of the health care delivery system, nurses are responsible for partial or total health assessment. With this in mind, *Introduction to Health Assessment* is designed for students in clinical and didactic courses on health assessment. The beginning student will find the organization of the text helpful in mastering this new knowledge. The more advanced student will find the depth of concepts discussed and the charts for abnormal findings helpful in synthesizing the health assessment process into clinical performance.

The organization of the book is by body regions and systems utilized in a total health assessment. Several unconventional chapters for a book on health assessment are included. These chapters include fluid and electrolyte balance and acid–base balance, as well as nutritional, hematological, and psychosocial assessment. These areas are fundamental in the regulation and promotion of health.

Most chapters follow a standard organization for easy reference. The first section, Anatomy and Physiology, includes those concepts relevant to the physical manifestations of health and illness. This information provides a foundation for learning health assessment skills.

Each chapter has a section on preparation for both the client and examiner. Any special position or clothing for the client is discussed. Also included is a list of the equipment necessary for performing the examination.

The standard assessment modalities (inspection, palpation, percussion, and auscultation) are discussed in their order of use. Any additional modalities or techniques are also discussed in this section. For example, in Chapter 7 on the eye, testing of visual acuity is presented.

The text is written in terms of a middle aged adult, and each chapter includes a section on life cycle variations. This section presents the changes in findings that occur during the other developmental stages (childhood, adolescence, pregnancy, and late adulthood). Assessment techniques used specifically with particular age groups are discussed here.

The content of the chapters includes the range of normal, or the healthy state. Throughout the chapters various charts are presented showing abnormal findings, their various causes, and a description or explanation of the finding. It is through these charts that the student's knowledge of normal can be applied to define and identify abnormal. Discussion of pathophysiology and psychopathology is beyond the scope of this text. *Introduction to Health Assessment* is limited to a discussion of normal and an identification of abnormal.

According to *The Living Webster Encyclopedia Dictionary of the English Language,* a client is "one who resorts to another for professional . . . services." A patient is a "person who is under medical treatment." Based on these two definitions, we chose to use "client" when the receiver of the examination is a healthy person in an out-patient facility. The word patient is used when we are referring to an ill person in a hospital setting who is being examined to follow the course of the treatment or illness. Of course, there is an overlap in the two definitions.

We wish to acknowledge those individuals who assisted us in preparing this book. Their suggestions and encouragement were most valuable:

Clyde Beck, M.D.; Joanne Butler, R.N., C.N.P.; Mary Jane Coombs, R.N., M.S.N.; Ginny Deutsch, R.N., A.N.P.; Victoria DiCicco, Ph.D.; Dean Echols, M.D.; Donna Ehrenreich, R.N., M.N., C. S.; Richard Hall, M.D.; James Hanson, M.D.; Benjamin Hourani, M.D.; Martin Le Winter, M.D.; Geoffrey McPherson, M.D.; Donley McReynolds, M.D.; Stuart Menn, M.D.; John Meyers, M.D.; Eli Miller, M.D.; LeRoy Miller, M.D.; Vicki Miller, R.N.; Bonnie Omara, R.N.; Sandra Pflaum, R.N., M.S.N.; Sheila Pickwell, R.N., M.N., C.F.N.P.; Paul Raffer, M.D.; Harold Richards, M.D.; David Roseman, M.D.; Jeffrey Schaeffer, M.D.; Fred Schnepper, M.D.; Frances Selder, R.N., C.N.P.; Edward Singer, M.D.; Marcie Smith, R.N., B.S.N.; William Smith, M.D.; Rita Solberg, R.N., M.N.; Sandra Buffington Sucek, R.N., C.N.P.; Roger Tibbetts, D.D.S.; Geneal Walton, R.D. Jane Malloy and Kathy Stevenson, our typists, were always available when we needed them.

Introduction to
Health Assessment

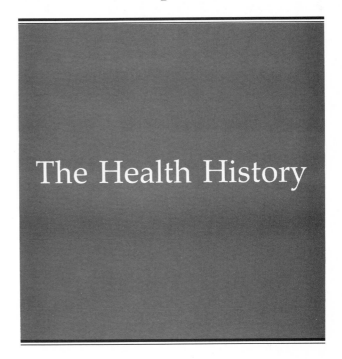

Chapter 1

The Health History

The health history is a collection of subjective data provided by the client (historian) and compiled by the health professional (interviewer). It is usually obtained during an interview prior to the physical examination. The history contains information pertaining to the client's present health and health practices, past health, perceptions of relationships with others, knowledge of and concerns about the health of family members, and feelings and reactions toward developmental stages. The history is an essential component in health assessment. It contains information that illuminates individual strengths and weaknesses, that is, past and present susceptibility and resistance to psychologic as well as physical stresses. The history also identifies health risks such as hereditary and environmental factors and indicates potential or existing problems such as disease.

The information obtained in the history is highly personal; therefore, the client must feel comfortable with the interviewer before this private information can be divulged. Since the comprehensive history most frequently is taken during the initial interview, the interviewer and client are usually strangers. The interviewer therefore, has the challenge of establishing rapport in a minimal amount of time.

Compiling an accurate and thorough history is a difficult health assessment skill to master and is an essential prerequisite to the physical examination. Some experts approximate that 80 percent of assessment is based upon historical data and that the physical examination derives much of its importance from validating the information elicited during the interview.

The dialogue between client and interviewer is termed the *interview*. Optimally the health history is completed during the initial interview; however, in many situations this is not possible, and additional data are obtained at subsequent encounters. For example, individuals who require emergency care are asked to provide information regarding only the immediate problem. Completion of the history is delayed until after resolution of the immediate crisis.

The history is an ongoing collection of information. Each time a client presents, additional life experiences have occurred that have had some effect on health or the perception of health; this additional information is added to the history.

Objectives

The interviewer will be able to do the following:

1. Provide a private, comfortable environment for the interview
2. Individualize interviewing techniques to maximize the client's ability to share information
3. Obtain a comprehensive health history
4. Record a comprehensive health history

Interviewing Skills

Interviewers should strive to improve interviewing skills in all encounters with patients and clients whether for comprehensive or limited data collection.

Each session increases the interviewer's skill in dealing with the personal and often emotional aspects of the health history.

Questionnaires. Many health history questionnaires are available. They are completed by clients prior to the interview. They range from comprehensive history forms to forms for specific situations, such as questionnaires for people experiencing gastrointestinal problems. Some are as short as 1 page, while others run more than 50 pages and require considerable time and interest on the part of the client. The forms may contain a variety of types of questions, such as fill-in-the-blank or multiple-choice. Although there is tremendous variety among forms, all are designed for the interviewer to review with the client and seek clarification of certain points.

Questionnaires are certainly timesaving devices, but they have some major drawbacks. They are often confusing to clients and lack specificity and detail. Forms that ask branching questions to provide specificity are often too complex and frequently bore or confuse clients. Also, since some questionnaires are comprehensive, they require many hours to complete. Questionnaires are best utilized as an adjunct to the interview process.

Communication Skills

General Considerations

Many students new at obtaining histories have the experience of questioning a client and feeling somewhat confused, as if the client is "holding back" useful information. To complicate matters further, upon returning to the same client with an instructor or more experienced interviewer, the student observes an entirely different scenario. The client is talkative, elaborates on certain key points, and may even seem to contradict some previously obtained data. Expertise at assisting clients to feel comfortable and speak freely accompanies practice of basic communication skills.

Listening. It cannot be overemphasized that the interviewer's primary role in history taking is listening. The history is the client's story. The interviewer listens intently to convey interest and facilitate communication, which in turn maximizes information gathering. Often an interviewer is concerned with the next question and does not listen fullly to what the client is saying.

Individualizing. Because of vastly differing physical, educational, social, psychological, and experiential factors among clients, the interviewer's major concern is to individualize the approach in order to facilitate client comfort and to establish rapport.

Flexibility. Flexibility is easier for the more experienced interviewer due to familiarity with the history format. New interviewers frequently fear that they will forget an important question or area of inquiry and therefore attempt to adhere to a rigid method of gathering data. Although the history is recorded in a standard format, the actual order of topics discussed during the interview is varied to address the individual client's needs. For instance, if during a routine examination a woman expresses concern over her child, she would perceive the interviewer as interested if this topic were pursued first. After the client's most important issues are fully discussed, the interviewer proceeds with the portions that were temporarily bypassed.

Genuine Interest and Trust in Clients. Genuine interest and trust can be conveyed only when the interviewer firmly believes that clients are interested in and responsible for their own health. Genuine interest and trust are also conveyed by nonverbal communication such as body language and voice intonations. The interested interviewer sits in a relaxed, alert, and attentive position; leans slightly forward; and maintains eye contact.

Personal space is an aspect of body language with cultural and individual variables. It refers to the distance an individual maintains from another person. In general, people of Hispanic and Middle Eastern origin are comfortable with less personal space than people of Asiatic and Northern European origin. Touching is generally more appropriate with the former. For example, the interviewer can convey empathy for a profound emotional experience such as death with a touch on the shoulder, back, or hand. The interviewer modulates the voice appropriately by following the client's cues.

Ability to Put Clients at Ease. To help a client feel at ease, it is essential to respect the individual, provide privacy, and maintain confidentiality. It is always desirable to obtain the history in a separate room with a closed door, free from interruptions by phone calls, and other people. Sometimes the history must be obtained in a hospital room while other patients and staff are present. Even in these cases, asking visitors to leave during the interview and drawing the curtains around the bed contribute toward patient privacy. Another approach is to plan the interview outside visiting hours and while the patient's roommates are in another department.

Sensitivity. Proceeding from less emotionally charged items to more emotionally charged items is helpful since it gives the client an opportunity to establish a sense of trust in the interviewer. For example, the history usually begins with a collection of biographical data. Later in the interview the interviewer asks about more personal areas such as sexuality. However, if the client expresses concern over a sexual matter and is eager to discuss it, delaying discussion to the end of the interview could convey disinterest or disapproval on the part of the examiner.

Language. Another consideration involves judging the client's language ability and adapting to it. Frequently examiners use professional jargon, which tends to frustrate, confuse, belittle, or anger clients. On the other hand extremely simplistic phraseology appears condescending to a person who understands professional terminology.

When interviewing a non-English-speaking person, an interpreter is necessary if the examiner is not fluent in that language. Interviewers who work with largely non-English-speaking populations should make an effort to learn some phrases in those languages. However, it is important to recognize one's own limitations and obtain the help of an interpreter when necessary, in order to assure an accurate and complete history. Regardless of language, all persons respond to nonverbal communication, such as eye contact, voice intonations, and personal space considerations. A gesture that can demonstrate genuine interest in the client is using at least a few introductory remarks and general questions in the client's language before proceeding with an interpreter. This can convey to the client that the interviewer respects the native tongue and culture.

Writing During the Interview. Many clients find it distracting to talk while the interviewer writes. Also, it is difficult to listen fully while concentrating on writing. Therefore, it is best to listen with only an occasional note as a reminder. It is generally possible to review forgotten details with the client.

Client Variables. A client's willingness and ability to give an accurate health history are influenced by the level of anxiety, language ability, perceptions and expectations of health professionals, interest in health, comfort with strangers, previous experiences with health care, trust in the interviewer, and physical and psychological well-being (Table 1-1).

Communication Techniques

Beginning with a self-introduction, the interviewer calls the client by name and explains the purpose of the history. For example,

Hello, my name is Mrs. Carter. I'm a nurse practitioner at the clinic, Mr. Boyd. I'll be asking you some questions about your present and past health. After this interview and a physical examination, you and I will review what I've learned about you and discuss areas of concern.

The interviewer's role is threefold: to direct the communication process in order to incorporate all important data; to organize information into a meaningful whole; and to record the history accurately.

Open-ended Questioning. Nondirective or open-ended questioning encourages a free flow of ideas by the client. It minimizes interviewer verbalization and fosters maximal client involvement. For example, the client is asked, "How would you describe your sleeping habits?" In answering this question, the client might respond, "Well, I live in a noisy apartment so I usually sleep a restless four hours at night, but I usually nap soundly for three to four hours in the afternoon."

The opposite of open-ended questioning is forced-choice questioning. An example is, "How many hours a night do you sleep?" To this question the client responds, "Four hours." Forced-choice questioning encourages client passivity, and often the client perceives the examiner as interested only in short answers with no description.

Another type of question in contradistinction to the open-ended question is the biased question. With this line of questioning the interviewer implies the expected answers. For example, if the interviewer asks, "You attend a church regularly, don't you?" that implies an expected affirmative answer. The client may feel that it would be unacceptable to the interviewer's values to hear the real situation. A better way to ask about religious background is the following: "Can you tell me how religion influences your life?"

Controlling the Interview. Through open-ended questioning the client is encouraged to use the client's own words. However, the interviewer controls the interview by guiding the discussion to include a thorough investigation of each aspect of the history prior to proceeding to a new topic. Discussion is limited to relevant information, and the client is redirected to the topic at hand when the subject is changed. For instance, sometimes clients ask examiners about their personal lives. In the following example the professional redirects the discussion.

INTERVIEWER: You're a steelworker, I see. How would you describe your feelings toward your job?

Table 1.1.   Effects of Certain Client Variables on Interview

Variable	Client Reaction	Possible Outcome
Level of anxiety	High anxiety: unsure of what to expect from history and physical.	Extremely talkative with frequent attempts to change topic or talk about other matters.
	High anxiety: fears diagnosis of cancer or other terminal illness.	Denial of symptoms.
Language ability	Fluent in a foreign language only, limited use of English.	Quiet, persistent yes-no answers.
	Limited education.	Intimidated by examiner, afraid to say "wrong" thing.
Perceptions of health professional	Sees interviewer as interested.	Feels important and therefore sees own input, the history, as highly important; strives to provide accurate answers.
	Sees examiner as condescending and hurried.	Feels embarrassed to talk about self; fears may say something stupid.
Interest in health	Great interest, reads extensively in lay literature, and applies this knowledge.	Highly motivated to give history. One important point to emphasize is that although highly motivated, this kind of client may be operating on some basic misconceptions; therefore it is essential to maintain an investigative attitude as opposed to relying on the client's self-diagnoses.
	Little interest.	Unwilling to provide clarifying information spontaneously.
Comfort with strangers	Shy, uncomfortable.	Quiet, anxious to get interview over with, provides hurried answers
	Outgoing, comfortable with strangers.	Readily provides information.
Expectations of health professionals	Unrealistically high, prefers to leave everything up to the interviewer, will let interviewer worry about it (health): It's too complicated for me. I'm not a doctor."	May feel that it is the interviewer's sole responsibility to find out "what's wrong."
	Realistic.	Views interviewer's and own roles as complementary.
	Unrealistically low.	Little confidence in interviewer's ability: "Are you sure you're getting all this?"
Previous experience with health care	Has traditionally had vital interest in health and has felt that health professionals respected this interest and worked in a complementary fashion.	Willing and able to provide thorough responses.
	Has felt that client input was not important.	Little desire to provide information.
Trust in the interviewer	Feels interviewer is interested and will try to help.	Willing to provide a comprehensive health history.
	Little trust in the interviewer.	Attitude of "What's the use?" Unwilling to speak freely.
Physical well-being	Experiencing pain.	Preoccupied, anxious for relief of pain, fearful of meaning of pain.
	Physically comfortable.	Able to focus on history.
Psychologic well-being	Depressed.	Disinterested in interview and provides inconsistent and vague responses.
	Well-integrated personality, coping with stress.	Willing and able to provide thorough responses.

CLIENT: It's okay. What are your hours like here? Do you like this sort of work?

INTERVIEWER: Yes, I enjoy my work, but I prefer to limit our discussion to your work so that we can complete your history.

Frequently clients have several problems and discuss them in a haphazard manner. This occurs because they are usually unaware of pathophysiology and want to be sure to include everything. In these cases it is often helpful to write a list of problems and assure the client that each area will be explored in depth. Throughout the interview, if other problems are uncovered, they can be added to the list. For example, a woman relates the following:

> I have headaches a lot, well, probably because of our marriage problems. My husband and I fight a lot since he has been out of work. He gets mad at me all the time because I don't want to make love anymore. We have money problems and have four kids already.

The astute interviewer appreciates that this person has many problems. Although open-ended questioning facilitates the client telling her story in her own words, the interviewer, as an objective listener, is challenged to direct the conversation in an organized manner. In the preceding example the interviewer could say the following:

> Mrs. X, it seems that you have quite a few things on your mind. Let me make a list of the things you have mentioned so that we don't overlook any of them. Then it would be less confusing to me if you could tell me all about one item at a time. Which of these would you like to explain first? [Interviewer shows client the list: husband unemployed, fearful of another pregnancy, financial difficulties, headaches, disagreement over sexual life, marital problems.]

Seeking Clarification. Although the order among topics is not important—except that related ones usually follow one another—discussion of each one should proceed from general to specific information. After the client gives a general description of a particular item, the interviewer directs the discussion to provide increasingly detailed information.

Reflecting Feelings. The interview provides nonverbal as well as verbal information. Because these nonverbal cues may sometimes be misinterpreted just as words can be misunderstood, it is often helpful for the interviewer to reflect the client's feelings. Reflecting feelings involves making a statement about the interviewer's perceptions of what the client is experiencing.

The following statement can have different meanings when made with a variety of voice intonations, mannerisms, and facial expressions: "I haven't been sick much in my life." The emotional state conveyed if the client emphasizes the word *much*, while rolling the eyes and lifting the head, could mean sarcasm as if to ask the interviewer, "Are you really listening to what I am saying?" On the other hand the client could be exasperated with past health and fearful of the future. To this the interviewer responds, "As I understand it, you have had quite a few illnesses, and you're really down about that and afraid of what will happen next." If the client emphasizes the words *I* and *my* and talks in a relaxed manner, the client might be affirming a long history of good health and looking for some positive feedback. An appropriate response by the interviewer is the following: "You seem to have remained very healthy, and that makes you happy and proud."

Summarizing. Often it is desirable to state in the interviewer's own words a summary of what the client has said. In summarizing, the interviewer is assured that the message received is the message sent. Occasionally the client modifies the description after hearing the interviewer's account. The following example illustrates this phenomenon.

INTERVIEWER: So you say it is a sharp, stabbing pain—like a knife—that starts about 30 minutes after eating. . . .

CLIENT: Well, it's not really sharp—maybe more like a severe burning feeling. . . .

Components of the Comprehensive Health History

The health history is recorded in a standardized format to facilitate use by various members of the health care delivery system. However, the order of topics discussed during the interview corresponds with the patient's or client's priorities. Frequently the physical condition of clients or time limitations dictate that partial histories be taken, with information relevant at the moment only. However, since this necessitates a high level of clinical judgment, beginning students are encouraged to practice taking and recording the *complete* health history.

The format of the comprehensive health history is as follows:

1. Identifying data (client profile)

2. Chief complaint (reason for presenting for health care)

3. History of present illness (present state of health)

4. Past health history

5. Family history

6. Psychosocial history

7. Socioeconomic history

8. Nutritional history

9. Review of systems

Identifying Data

The history begins with detailed biographical information. Frequently clients themselves provide this information by completing a questionnaire (Table 1-2).

Chief Complaint or Reason for Presenting for Health Care

Traditionally a brief description in the client's own words of why health care is sought has been called the *chief complaint* (CC). This term is appropriate when

Table 1-2. Identifying Data

Item	*Rationale*
A. Full name (includes maiden name)	Assures exact identification and reduces likelihood of confusion with another person.
B. Address and telephone number at home and at work (includes client's information and the same information about a contact person.	Facilitates contacting client if necessary. Upon subsequent visits the interviewer inquires if there are any address or phone number changes.
C. Birthdate in full	Facilitates interviewer's awareness of age-related health risks.
D. Sex	Facilitates interviewer's awareness of sex-related health risks.
E. Race	Facilitates interviewer's awareness of racially related health risks.
F. Religion	Increases interviewer's sensitivity to and awareness of client's life style.
G. Marital status and number of children	Establishes a basis for later description in family, psychosocial and socioeconomic histories.
H. Social Security number	Increases precision of identification.
I. Occupation	Increases interviewer's awareness of environmental health risks, level of activity, and job-related stress.
J. Birthplace	Assists in identifying health risks and increases interviewer's understanding of the social history.
K. Referral source	Lays a foundation for understanding the client's role with health care professionals and facilitates interviewer's awareness of any existing data available at another facility.
L. Informant and reliability	Establishes the validity of the data collected and increases the interviewer's awareness of the client's relationship with significant others. The interviewer's perceptions of the informant's reliability are important. Frequently the client is disoriented because of illness or drugs, and the data are conflicting or confusing. Although it is best to obtain the history from the client, sometimes it is necessary to obtain the history from another informant. Whenever possible, the accuracy is validated and the history is supplemented at a later date by rechecking with the client.
M. Date of interview	Establishes information in a time frame as a reference point for later comparisons.

the client presents with symptomatology. Since health care is a service provided to maintain optimal health and prevent illness, this section is more appropriately entitled the reason for presenting for health care, when the client is asymptomatic. Whenever possible the duration is included in this statement. The interviewer asks the client, "What brings you here today?" The following are examples of client responses:

Chief complaint: Stomachaches and diarrhea for three weeks

Reason for presenting: Desires yearly checkup and pre-employment physical

This section is confined to what the client is experiencing. It is not a diagnostic statement, such as asthma for 12 hours. If a diagnosis is given as a chief complaint, the client is questioned as to what specifically has been happening. For example,

INTERVIEWER: You've had an asthmatic attack for 12 hours? What has been happening during this attack?

CLIENT: I've been wheezing and I can't seem to catch my breath.

The chief complaint is then recorded as "wheezing and can't catch breath for 12 hours." It is important to avoid the use of diagnostic nomenclature in this section for several reasons. First of all, the patient frequently misdiagnoses the condition and might omit useful contributory information. Second, it undermines the investigatory nature of the interview. For the same reason the interviewer must avoid jumping to diagnostic conclusions at the outset. Once a problem is diagnosed, the tendency may be for the interviewer to reflect the client's assumptions rather than maintain objectivity.

History of Present Illness or Present State of Health

This section contains a thorough investigation of the chief complaint or a more detailed description of the well client's health status. The components of the history of present illness (HPI) or present state of health are as follows:

A. Introduction
   1. Description of client
   2. Usual health
B. Chronological investigation of symptoms
   1. Course of symptomatology: incidence, duration, and manner

   2. Symptom analysis: aggravating, alleviating, and associated factors; location; quality; quantity; and setting
C. Pertinent negatives
D. Relevant family history, psychological and social data
E. Assessment of disability
F. Related medications including over-the-counter medications

Introduction. The introduction is a brief biographical section including age, sex, marital status, occupation, and employment status. It also includes the number of visits to the interviewer's facility and the number of hospital admissions for the problem identified in the chief complaint section, or for any other problem related to it. In addition, it contains information about the client's usual health status and any previous or present health problems. Several examples are the following:

Introduction. This is the first visit for this 17-year-old, unmarried, black female high-school-student, who is healthy and has never had serious health problems.

Introduction. This is the first hospital admission for this 30-year-old Mexican-American, a separated father of four, a self-employed brick layer. Health has always been good until two years ago, when burning in stomach began. Was unable to go to work today because of weakness, vomiting, and severe stomach pain.

Chronological Investigation of Symptoms. In this section the interviewer investigates the course of each symptom and uses clarification for symptom analysis. The course of symptomatology refers to chronology and includes onset, incidence, duration, and manner.

Onset describes when the symptom first occurred and may be sudden or gradual. *Incidence* refers to the frequency of the symptom. *Duration* applies to the amount of time the symptom lasts. All are documented in standard terms, for example, *upon awakening in the morning, 30 minutes after meals, twice a day,* and *for three hours.* Terms such as *frequently, a lot,* and *often* are inexact and confusing. *Manner* describes the nature of the symptom over time, for example, *intermittent, constant, continually worsening,* and *crescendo-decrescendo* (increasing for a specific amount of time and then decreasing).

In symptom analysis the interviewer seeks to identify seven dimensions: aggravating, alleviating, or associated factors; location; quality; quantity; and setting.

An *aggravating factor* seems to increase the intensity of a symptom, while an *alleviating factor* seems to produce a lessening effect. An *associated factor* appears to be related to the feeling being discussed or seems to occur at the same time. For example,

INTERVIEWER: Did you notice any other changes during the headache?

CLIENT: Well, as a matter of fact, I felt sick to my stomach and was afraid that I would vomit.

The *location* applies to the specific place where a symptom is experienced. Most frequently it is used for pinpointing an area where pain occurs and includes the origin and any radiation to other areas.

The *quality* of the symptom is described in the client's words as specifically as possible. Sometimes it is helpful to ask the client if it feels like anything experienced before. An example is the feeling of pressure or chest constriction during a myocardial infarction. Patients often describe this feeling as if the weight of an elephant were sitting upon the chest. There are at least 50 descriptive words in the English language for pain; however, the most commonly used ones are *aching, burning, dull, sharp, stabbing, stinging,* and *throbbing.*

The *quantity* is the amount experienced in concrete, measurable terms, such as minutes, hours, days, or weeks. For instance, the client relates, "My heart was racing. My pulse was up to 200 for 15 minutes."

The *setting* refers to the circumstances surrounding the symptom. This applies to who was present, where it occurred, and during what kind of activity. The following is an example of the family counselor's process of seeking clarification of a general statement.

CLIENT: My husband and I are having marital problems.

INTERVIEWER: Tell me more about that.

CLIENT: We fight a lot.

INTERVIEWER: You're fighting more than you used to?

CLIENT: It seems like we fight all the time. Whenever we are in the same room, one of us seems to get mad at the other.

INTERVIEWER: Is there anything else going on that seems related to these fights?

CLIENT: Well, my husband lost his job three months ago, because of a big funding cut. I guess we're both worried about finances more than anything else.

INTERVIEWER: Anything else?

CLIENT: I'm afraid I'll get pregnant again, so I haven't been too interested in bed.

INTERVIEWER: Does anything seem to help?

CLIENT: We used to go out once a week until the job layoff. That gave us a chance to talk alone without the kids. Now we can't afford it.

Of course, for the well client the chronological investigation of symptoms is usually omitted. If later in the interview, usually during the review of systems, a symptom is uncovered, it would most appropriately be discussed then. For example, when a client presents for a routine checkup and later mentions amenorrhea for two months, this symptom is fully investigated, and recorded in the present illness section, proceeding from the most remote to the most recent symptoms as follows:

Five years ago: Menarche—age 13—menses every 29–31 days, lasting 4–5 days of moderate blood flow (saturates 5–6 tampons/day). Mild cramping on second day that usually responds to aspirin, grains 10, bid.

Two years ago: Began having unprotected sexual relations with steady boyfriend about twice/month. Has never practiced contraception because it would "ruin the naturalness."

Two months ago: Last menstrual period (LMP)—December 4, period different than usual—lighter flow and lasted two days.

One week ago: Noticed breast tenderness and fullness and began to experience nausea every evening.

The chief complaint is changed to say, "desires routine checkup and thinks she is pregnant (LMP—December 4)."

Pertinent Negatives. A negative response to certain questions about symptoms is just as important as a positive response in assessment. This is referred to as a *pertinent negative.* The items can be symptoms, as well as information from any other section of the history (family history, psychosocial history, socioeconomic history, or nutritional history) that could have significance in the overall course of health or illness. Hence the descriptive word *pertinent* is used. Some relationships are obvious; for example, persons with any respiratory system symptoms are asked about their smoking history and persons with vascular changes such as cold extremities or intermittent claudication are asked about family history of angina, arrhythmias, arteriosclerosis, hypertension, and myocardial infarction. A good rule of thumb for beginning interviewers is to ask all of the review of system questions for a given system or region when symptoms of that system or region are mentioned in the history of present illness.

Disability. An assessment of disability indicates what changes in life style the client has made as a result of the symptoms discussed in the history of present illness. For example, a client who relates recent difficulties in walking to work (a distance of 1 mile), due to shortness of breath and fatigue has made a quantitative statement about the effects of declining health on life style. Disability also includes financial constraints and physical limitations imposed by illness or injury.

Medications. All medications taken by the client are recorded in this manner: drug's name, dosage, frequency of administration, and description of the effect of the drug and any untoward reactions. Over-the-counter drugs including vitamins, aspirin, and cold remedies are also listed.

This additional information in the history of present illness is written in prose. The following is an example of a completed history of present illness for a client with burning pains in the stomach.

Pertinent negatives: Denies diarrhea, melena, belching, nausea, jaundice, dysphagia, bloating, constipation, and hemorrhoids.

Family history: Paternal grandfather died of stomach hemorrhage at age 45. Father—age 64—three hospital admissions for bleeding peptic ulcers. Well since ulcer surgery 5 years ago.

Socioeconomic history: Smokes two packs of cigarettes/day for 15 years. Stopped drinking coffee and cola drinks 2 years ago. Drinks beer with buddies—about a six-pack every Friday night. Still fights with wife about twice/week over children. Business slow.

Medications: Maalox, two tablets, 30 minutes after meals and between meals, about 20/day, provides relief for 30 minutes.

Disability: Uninsured. Worried about loss of income during hospitalization and about ability to pay for medical expenses.

Past Health History

The past health history is a record of all major health problems that the client has experienced and possible sources of problems. The following items are included:

A. Past illnesses
   Childhood diseases
   Serious injuries, accidents, and disabilities
   Hospitalizations (medical and psychiatric)
   Surgical procedures
   Transfusions
   Major illnesses (medical and psychiatric)
B. Allergies
   Food
   Drug
   Environmental
C. Immunizations
D. Military service
E. Foreign travel
F. Diagnostic procedures

Past Illnesses. Most clients know whether they have had the childhood diseases. At this point, they are asked specifically about measles, mumps, rubella, and chicken pox. Occasionally clients forget about injuries; asking about accidents, broken bones, or serious burns serves as a reminder. Hospitalizations are listed with date, name of hospital, name of attending physician or practitioner, reason for admission, and discharge diagnosis. Surgical procedures are itemized with dates and descriptions. Clients may be confused when asked whether they have ever had any major illnesses. Most clients are not aware which diseases are considered major, nor do they appreciate the significance of screening for them. The examiner asks, "Have you ever been told that you have any of the following conditions or received treatment for them: alcoholism, arrhythmias, arteriosclerosis, asthma, blood diseases, cancer, coronary artery disease, depression or other emotional problems, diabetes, gout, hepatitis, hypertension, kidney stones, urinary tract infection, rheumatic fever, scarlet fever, tuberculosis, and venereal disease."

Allergies. The interviewer inquires about food, environmental, and drug allergies and their reactions.

Immunizations. All immunizations are listed with dates and specific mention of most recent boosters for polio, tetanus, diphtheria, and pertussis.

Military Service and Foreign Travel. Documentation of the dates and locations while in the military service and during foreign travel can sometimes provide useful clues in detecting conditions uncommon in this country.

Diagnostic Procedures. The interviewer asks about past diagnostic procedures including head X-ray, electroencephalogram, chest X-ray, electrocardiogram, and intravenous pyelography. Clients sometimes forget that they have had major illnesses or trauma but remember having related diagnostic procedures and their results.

Family History

The family history comprises two major sections: an investigation into the health of the client's relatives and a search for the existence of certain illnesses within the living unit. These are the illnesses suspected or known to have familial tendencies whether for genetic or environmental reasons. The client is questioned about the health and ages of the spouse, children, parents, siblings, maternal and paternal grandparents, uncles, and aunts. In the case of deceased relatives, the interviewer obtains the age and cause of death whenever possible. This section is recorded in outline form as follows:

Spouse—52, healthy except for being 20 lbs. overweight.
Children: Son—19, healthy
           Daughter—16, multiple environmental allergies (dust, mold, and pollen), asthma until age 12, undergoing desensitization since then, and asymptomatic
Brother—48, heavy drinker
Sister—44, healthy

Mother—74, mild arthritis, uncomfortable but can perform all previous activities
Father—73, healthy
Maternal grandfather—94, healthy
Maternal grandmother—94, healthy
Paternal grandfather—deceased at age 74, heart attack
Paternal grandmother—deceased at age 58, breast cancer

An alternate method of recording the family history is the family tree (Figure 1-1). Frequently clients forget about the existence of certain conditions unless specifically questioned about them. This part of the family history includes questioning the client about the following diseases: alcoholism, allergies, anemia, angina, arrhythmias, arteriosclerosis, asthma, birth defects, blood diseases, cancer, coronary artery disease, depression, diabetes, emotional disturbances, epilepsy, glaucoma, gout, Huntington's Chorea, hypertension, neuromuscular disorders, renal disease, schizophrenia, suicide, and tuberculosis. If negative, this information is recorded as a statement of denial of these conditions. If positive, that information is added to the outline or the family tree of family members' health.

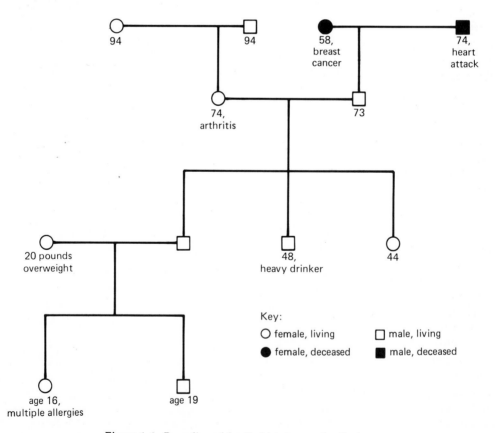

Figure 1-1. Recording of family history on a family tree.

Psychosocial History

See Chapter 3 for a complete discussion.

Socioeconomic History

The socioeconomic history is a composite of the client's life style and includes cultural, environmental, and economic considerations; information regarding how the client functions on a daily basis; and the client's health practices. It contains the following information:

A. Cultural considerations
   1. Members of household
   2. Role and position in household
   3. Position in extended family

B. Environmental factors
   1. Description of neighborhood
   2. Pattern of moving
   3. Description of home
   4. Occupational health risks

C. Economic profile
   1. Existence of health insurance
   2. Effect of health on finances
   3. Effect of finances on health

D. Activities of daily living
   1. Example of a normal day
   2. Sleep and activity patterns
   3. Identification of unhealthy habits
   4. Hobbies and recreational interests

E. Health practices
   1. Orientation to and philosophy of health care
   2. Hygiene facilities
   3. Sanitation, refrigeration
   4. Safety precautions
   5. Source of health care
   6. Emergency readiness

Cultural Considerations. It is always important for the interviewer to attempt to remove cultural biases from the line of questioning, but it is particularly important in the socioeconomic history. It is better to inquire about household members rather than family members as not all clients live in a traditional family setting, for example, homosexual couples, commune members, and boarding house dwellers.

The *role in the household* refers to the tasks and responsibilities assumed by the client, while the *position* refers to placement in the structure of the household unit. For example, many women have the combined roles of breadwinner, mother, and homemaker, and have the positions of heading single-parent families. It is becoming increasingly common for couples to combine the roles of parenting while both work outside the home. Insight into role definitions and positions within the household illuminates who is responsible for health care and for decision making.

Role and position in the extended family, which includes grandparents, aunts, and uncles, are also significant. For instance, the adult client who has no siblings might feel sole responsibility for the health and safety of aging parents. Significant others include close friends, day care personnel, and child care providers. A statement about the role and position of significant others also indicates existing relationships.

A brief description of interpersonal crises, for example, divorce or death, often indicates the strengths and weaknesses of the client and significant others, an indication of how they might be expected to cope with a major illness, an emergency, or a chronic illness.

Environmental Factors. A description of the neighborhood highlights the proximity of neighbors, relationships with neighbors, and any environmental risk factors. Risk factors include contact with industrial waste, incidence of violence, and handling of sewage and waste (of particular importance for those who drink well water). Identification of the client's pattern of moving may be significant. Transient groups tend to have less opportunity for establishing support systems and using community resources. A description of the home setting includes a statement about comfort, adequacy of heating and light, and provisions for privacy. Occupational health risks are also identified. Examples are inhalants, chemicals, pollutants, large equipment, excessive hours on the job, inadequate rest periods within shifts, and temperature extremes.

Economic Profile. Health and finances have an interdependent relationship. Generally, the more financially secure a client is, the wider is the range of services available. However, a major illness or catastrophic accident can quickly deplete the reserves of a financially secure person. A person with limited finances or a fixed income often fears not being able to afford adequate health care or to pay for services rendered. It is important for the interviewer to inquire about the existence of health care insurance and also to make an assessment of the client's understanding of coverage. It is not uncommon for people to misunderstand the terms of insurance policies and involvement in health maintenance organizations.

Activities of Daily Living. An inquiry into the client's actions in a 24-hour period identifies habits that either facilitate or thwart healthful living. A history of the client's sleep and activity patterns may indicate the reason for some symptoms. For example, fatigue may indicate the client's inability to cope with stress. Unhealthful habits that place clients at risk are smoking cigarettes, drinking alcoholic beverages, ingesting caffeine-containing substances, and using illicit drugs. These data are quantitative, that is, listed as cigarette packs smoked per day for the number of years the habit has persisted; cups or ounces of coffee, tea, or cola per day; and ounces of beer, wine, or liquor per day.

Health Practices. A summary of health practices beginning with the individual's orientation to health and philosophy of health care may illuminate previous information and predict future practices. For instance, clients are asked about the frequency and findings of self-examination of the head and neck, breasts (women), and testes (men). Clients who practice preventive health care organize their lives differently than those who enter the health care system only when problems develop, for example, for episodic illness or trauma. The interviewer records the usual source and pattern of health care and includes whether it is in the private or public sector and vacillating, constant, or searching among various agencies and offices.

Safety precautions are discussed to elicit information regarding fire evacuation plans, use of seat belts in automobiles, posting of poison control information, use of pool covers, availability of fire extinguishers, use of decals pasted on glass doors, rapid and safe disposal of waste, and proper storage and care of firearms, if any. Professionals are again cautioned to discard their own cultural biases whenever possible and ask whether sanitation and refrigeration exists. The client's water source may be significant, for example, if vitamins with fluoride are taken and the water supply is fluoridated.

Emergency readiness includes first-aid training, cardiopulmonary resuscitation certification, posted emergency numbers, and emergency kits in the home and car.

Nutritional History

See Chapter 4 for a complete discussion.

Review of Systems

The last and most rigorous part of the health history is the review of systems (ROS). In this section the client responds to a series of questions about symptoms pertaining to each body system and region. The interviewer records the review of systems in medical terminology but phrases the questions in lay terminology. Whenever the client gives an affirmative answer to one of the questions, the interviewer investigates that symptom further by using branching questions for clarification. The interviewer records each symptom so that others reading the chart can use this information as a point of reference. Frequently information contributing toward the history of present illness and past history is uncovered during the review of systems. The review of systems serves to jar the client's memory and facilitates collection of a thorough health history (Table 1-3).

Table 1-3. Review of Systems

Questions in Lay Terminology (Medical Terminology)	Rationale-screening for the following
General Health	
Have you had any recent fever or chills?	Infection
Have you been tired for no apparent reason? (fatigue)	Generalized complaint found in many conditions
Have you felt badly, just not felt up to par? (malaise)	Generalized complaint found in many conditions
Has your appetite changed?	
Increased appetite (polyphagia)	Diabetes mellitus
Loss of appetite (anorexia)	Generalized complaint found in many conditions
Have you noticed excessive thirst? (polydipsia)	Diabetes mellitus or insipidus
Have you had any unexplained weight loss?	Malignancy
Have you had any unexplained weight gain?	Endocrine disorders
Have you noticed any changes in your tolerance to temperature? For example, are you the first one in a group to be too hot (heat sensitivity) or too cold (cold sensitivity)?	Thyroid disorders
Have you noticed any change in your hat, glove, or shoe size?	Acromegaly
Skin	
Have you had any unexplained changes in skin color?	Cardiovascular disorders
Increased color (hyperpigmentation)	Endocrine disorders
Decreased color (hypopigmentation)	Fungal infections
Yellowing (jaundice)	Liver disease, hematologic disorders
Have you had any excessive skin dryness?	Climate, fluid volume deficit, endocrine disorders, hematologic disorders
Have you noticed any changes in skin texture?	Actinic keratoses, endocrine disorders
Have you had any rashes or itching? (pruritus)	Dermatoses
	Liver disease
Have you had any unexplained bruises? (ecchymoses)	Hematologic disorders
Have you noticed any changes in moles? (nevi)	Melanoma
Do you have any acne or pimples?	Acne vulgaris
Do you have any skin sores (lesions), infections, or lumps? (nodules, tumors)?	Generalized complaint found in many conditions
Do you have any stretch marks? (striae)	Pregnancy
	Endocrine disorders
Have you noticed any changes in your nails?	Endocrine disorders
Have you noticed any loss of hair? (alopecia)	Male pattern baldness
	Postpartum hair loss
	Endocrine disorders
Have you noticed any growth of hair in unusual places? (hirsutism in females)	Endocrine disorders
Head and Neck	
Have you ever had a head injury? (trauma)	Sequelae following trauma
Have you had any headaches?	Psychologic stress
	Neurologic disorders
Have you had any sensations of loss of balance—objects seem to move around you or you seem to move in space? (vertigo)	Neurologic disorders
	Middle-ear disorders
	Infectious disease
	Postural hypotension
	Alcohol or other drug toxicity
Have you had any dizziness, lightheadedness, or faintness? (syncope)	Cardiovascular disorders
	Neurologic disorders
Have you noticed any swollen glands? (lymphadenopathy)	Infections
	Lymphomas
	Metastatic carcinoma
Have you noticed any lumps in the head or neck? (tumors)	Malignancy
Have you had any neck pain or limitation in movement?	Trauma, arthritis
Have you noticed a swelling in the front of your neck? (goiter)	Thyroid disorders

Table 1-3.   Review of Systems (*continued*)

Questions in Lay Terminology (Medical Terminology)	Rationale-screening for the following
Eyes	
Do you use glasses or contact lenses? If so, when and how well do they work?	Visual problems
Do you use an artificial eye? (prosthesis)	Trauma Malignancy
Have you had any eye pain?	Eye strain
	Glaucoma
Do you ever see haloes around lights?	Glaucoma
Have you had any redness? (inflammation)	Infection
	Glaucoma
Have you noticed any tunnel vision?	Glaucoma
	Neurologic disorders
Have you lost any areas in your field of vision? (scotomata)	Retinal detachment
	Neurologic disorders
Do you have any blurring of vision?	Cataracts
Have you noticed any spots in your vision?	Cataracts
Have you noticed any double vision? (diplopia)	Neurologic disorders
Do you wake up with your eyelids or eyelashes matted together?	Infection
Have you had any drainage from your eyes? (discharge)	Infection
Have you noticed any drying of the eyes? (lack of lacrimation) or excessive tearing (lacrimation)	Collagen vascular disease
	Blocked nasolacrimal duct
Ears	
Have you had any earaches?	Infection
Have you noticed any drainage from your ears? (discharge)	Infection
Have you noticed any loss of hearing? (deafness)	Conductive and neurologic hearing disorders
When was your last hearing test? Do you know what the results were?	
Have you noticed any ringing in the ears? (tinnitus)	Aspirin toxicity
	Neurologic disorders
	Infection
Do you use a hearing aid? If so, how well does it work?	Evaluate progression of hearing loss.
Nose and Sinuses	
Have you had a persistent runny nose? (rhinitis)	Upper respiratory infections
	Allergy
Have you had any drainage from the nose? (discharge)	Infection
	Foreign body
Have you had frequent or prolonged sneezing?	Upper respiratory infections
	Allergy
Have you had a stuffy nose?	Upper respiratory infections
	Allergy
Have you had any severe nosebleeds? (epistaxis)	Hematologic disorders
Have you noticed any changes in your sense of smell (olfaction) or taste (gustation)?	Neurologic disorders
Have you had painful sinuses or postnasal drip?	Sinusitis
Mouth and Throat	
Have you had any tooth pain?	Dental caries
Have you had any gum pain or bleeding?	Periodontal disease
Do you wear dentures? If so, how do they fit?	Nutritional deficiencies
Have you had any mouth pain?	Periodontal disease
Have you had any unusual mouth odors or tastes?	Periodontal disease
Have you noticed any changes in your ability to taste?	Periodontal disease
	Endocrine disorders
Have you had any mouth dryness?	Endocrine disorders
Have you noticed any change in your voice? Any hoarseness?	Carcinoma of the larynx
Have you had a recent cough or sore throat?	Upper respiratory infection
Have you had any difficulty swallowing your food? (dysphagia)	Neurologic disorders
	Malignancy

Table 1-3. Review of Systems (*continued*)

Questions in Lay Terminology (Medical Terminology)	*Rationale-screening for the following*
Breasts and Axillae	
Have you ever had a breast lump? (mass)	Polycystic disease, malignancy
Have you had any breast pain or fullness?	Menstrual cycle variations
Have you had any nipple drainage? (discharge)	Pregnancy, lactation, malignancy, infection
Respiratory	
Have you had a persistent cough?	Upper respiratory infection
If so, do you cough up any phlegm? (sputum)	Malignancy
	Cardiovascular disease
Have you coughed up any blood? (hemoptysis)	Malignancy
	Lung infection
Have you had any wheezing?	Pulmonary disorders
	Allergy
Have you had any trouble with your breathing? (dyspnea)	Pulmonary disorders
	Cardiovascular disorders
Have you had any pain in your chest with deep breathing?	Pleuritis
Have you ever had a chest X-ray? If so, what were the results?	Tuberculosis, malignancy
Cardiovascular	
Have you had any difficulty breathing when lying down? (orthopnea)	Congestive heart failure
Have you awakened suddenly with breathing trouble? (paroxysmal nocturnal dyspnea)	Congestive heart failure
Have you ever had any chest pain?	Angina
	Myocardial infarction
Have you ever had palpitations or been aware of your heart skipping a beat? (arrhythmias)	Musculosketal disorders
	Heart disease
Have you ever been told you have a heart murmur?	Heart disease
Have you ever been told you have high blood pressure?	Hypertension
Have you noticed any change in your ability to exercise or to perform your daily activities?	General complaint in many disorders
	Heart failure
Have you ever noticed that your feet are swollen? (edema)	Congestive heart failure
	Liver disease
Have you ever noticed that your hands and feet were blue? (cyanosis)	Heart disease
	Hematologic disorders
Have you had any unexplained coldness of your hands and feet?	Peripheral vascular disease
When walking, have you had any sharp pains or cramps in your legs that made you stop and rest? (intermittent claudication)	Arteriosclerotic vessel disease
Do you have any varicose veins?	Venous disease
Gastrointestinal	
Have you been unable to eat certain kinds of foods? (food intolerance)	Allergies
Have you had any nausea or vomiting?	General complaint in gastrointestinal disorders
Have you had any vomiting of blood? (hematemesis)	Peptic ulcer
Have you had any heartburn? (pyrosis)	Peptic ulcer
Have you had any persistent belching or burping? (eructation)	Malabsorption syndromes
Have you had any pain in your abdomen?	General complaint, acute abdomen
Have you had any bloating in your abdomen? (distention)	General complaint, obstruction, malabsorption syndromes
Have you had any swelling or fluid in your abdomen? (ascites)	Liver disease
Have you had any problem with passing a lot of gas? (flatulence)	Malabsorption syndromes
Have you noticed any changes in your bowel habits?	Malignancy
Frequent stools (diarrhea)	Malignancy, colitis, malabsorption syndromes
Infrequent, difficult to pass stools (constipation)	Insufficient dietary bulk or water, psychologic disturbance
Passage of blood in the stools (melena)	Malignancy
	Hemorrhoids
Have you had any rectal burning or pain?	Hemorrhoids, malignancy

Table 1-3. Review of Systems (*continued*)

Questions in Lay Terminology (Medical Terminology)	*Rationale-screening for the following*

Urinary

Have you had any change in the color or smell of your urine?	Infection, hepatitis
Have you noticed any blood in your urine? (hematuria)	Infection, malignancy, calculi
Have you had the desire to urinate small amounts of urine frequently? (frequency)	Infection, enlarged prostate
Have you had any pain or burning when urinating? (dysuria)	Infection
Have you had the feeling that if you don't urinate right away, you won't make it? (urgency)	Infection
Have you been unable to control urination—dribbling or wetting yourself unconsciously or when coughing or sneezing? (stress incontinence)	Pelvic floor relaxation
Do you get up in the middle of the night to urinate? (nocturia)	Congestive heart failure
Do you seem to be urinating the same amounts more frequently? (polyuria)	Diabetes mellitus
Have you had any pain in your sides? (flanks)	Pyelonephritis
Have you had a decrease in the amont of urine passed? (oliguria)	Renal failure, fluid volume deficit
Have you felt unable to empty your bladder completely? (retention)	Enlarged prostate

For males, in addition to the preceding questions, the interviewer asks the following:

Have you noticed a decrease in the size (caliber) of the stream?	Enlarged prostate
Have you had any trouble starting to urinate? (hesitancy)	Enlarged prostate

For men only ,the interviewer asks the following questions:

Genital

Have you had any drainage from your penis? (discharge)	Infection
Have you had any sores on your penis? (lesions)	Infection
Have you felt any lumps in your scrotum? (masses)	Malignancy
Have you had any problems with getting your partner pregnant? (infertility)	Reproductive disorders

Sexual

What is your usual pattern of sex? (sexual expression)	Sexual disorders
Have you had any problems with getting or keeping an erection? (impotence)	Sexual disorders
Have you had any difficulty with climaxing before you wanted to? (premature ejaculation)	Sexual disorders

For women only, the interviewer asks the following questions:

Gynecologic

At what age did you begin to menstruate? (menarche)	Primary amenorrhea
When was the first day of your last menstrual period?	Pregnancy, menstrual disorders
What is the pattern of your periods?	Menstrual disorders
Interval between cycles _____	
Duration of flow _____	
Description of flow _____	
Have you had any pain during your period? (dysmenorrhea)	Menstrual disorders
Have you had any bleeding between periods? (metrorrhagia)	Menstrual disorders
Do you usually have bloating before your periods?	Premenstrual tension
Do you usually have irritability before your periods?	Premenstrual tension
Have you missed any menstrual periods? (amenorrhea)	Menstrual disorders, menopause
Have you had any vaginal pain or drainage? (discharge)	Infection
Have you had any vaginal itching? (pruritus)	Infection, infestation
Have you had any genital sores? (lesions)	Infection, infestation
Have you had any cramping?	Menstrual disorders
Have you had any pain during sexual intercourse? (dyspareunia)	Vaginal disorders, pelvic mass, endometriosis, psychological disorders
Have you had any difficulty becoming pregnant? (infertility)	Menstrual disorders

Table 1-3. Review of Systems (*continued*)

Questions in Lay Terminology (Medical Terminology)	Rationale-screening for the following
Obstetric	
How many pregnancies have you had? (gravida)	Obstetric disorders
How many of your pregnancies were full-term? (para X _ _ _)	Obstetric disorders
Did any of your pregnancies end in a premature delivery? (para _ X _ _)	Obstetric disorders
Have you had any miscarriages (spontaneous abortions) or therapeutic abortions? (para _ _ X _)	Obstetric disorders
How many living children do you have? (para _ _ _ X)	Obstetric disorders
For each pregnancy, the examiner asks the following:	
How would you describe your pregnancy?	Obstetric disorders
Did you have any complications during pregnancy? Did you have any high blood pressure? Excessive weight gain? Toxemia? Bleeding?	
Where did you have the baby and how long were you there?	
How long was your labor and how would you describe it?	
How would you describe your delivery?	
Did you have any anesthesia?	
Were there any problems with the delivery? Forceps? Excessive bleeding? Birth defects?	
What was your baby's condition? (Apgar)	
Did you have the "baby blues"? (postpartum depression)	
Sexual	
What is your usual pattern of sex? (sexual expression)	Sexual disorders
Are you able to reach a climax? (orgasm)	Sexual disorders
Have you had a decrease in your desire for sex? (libido)	Generalized complaint
What do you use for contraception?	Menstrual disorders
Musculoskeletal	
Have you had any joint pain or stiffness?	Arthritis
Have you had any joint swelling? (edema)	Arthritis
Have you noticed any change in your ability to move your joints? (range of motion)	Arthritis
Have you noticed any change in your ability to use your muscles? (limitation of movement)	Neuromuscular disorders
Have you had any decrease in the size of your muscles? (wasting, cachexia)	Dietary protein deficiency, malignancy, neuromuscular disorders
Neurological	
Have you had any convulsions? (seizures)	Neurologic disorders
Have you had any muscle weakness (paresis) or paralysis?	Neurologic disorders
Have you had any numbness or tingling? (paresthesia)	Neurologic disorders
Have you had any loss of feeling or sensation? (hypoesthesia, anesthesia)	Neurologic disorders
Have you had any unusual sensitivity to touch? (hyperesthesia)	Neurologic disorders
Have you had any difficulties with your speech? (dysphasia)	Neurologic disorders
Have you had any difficulties with walking? (ataxia)	Neurologic disorders
Have you had any shaking? (tremors)	Neurologic disorders

Table 1-3. Review of Systems (*continued*)

Questions in Lay Terminology (Medical Terminology)	Rationale-screening for the following
Psychosocial	
Have you had any major changes in your behavior?	Psychiatric disorders
Do you have spells of emotional highs and lows? (mood swings)	Manic depressive disorder
Have you had any nervousness?	Psychiatric disorders
Have you had periods of anxiety?	Psychiatric disorders
Have you had nightmares?	Psychiatric disorders
Have you had difficulty with sleeping? (insomnia)	Psychiatric disorders
Have you seen or heard things other people have not? (hallucinations)	Schizophrenia, organic brain syndrome
Have you had feelings that others are out to get you? (delusions)	Schizophrenia
Have you had trouble with your memory?	Organic brain syndrome, depression
Have you had any trouble with your thinking? (intellectual impairment)	Mental retardation, organic brain syndrome (dementia)
Have you had any crying spells?	Depression
Have you had any severe sadness or depression?	Depression
Have you had any thoughts of suicide or homicide?	Depression
Have you attempted suicide or homicide?	Depression

Life Cycle Variations

Childhood

The most striking difference in interviewing children is that some of the information is provided by a third party. The informant is usually one or both parents. Although infants are incapable of speaking for themselves, they as well as all children are addressed by name and given the respect afforded adults. Children of all ages are involved in the interview as much as possible. For example, a wise interviewer engages the young baby in a few minutes of play, which establishes a pleasant memory of early contact with health professionals. Early interactions with health professionals frequently set the stage for lifelong expectations. Once children begin to converse, the interviewer can direct several simple questions to elicit their participation; possibilities are, "What's your name?" "How old are you" "What are your favorite foods?" Since the attention span is limited among children and the initial interview is time consuming, several toys such as blocks, balls, crayons and paper, and books are available for diversion. Also allowing the child to hold and play with the stethoscope makes one more aspect of health care familiar.

The interviewer has the additional challenge of putting two or more people at ease when working with an adult/child dyad. Parents are afforded respect, and their stories accorded interest since they are the spokespersons for young and shy or quiet older children (Figure 1-2).

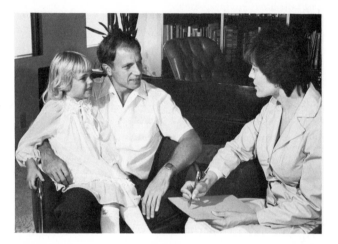

Figure 1-2. *Interviewer obtaining the health history of a 4-year-old.*

The child's perception of health or illness is highly informative. For example, the eight-year-old who is being admitted for a tonsillectomy and recently experienced the death of a hospitalized grandparent might also fear death in the hospital.

In addition to establishing the reliability of the informant, the apparent relationship between the parent and child is significant. For example, if the parent continually interrupts and answers questions directed at a 12-year-old daughter, the interviewer records that the informant seemed unwilling to allow the child to speak for herself.

When interviewing older children (over age eight) and children in whom parental neglect or abuse is suspected, the interviewer begins the initial introduction with a statement indicating that it would be helpful to talk with the child alone. When alone with the child, the interviewer attempts to clarify any confusing areas.

The perinatal history is included with the health history during childhood. The goals of the perinatal history are to identify risks for later developmental lags and to establish the origin of any existing problems. The perinatal history includes the following information:

Course of pregnancy

Difficulties during pregnancy, such as prolonged anorexia, nausea, and vomiting; excessive weight gain; toxemia; illnesses; trauma; bleeding; exposure to rubella without immunization or history of actual disease during pregnancy

Attendance at prenatal classes

Mother's dietary habits

Mother's weight gain

Mother's use of alcohol, cigarettes, caffeine, medications (prescription, over-the-counter, and illicit)

Length of pregnancy

Labor
   Length
   Description
   Problems during labor

Delivery—vaginal or caesarean
   Location
   Anesthesia
   Complications—hemorrhage, forceps
   Birth weight, length
   Length of hospital stay for mother and baby
   Apgar score—any difficulty in starting to breathe
   Any difficulties in hospital

The socioeconomic history is expanded to include inquiry about specific safety practices as follows:

Does the child use seat belts in the car?

Are stairways in your home blocked?

Are electrical outlets in your home covered?

Is there a pool? If so, is a pool cover used?

Has the child taken swimming lessons?

Are medications, chemicals, and cleaning solutions stored beyond the child's reach?

Are sharp and pointed tools and breakable objects stored beyond the child's reach?

The immunization section of the past health history includes specific questioning regarding diphtheria, pertussis, tetanus (DPT); measles, mumps, and rubella (MMR); and the oral polio vaccines and boosters and the dates administered. Many parents have immunization history records or know where they are recorded and can be obtained.

Adolescence

By adolescence the client deserves a private interview. If a parent or guardian insists on providing information, the adolescent is asked if there are any objections. Adolescence is a time of many ambivalent feelings. The young person desires to give up childhood, yet is unwilling to assume all the responsibilities of adulthood. This is frequently a time of family turmoil; the adolescent may feel that the parents do not give enough freedom, and the parents may feel that the young person is not mature enough to handle the desired freedom. The interviewer frequently is the only person whom the adolescent perceives as being an objective, unbiased listener.

The physical changes that occur during adolescence produce a wide variety of psychosocial responses dependent on familial and peer attitudes and cultural biases. Also many adolescents are fearful that they are not developing normally. The interviewer asks the adolescent about feelings toward school, achievement in school, extracurricular activities, hobbies, sports, ways of earning money, importance of friends, membership in groups, peer group interests, relationships with parents, teachers, and other authority figures, ways of reducing stress, and sexuality.

Working with members of this age group challenges the sensitivity and flexibility of the most experienced interviewer. It is often helpful to initiate questions about sensitive areas such as sexuality and the functioning of the sex organs with a statement about normalcy. For example,

INTERVIEWER: It is normal for most girls to begin to have monthly bleeding, menstrual periods, between the ages of 10 and 16. Have you started to menstruate?

INTERVIEWER: Most professionals consider masturbation, or playing with yourself, a normal activity. Frequently patients tell me they are worried about themselves for masturbating. How do you feel about this?

Some adults believe that sexuality should be discussed only if the patient or client introduces the topic. That expectation is unrealistic for most members of a group who are confused and embarrassed about this vital subject. With teenage pregnancies, venereal disease, and family dissolutions on the increase in this country, health professionals must be willing to introduce the topic of sexuality and proceed at the client's pace in their discussion. The interviewer asks the sexually active adolescent about methods of contraception, function, and effectiveness.

Late Adulthood

Although all clients deserve to be comfortable and to have an interviewer who speaks clearly and maintains eye contact, these considerations acquire additional significance among the aged. With aging, there is a decrease in muscle mass and subcutaneous tissue; therefore, comfortable seating is essential for the ambulatory client. The bedridden patient is assisted in changing positions frequently. The body becomes less efficient in perceiving, processing, and responding to external stimuli; therefore, the interviewer strives to reduce extraneous noise and to speak clearly and maintain eye contact.

Recording of a Normal History

Identifying Data

Client: Maria (Ramirez) Martinez
Address: 3715 Oak Street
        San Diego, California 92002
Phone number: (714) 267-4410
Contact: Mrs. Luz Connolly (sister)
Address: 411 Pine Street
        Los Angeles, California 90803
Phone number: (213) 762-0144
Birthdate: October 9, 1951
Birthplace: Los Angeles, California
Sex: Female
Race: Caucasian
Religion: Latter Day Saints
Marital status: Married
Social Security number: 474-74-7474
Occupation: Housewife and mother; worked as a R.N. in Navy in O.R. until 5 years ago.

Referral source: Dr. James Tinmore
        375 N. Snow Avenue
        San Diego, California 92011
(Family practice doctor who no longer provides obstetric care)
Informant: Client, reliable and cooperative
Date: October 12, 1982

Reason for Presenting

To establish relationship at Women's Health Care Foundation for future pregnancy. Family physician no longer provides obstetric care.

Present Health

This 28-year-old Gravida 1, Para 1-0-0-1, Mexican-American married, unemployed R.N. has enjoyed good health throughout her life. She is strongly supportive of preventive health care and presents for the first time at the foundation to begin services and establish her record. She plans to become pregnant for the second time this spring.

Takes no medications (prescribed, OTC, or illicit).

Past Health History

Illnesses. Measles and rubella, mumps, and chicken pox before age 10. Denies serious injuries, accidents, disabilities, alcoholism, arrhythmias, arteriosclerosis, asthma, blood dyscrasias, coronary artery disease, depression, diabetes, hepatitis, hypertension, kidney disease, obesity, rheumatic fever, scarlet fever, tuberculosis, and venereal disease.

Hospitalizations. December 1977—one day for uncomplicated childbirth; 1955—Tonsillectomy

Allergies. None known. Has taken penicillin during childhood without problems.

Immunizations. Completed full course of DPT and oral polio during childhood; 1973—DT and oral polio boosters, tetanus toxoid

Military Service. Navy Nurse Corps—1971–1973 (Villanova University), 1973–1976 (Corpus Christi Medical Center)

Foreign Travel. Travels to Mexico City about once/year to visit maternal grandparents

Family History

Spouse—36, healthy except for multiple allergies (mold, cats, ragweed), asymptomatic for past 2 years while undergoing desensitization

Child—daughter, 25 months, healthy

Sisters—27, healthy
—26, healthy
—24, healthy

Brother—16, healthy

Mother—51, healthy

Father—50, healthy

Maternal grandmother—73, rheumatoid arthritis

Maternal grandfather—75, healthy

Paternal grandmother—deceased at 47, breast cancer

Paternal grandfather—deceased at 69, CVA

Denies family history of alcoholism, anemia, angina, arrhythmias, arteriosclerosis, asthma, birth defects, blood dyscrasias, coronary artery disease, depression, epilepsy, glaucoma, gout, Huntington's Chorea, hypertension, neuromuscular disorders, renal disease, and tuberculosis.

Socioeconomic History

Cultural. Lives with husband and daughter in comfortable three-bedroom home. Content with role as wife and mother. Extended family live within 25 miles of one another and visit frequently. Keeps in touch with professional friends by attending monthly interest group meetings and socials. Belongs to play group of young mothers and their children under three. Has strong involvement in church activities.

Environmental. Client's spouse and she have lived in present home for five years and they value their friendships with their neighbors. They live on a cul-de-sac in a "family-oriented" neighborhood in a comfortable home with many modern conveniences.

Economic. Husband is a tenured university associate professor in history and has family health benefits (major medical and catastrophic) as well as adequate life insurance and disability. Client feels financially secure and could return to work if necessary.

Activities of daily living. Sleeps between 7 and 8 hours/night. Jogs 3 miles/day. Likes to hike and backpack with family. Bikes or walks with daughter daily. Cares for daughter throughout day, stimulating her in the areas of language, motor development, cog-

nitive development, and socialization. After family dinner spouse and she play with child for about 1 hour. Reserves most evenings for interacting with spouse. Attends church weekly and is involved in other church activities.

Health Practices. Strongly committed to preventive health care. Denies smoking and ingestion of alcoholic and caffeine-containing substances. Regular annual health checkups with family physician, Dr. James Tinmore, for self, spouse, and child. Sees family safety as a priority—home is "childproofed" (medicines and chemicals are beyond baby's reach), child's car seat and seat belts are used, family has fire evacuation plans and fire extinguishers are in the home. Has CPR instructor's certificate and teaches CPR about twice/year. Keeps emergency phone numbers and first-aid kits accessible.

Review of Systems

General. Usually healthy. Denies chills, fatigue, fever, polydipsia, polyphagia, polyuria, anorexia, malaise, temperature intolerance, or change in weight.

Skin. No color changes, infections, ecchymoses, lesions, pruritus, petechiae, changes in pigmentation, nevi, temperature or texture changes.
  Nails: No changes in texture or appearance.
  Hair: No changes in texture or appearance. Denies use of dyes or permanents.

Head and Neck. No headaches, vertigo, trauma, syncope, dizziness, lymphadenopathy, goiter, or masses.

Eyes. Vision last checked June 1982—20/15 OU. Denies pain, haloes, scotomata, diplopia, inflammation, discharge, and excessive lacrimation.

Ears. No pain, hearing loss, discharge, tinnitus, vertigo.

Nose and Sinuses. No epistaxis, discharge, loss of sense of smell, trauma, stuffiness, postnasal drip, sinusitis, sinus pain, sneezing.

Mouth and Throat. Last dental checkup 3 months ago, teeth in good repair. Denies pain, decreased ability to taste, dentures, bleeding gums, dryness, odors, hoarseness, soreness, or dysphagia.

Breasts and Axillae. Performs self-examination monthly. No masses, tenderness, nipple discharge.

Breast-fed daughter December 1977—December 1978, without problems.

Respiratory. Denies cough, sputum production, wheezing, hemoptysis, recurrent respiratory infections, and pain. Last chest X-ray in 1976, normal.

Cardiovascular. Denies dyspnea, orthopnea, paroxysmal nocturnal dyspnea, chest pain, palpitations, arrhythmias, edema, varicosities, murmurs, cyanosis, hypertension, syncope, intermittent claudication, or wheezing. Last ECG in 1976, normal.

Gastrointestinal. Appetite is "too good." Denies anorexia, ascites, abdominal pain, belching, constipation, diarrhea, flatulence, heartburn, nausea, vomiting, change in bowel habits, hematemesis, melena, hemorrhoids, hernia, pyrosis, or rectal discomfort.

Urinary. No history of urinary tract infections, dysuria, frequency, urgency, calculi, incontinence, suprapubic pain, nocturia, polyuria, oliguria, or flank pain.

Gynecologic. LMP = September 22, 1982. Menarche—13. Menses every 31–33 days, duration of 4–5 days, moderate flow—saturates 6–7 tampons/day. Denies amenorrhea, cramps, vaginal discharge, and pruritis. Last Pap smear in June 1982, normal.

Obstetric. Gravida 1. Para 1-0-0-1.

Previous pregnancy:

Course—healthy, no bleeding, infections, discharge, excessive weight gain, toxemia, nausea, or vomiting. Positive attitude with supportive husband. Attended childbirth education classes. Jogged and worked until delivery day. Weight gain = 31 pounds.

Labor and Delivery:

Labor = 7 hours. Ambulatory until fully dilated. No analgesia necessary

Delivery = uncomplicated. No anesthesia except local for episiotomy.

Apgars = 9 and 10.

Sexual. Contraception—diaphragm, last fitted June 1982. Libido active, orgasmic with each intercourse, about 4 times/week.

Musculoskeletal. Full range of motion, denies back or joint pain, weakness, heat, joint stiffness, or atrophy.

Neurological. No headaches, seizures, paresis, paralysis, tremors, paresthesia, or ataxia.

Psychosocial. No emotional lability, anxiety, nervousness, insomnia, amnesia, depression, suicidal or homicidal ideation, or nightmares.

Chapter 2

In all clinical settings the assessment process is enhanced when the examiner provides environmental conditions such as a warm, private, quiet, and well-lit area. The client's body parts are exposed only when necessary; otherwise blankets and drapes are used to maintain warmth and privacy. In addition, the examiner uses privacy screens and curtains in acute care settings and informs visitors and other health care staff of the need for no interruptions during the examination. In the home the examiner conducts the assessment in a room that can be isolated by a closed door when possible. An additional light source such as a gooseneck lamp enhances illumination when available.

Four classic techniques are used during the physical examination: inspection, palpation, percussion, and auscultation. This chapter focuses on how each of these is used in the assessment process.

The general survey is an overview or composite picture of the client and is part of inspection. As part of the general survey the examiner usually obtains the vital signs and the height and weight measurements prior to other assessment techniques of individual body systems and regions.

Introduction to Assessment Techniques and the General Survey

Inspection

Inspection is derived from the Latin word *specere,* to look. This aspect of examination encompasses visual as well as auditory and olfactory observations. From the first moment the examiner sees the client, throughout the interview, and during the entire examination, inspection is used to ascertain the client's state of wellness and reactions to the assessment process. Inspection is of paramount importance during the general survey. The general survey constitutes an overview of health and includes physical, mental, and emotional characteristics and measurements of body size and vital signs.

Physical characteristics include apparent age, sex, race, general state of health and hygiene, nutritional status, body build, stature, posture, gait, motor activity, respiratory pattern, and skin integrity. Mental characteristics include level of consciousness, interest and degree of cooperation in the assessment process, speech, attention span, ability to understand the examiner's directions, and speed of reaction time in following them. Emotional characteristics include affect, mood, facial expressions, ease with which the client is able to relate with the examiner, appropriateness of clothing, punctuality, amount of eye contact, tone of voice, anxiety, and the client's apparent expectations of the examiner.

Objectives

The examiner will be able to do the following:

1. Use inspection to complete the general survey
2. Recognize five distinct qualitites of percussion
3. Obtain vital signs
4. Palpate peripheral pulses
5. Obtain height and weight measurements
6. Obtain head circumference measurements on children under two years of age
7. Obtain serial measurements of the height of the uterine fundus in pregnant women
8. Recognize abnormalities
9. Record the information obtained

Certain observations cause the examiner to vary the order of examination and defer certain aspects until a future visit. For example, if respiratory distress is apparent, attention is immediately focused on identification and resolution of the respiratory problem. In addition, when the examiner perceives pain or anxiety, an attempt is made to manage those conditions prior to the traditional history taking and physical examination sequence.

In recording the general survey the examiner uses descriptive terminology. This provides supporting documentation for judgments that are particularly informative to other professionals who work with the client. For example, in describing a client in respiratory distress the examiner might record one of the following:

1. Client exhibits stridorous breathing pattern, respiratory rate = 38/minute, color—ashen, skin—cold and clammy.

2. Client breathing through pursed lips, leaning forward with elbows resting on overbed table, experiencing difficulty with talking, prolonged expiratory phase of respirations, color—ruddy.

Palpation

The Latin word *palpare,* to touch, is the root word for *palpation,* examining by touching. Palpation provides information about contour, size, consistency, texture, moisture, motility, pulsatility, vibration, and tenderness. Different areas of the hands are more specialized for certain types of information. The dorsal aspects of the hands and fingers are more receptive to temperature while the fingertips are more sensitive to discrimination of fine tactile stimuli. In addition, the palmar surfaces of the fingers are best for perception of vibratory motions such as thrills while use of the fingers in a grasping manner provides information about consistency and position.

The three major types of palpation are light palpation, deep palpation, and ballottement. Light palpation requires minimal pressure as the fingers are applied to the skin and always precedes deep palpation. It is essential in examining the superficial tissues and facilitates maximal sensitivity to touch.

Deep palpation necessitates more pressure and is useful in assessing organs more deeply located, for example, the abdominal organs. However, heavy pressure and continued pressure may dull the sensitivity of the fingertips; therefore, when deep palpation is used, the preferred technique calls for pushing downward and releasing several times rather than

sustaining pressure. Deep palpation is usually a bimanual technique in which the fingers of one hand are placed over the area to be palpated and the fingertips of the other hand are placed on top of the fingers of the first hand. The lower hand is used as the sensitive one while the upper hand exerts most of the pressure. Light and deep palpation are used in examination of the abdomen (Figure 2-1).

Ballottement is derived from the French verb *baloter,* to toss or bounce a ball. As the name implies, it is a type of palpation in which the fingertips move in a bouncing motion. In the bimanual pelvic exam it is possible to ballotte the uterus (Chapter 15).

Each of these techniques has advantages. Their application to individual body systems is covered in detail in the appropriate chapters.

Palpation is often most useful in confirming or further illuminating the findings made during inspection and history taking. Sometimes it identifies things previously unsuspected. An important consideration prior to the "laying on of hands" is to ask whether the client is experiencing any kind of discomfort and if so,

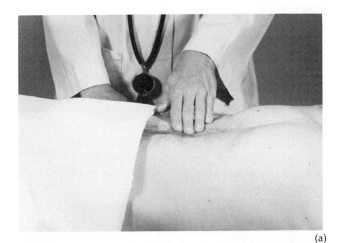

(a)

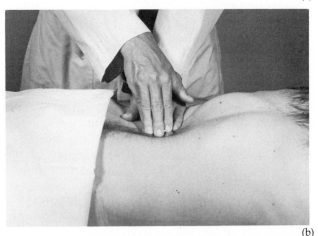

(b)

Figure 2-1. *(a) Light palpation of the abdomen; (b) deep palpation of the abdomen.*

where it is located. This enables the examiner to minimize painful stimuli and reserve palpation over painful areas until last. Another important question is whether the client has noticed any changes, for example, lumps or masses. The examiner then begins palpation distally and contralaterally to the potential problem area. As an illustration, if a client relates that he discovered a lump near his right testis, the examiner begins by examining the left testis. Then when examining the right testis, the examiner begins away from the area in question and works toward it starting with gentle light palpation.

Another bimanual technique involves using one hand to lift or steady an organ or mass away from the surrounding tissues while using the other to palpate. This technique is used during examination of the thyroid gland (Chapter 6).

Percussion

The word *percuss* stems from the Latin *percutere,* to strike or to beat. Percussion is clinically important because in striking or tapping over different body structures, a variety of qualities of sound is produced. These sounds vary according to the degree of vibration produced. The underlying principle is that objects vibrate in inverse proportion to their density; that is, the more dense a tissue or organ is, the less it vibrates in response to being struck. Conversely, the less dense a tissue or organ is, the more it vibrates. Therefore, percussion is useful in locating and identifying structures, particularly those of the chest and abdomen, as well as eliciting sensation, as normal organs are nontender when percussed.

There are two types of percussion: immediate (blunt) and mediate. Immediate percussion is useful in eliciting tenderness. It involves delivering a blow directly against the body with either a fisted hand over a large area such as the costovertebral angle (over the kidneys) or the tip of the middle finger over a smaller area such as the paranasal sinuses (Figures 2-2 and 2-3). Mediate percussion involves using the tip of the middle finger of one hand (plexor) to strike the middle finger of the other hand (pleximeter). The pleximeter rests firmly on the client's body with the distal interphalangeal joint making maximal contact. The plexor strikes over the same area with a sharp crisp blow achieved by rapid wrist flexion and extension. The forearm does not move (Figure 2-4). Medi-

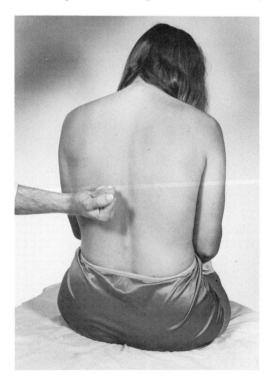

Figure 2-2. Immediate percussion over the costrovertebral angle.

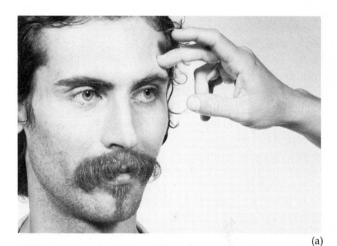

(a)

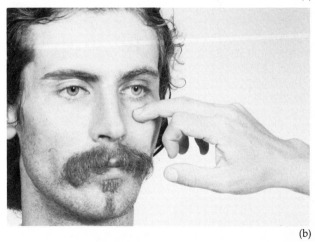

(b)

Figure 2-3. (a) Immediate percussion over the left frontal sinus; (b) immediate percussion over the left maxillary sinus.

area of one density to one of another and notes each point where the sound changes (Figure 2-5).

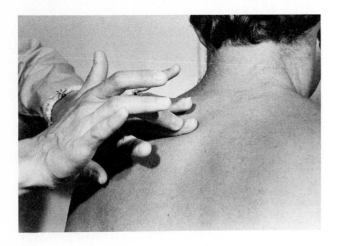

Figure 2-4. *Mediate percussion over the posterior chest.*

ate percussion uncovers findings up to a depth of 5 centimeters.

Since body structures differ in density, the qualities of sound produced when they are percussed also differ. The various percussion sounds are flatness, dullness, resonance, hyperresonance, and tympany. These different sounds arise from differences in vibrations produced by percussion.

The amount of vibration determines the intensity, pitch, duration, and quality of percussion sounds. *Intensity* is the amplitude or loudness of a sound and is related to tissue elasticity. The more elastic a tissue is, the greater the amplitude of vibration and the louder the sound. *Pitch* refers to the frequency of vibration and is related to tissue density. The denser or more solid a tissue is, the faster it vibrates, and the higher the pitch. *Duration* of sound is how long it lasts; it is related to the amount of air within a tissue and its elasticity. The more air a tissue contains and the more elastic it is, the longer its vibration. *Quality* is a subjective description of a sound and includes words such as thump, thud, hollow, booming, and musical (Table 2-1).

Percussion is also used in mapping the demarcations of an organ. The examiner percusses from an

Auscultation

The word *auscultate* comes from the Latin *auscultare,* to listen to. It applies to listening to a range of body sounds with and without the use of a stethoscope. This includes breath sounds, vascular sounds, joint sounds, bowel sounds, and voice characteristics. Auscultation without a stethoscope is termed *immediate* or *direct auscultation* and may necessitate placement of the examiner's ear directly on the body of the client. However, some abnormal findings are so noticeable that the examiner can hear them when standing at a normal social distance, for example, a pronounced cardiac murmur or a severe pulmonary wheeze.

The examiner attempts to minimize extraneous noise during auscultation. In the home setting, the examiner turns off the television or radio and asks others to lower their voices during the assessment. In hospital settings the examiner conducts the assessment in an examining room, if possible. Flexibility and perseverance are essential in critical care areas

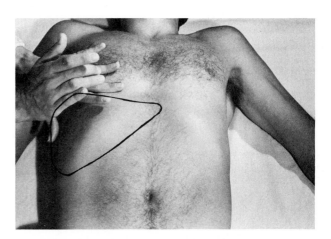

Figure 2-5. *Percussion over the right chest and abdomen demarcates the liver borders.*

Table 2-1.   Percussion Sounds

Sounds	Intensity	Pitch	Duration	Quality	Normal Location
Flatness	Soft	High	Short	Thump	Bone
Dullness	Soft	High	Moderate	Thud	Liver
Resonance	Moderately loud	Low	Long	Hollow	Normal lung
Hyperresonance	Very loud	Very low	Very long	Booming	Infant lung
Tympany	Loud	Low	Moderate	Musical	Air-filled stomach

where respirators, monitors, and other equipment produce noise.

Most auscultation is performed with the aid of a stethoscope. The stethoscope accentuates sound and screens out ambient noise. Although there are several varieties, the one in popular clinical use is the acoustical stethoscope, which consists of two ear pieces, binaurals, tubing, and combination chest piece (Figure 2-6).

The ear pieces should provide a snug but gentle fit. The largest size that fits comfortably functions most efficiently to occlude the ear from transmission of ambient noise. The binaurals are the metal tubes that connect the ear pieces to the tubing and are inclined anteriorly to conform to the direction of the normal ear canals. The two tubes join at the chest piece and are most efficient when they are no longer than 17 inches. In many stethoscopes the tubes join to form one tube for some distance proximal to the chest piece. While these models are useful in blood pressure determination, they are unsuitable for cardiac and pulmonary auscultation. Since the increased length of tubing results in decreased sound conduction, the examiner may miss subtle abnormalities. A combination chest piece contains a diaphragm and a bell. Stethoscopes with the diaphragm only are useful in blood pressure determination but are inadequate for thorough cardiovascular assessment.

The two heads differ in transmission of sounds. The diaphragm amplifies sounds and transmits higher-pitched sounds better than lower-pitched ones. This amplification is enhanced by firm placement of the diaphragm against the skin surface. When the diaphragm is applied without enough pressure, it sometimes slides across the skin during auscultation; this introduces artifacts. Artifacts are abnormal sounds that result from poor technique. The bell is better suited for low-pitched sounds as it filters out high-pitched noises. Since lung sounds are basically high-pitched, the diaphragm is used for pulmonary auscultation. However, the auscultation of the heart requires both chest pieces because cardiac sounds are both high- and low-pitched. The bell is placed lightly on the chest. Firm placement converts it to a diaphragm due to the taut skin within the contact area.

Vital Signs and Measurements

Vital signs and the other physical measurements provide valuable insight into the cardiovascular, pulmonary, gastrointestinal, neurologic, urinary, and endocrinologic systems.

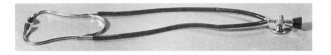

Figure 2-6. Parts of the stethoscope: earpieces, binaurals, tubing, bell, and diaphragm.

Body temperature is affected by biological rhythms, environmental factors, exercise, hormonal secretions, drugs, and age. Temperature has a diurnal pattern of fluctuation with variations of 1.0 to 1.5°F. Lowest temperatures occur in the hours before waking while highest temperatures occur in late afternoon or early evening. Saunas, hot baths, and whirlpools elevate body temperature while cold baths lower it. Exercise, thyroid hormone, and progesterone also elevate body temperature. Temperatures are highest among children and decrease with age.

Temperatures vary among individuals and in the same individual throughout the day. Normal oral temperatures range from 96.5 to 99.3°F. (33.7 to 37.8°C.) while rectal temperatures are generally 1° F. higher and axillary temperatures are generally 1° F. lower (Appendix 1). Rectal temperatures are considered most accurate while axillary temperatures are least accurate. Rectal temperatures are indicated in confused and comatose individuals, infants, and persons receiving oxygen therapy.

Although electronic thermometers are in widespread use and are faster and safer, they do occasionally malfunction and require periodic calibration. Therefore the astute examiner checks temperature readings against a mercury thermometer reading whenever in doubt. Careful inspection of skin color and warmth and the findings of other vital signs should support the actual temperature reading.

The pulse rate is routinely obtained by palpation over the radial artery; however, it may be determined at any pulse point over other arteries. Clients with cardiovascular collapse may have only the central pulses (carotid and femoral) palpable. The carotid pulse is the most accurate for timing cardiovascular activities. In palpation the pads of the middle and ring fingers are placed firmly over the pulse site, and the pulse rate is counted for an interval of at least 15 seconds (preferably 30 seconds). Pulse rates taken for shorter time intervals may cause the examiner to miss an arrhythmia. Whenever an irregularity is detected, the pulse is counted for a full minute.

During initial evaluations and thorough health assessments the examiner palpates the pulse at all peripheral pulse points and compares the symmetry, rhythm, quality, and strength of the right and left sides at each point.

The peripheral pulse points are as follows: brachial, radial, popliteal, posterior tibial, and dorsal pedal (Figure 2-7). The pulses are normally symmetrical and regular. The quality is described as rapid or slow rise, normal, or rapid or slow collapse. Rapid rise describes a pulse that has a booming quality and seemingly prolonged recovery phase (interval between pulsations). With the slow rise pulse the examiner feels the vessel filling prior to the tap of the pulse against the fingertips. The tap of the rapid collapse pulse fades more quickly than normal, while the tap of the slow collapse pulse precedes a period when the examiner is able to feel the blood emptying the vessel. The strength of the pulse is described by a numerical grad-

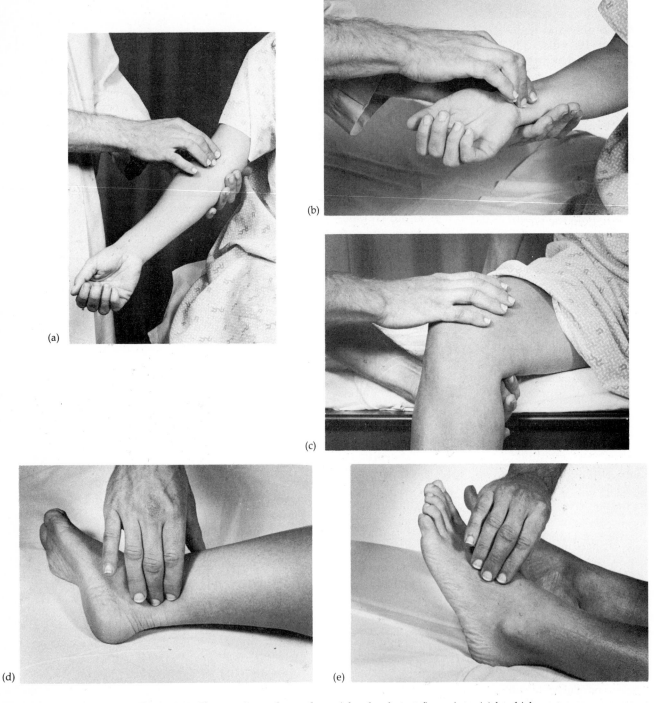

Figure 2-7. *The examiner palpates the peripheral pulses at five points: (a) brachial, (b) radial, (c) popliteal, (d) posterior tibial, and (e) dorsal pedal.*

ing system ranging from 0 to 4 as follows: 0 = no pulse; 1 = barely palpable pulsation; 2 = weak pulsation; 3 = strong pulsation; 4 = bounding pulsation. The normal pulse is 3+ at all points, although the popliteal pulses are sometimes not palpable in obese and muscular clients. This finding is insignificant when the distal pulses are palpable.

Pulse rates are influenced by biological rhythms, sex, age, activity, and conditioning. The pulse rate shows a diurnal pattern of variation. It is lowest in the early morning and highest in the later afternoon and evening. The pulse rates of women average 5 to 10 beats per minute faster than those of men. The pulse decreases from infancy through middle adulthood and increases slightly in late adulthood (Appendix 2). The pulse increases with increased activity but is lower than normal in athletically conditioned persons. The normal pulse rate among adults ranges between 50 and 100 beats per minute. The pulses are symmetrical, strong, and regular (Table 2-2).

The respiratory rate is usually taken immediately after obtaining the pulse while the examiner continues to hold the wrist as if taking the radial pulse. It is difficult to obtain an accurate respiratory rate when the client is cognizant that the breathing is being monitored, since voluntary control can override the normal involuntary process of inhalation and exhalation.

In counting respirations the client's chest is observed for inspiratory excursions for at least 15 seconds. When an irregular rhythm is detected, the respiratory rate is counted for a full minute. If the respirations are not readily discernible, the examiner gently places a hand upon the client's chest and palpates chest movement. In addition to the rate, the rhythm is also described. Respiratory rates vary with age, activity, and physiologic conditioning. The respiratory rate decreases from infancy through middle adulthood and increases slightly in late adulthood. It increases with activity but decreases with athletic conditioning. The normal adult respiratory rate ranges from 12 to 20 breaths per minute (Appendix 3).

The blood pressure can be measured directly and indirectly. Direct measurement is more accurate but is an invasive procedure necessitating cannulization of an artery. Indirect measurement is the preferred clinical method due to its ease, client acceptability, and lack of possible complications. It requires a sphygmomanometer and a stethoscope and involves a combination of inspection, palpation, and auscultation. There are two types of sphygmomanometers: aneroid and mercury (Figure 2-8). The aneroid sphygmomanometer consists of metal bellows connected to

Table 2-2   Abnormalities of the Arterial Pulse

Finding	Condition	Explanation
Small, weak pulses (slow rise and prolonged peak).	Congestive heart failure Shock	Diminished pulse pressure from decreased stroke volume.
	Aortic stenosis	Diminished pulse pressure from mechanical obstruction to left ventricular output.
Large, bounding pulses (rapid rise, rapid collapse).	Anxiety, exercise, fever, anemia, hyperthyroidism	Decreased pulse pressure from hyperactive states.
	Aortic regurgitation	Increased pulse pressure from rapid runoff of blood.
	Patent ductus arteriosus	
	Atherosclerosis	Increased pulse pressure from increased rigidity of aorta.
Pulse changes in amplitude from beat to beat—regular rhythm (pulsus alternans).	Left-sided heart failure	Ventricle pumps inefficiently.
Bigeminy. Normal beat alternates with premature beat of decreased amplitude.	Premature ventricular contractions	Diminished stroke volume of PVC results in early weak beat; pulse pressure alternates in volume.
Pulsus paradoxicus. Pulse diminishes in amplitude during inspiration (detected during blood pressure determination).	Obstructive lung disease Constrictive pericardial disease	Exaggeration of response to respiration in which the systolic pressure is inaudible for more than a 10 mmHg drop in cuff pressure.
Diminished, delayed femoral pulse in relation to radial pulse.	Coarctation of the aorta Occlusive aortic disease	With each systole, blood takes longer to reach lower extremities than upper extremities due to obstructed flow through aorta.

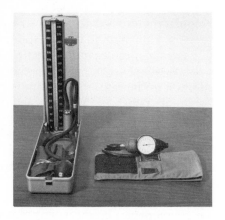

Figure 2-8. Aneroid and mercury sphygmomanometers.

a compression cuff. The bellows expand and contract as pressure within the apparatus increases and decreases. Movement of the bellows causes movement of an attached gear that moves a pointer across a calibrated dial.

The mercury sphygmomanometer consists of a straight glass tube attached to a mercury reservoir. The reservoir is connected to a pressure bulb. Increased pressure within the bulb pushes mercury from the reservoir up into the tube.

The technique of taking a blood pressure is the same for both types of sphygmomanometers. The underlying principle is that pressure is applied to a limb to cause temporary cessation of blood flow through an artery. A cuff is applied to an arm or leg. The cuff should be 20 percent wider than the diameter of the limb used and long enough to encircle it completely (Figure 2-9). Cuffs that are too small give falsely elevated readings while the converse is true for cuffs that are too large. When applied to the arm, the cuff is positioned approximately 2.5 centimeters (1 inch) above the antecubital fossa. When applied to the thigh, the cuff is applied the same distance above the popliteal space. The thigh is used when the arms are injured, are absent, or have therapeutic tubes or devices whose functioning could be hampered during

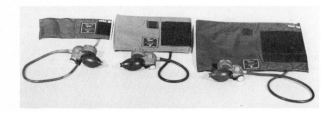

Figure 2-9. Infant, adult, and obese blood pressure cuffs.

cuff inflation. The thigh blood pressure determination is compared to the arm blood pressure in hypertensive clients to rule out aortic coarctation (Table 2-3). Thigh blood pressures are normally higher than arm blood pressures. The client is prone for determination of thigh blood pressures.

Within the cuff is a distensible bladder connected to a rubber hand bulb. After the cuff is applied, the examiner palpates the brachial or popliteal pulse and pumps the hand bulb approximately 30 mmHg above the point where the pulse is no longer palpable. The bladder pressure is gradually reduced at a rate of 3 millimeters of mercury per second until the pulse is again palpable. This represents the palpatory systolic pressure. Palpatory pressures are often falsely elevated up to 10 mmHg. Diastolic pressures cannot be obtained by palpation. The cuff is completely deflated.

The procedure is repeated with the diaphragm of the stethoscope placed over the pulse point (Figure 2-10). Auscultation of the blood pressure reveals several distinct changes in sound quality that reflect corresponding cardiac activities. These are called the Korotkoff sounds. The Korotkoff sounds consist of five phases: (1) loud, thumping beats; (2) swishing sounds; (3) crisper, sharper more intense sounds; (4) muffling of sounds; and (5) absence of sounds. Phase 1 reflects the point where pressure within the blood vessel is the same as the cuff pressure and is the systolic pressure. Phase 2 results from turbulent blood flow that vibrates the vessel wall. During Phase 3 the blood vessel is open fully during systole but closed during diastole. Phase 4 occurs when the cuff pressure falls below the pressure within the blood vessel; this is the first diastolic pressure. It signifies that the blood vessel is partially open during early diastole. Phase 5 occurs when the blood vessel re-

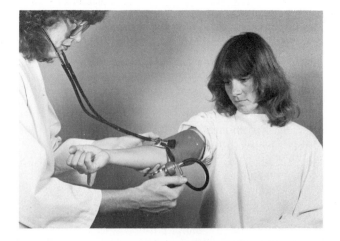

Figure 2-10. Procedure for taking blood pressure at the brachial artery.

Table 2-3. Selected Blood Pressure Abnormalities

Finding	Condition	Explanation
Elevated blood pressure	Anxiety	Increased circulating catecholamines cause increased total peripheral resistance and increased blood pressure.
	Hypertension	Blood pressure elevated on 3 separate visits; most prevalent form has unknown etiology. Risk factor for cardiovascular disease, cerebrovascular accidents.
Inaudible blood pressure	Shock (due to hemorhage, acute injury, surgery, burns, fluid volume deficit, infections, severe emotional disturbances, and drug toxicity)	Peripheral circulatory failure results in greatly diminished amount of blood pumped with each systole.
Variations in systolic pressure	Arrhythmias	Irregular rhythms cause variable amount of blood pumped with each systole (because ventricular filling times vary).
Auscultatory gap	Hypertension	Silent interval exists between systolic and diastolic blood pressures. If this situation is not recognized, the examiner can grossly underestimate systolic blood pressure or overestimate diastolic blood pressure
Blood pressure lower in the legs than in the arms	Coarctation of the aorta Occlusive disease of aorta	Narrowing of aorta causes decrease in volume of blood pumped to the legs with each systole.

mains open throughout systole and diastole. It is the second diastolic pressure (Figure 2-11).

Blood pressure is recorded as three values: the systolic blood pressure (loud, thumping beats), the first diastolic pressure (muffling of sounds), and the second diastolic pressure (disappearance of sounds). Pulse pressure refers to the difference between the systolic and second diastolic pressure.

New clients, those needing a general health assessment and those with suspected cardiovascular disease, require blood pressure readings on both arms in three positions: supine, sitting, and standing. The supine pressures are taken after the client has rested for five minutes; immediately afterward, the sitting and standing measurements are taken. The difference between the left and right sides and the difference between positions normally do not exceed 10 millimeters of mercury. Systolic blood pressure normally ranges from 95 to 140 mmHg with an average of 120 mmHg. The value for the second diastolic blood pressure normally ranges from 60 to 90 mmHg with an average of 80 mmHg. Blood pressure is age-related and reflects physiologic conditioning and emotional factors. In general, blood pressure increases with age or anxiety and decreases with athletic conditioning (Table 2-3, Appendix 4).

Other Measurements

Height and weight measurements provide baseline data for future comparisons and provide insight into general health, including nutritional status (Appendixes 5 and 6). Weight determinations are also necessary for planning some medication regimens.

In obtaining the height measurement, the client stands without shoes beside a standardized scale calibrated in centimeters or inches. The examiner lowers a bar along the axis of the scale to the level where it touches the client's head and records this as the height. For an accurate reading, the client must stand as upright as possible. The height of the bedridden patient is normally not necessary; however, an approximation is possible by using a tape measure for the distance from the top of the head to the heels.

The most accurate clinically useful method of obtaining the weight of ambulatory clients utilizes a balance beam scale. Home-variety spring scales usually do not provide consistently reliable readings. The client is weighed with an empty bladder and nude if possible. If this is impossible (most scales are located in hallways), minimal clothing is desirable and the amount of clothing is recorded with the weight. An

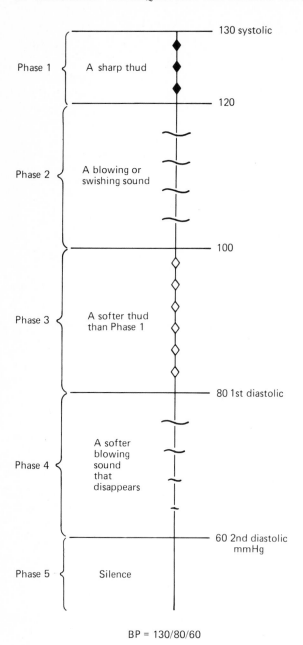

BP = 130/80/60

Figure 2-11. Korotkoff sounds.

weight determinations are most accurate if they are obtained at the same time each day.

Life Cycle Variations

Childhood

The examiner observes the child for the same physical, mental, and emotional characteristics as the adult. In addition, the interaction between the parent and child is assessed (Chapter 1).

Since children frequently are unfamiliar with most of the equipment used in physical examination, health assessment is expedited by involving the parent and child (the parent takes the temperature while the examiner asks history questions); introducing one instrument at a time; permitting the child to handle the instruments when possible (for example, a stethoscope); providing a brief explanation prior to beginning ("This is a stethoscope. I will use it to listen to your heart."); examining a doll first (Figure 2–12); proceeding in a confident and matter of fact manner; and reserving uncomfortable procedures for last (inspecting the throat with a tongue blade). Most children are inquisitive and interested in the assessment procedures if given some time to adjust to the presence of the examiner, a stranger. While the child sits on the parent's lap, some aspects may be covered, for instance, auscultation of the chest. One general rule of thumb is to begin with techniques requiring quiet, such as auscultation; however, in working with children the examiner demonstrates flexibility and willingness to alter routine in order to take advantage of alterations in mood.

attempt to obtain serial weight determinations with the client wearing the same clothing facilitates greater accuracy. It is important that the client stand with hands free during the measurement. If debilitated, another person can stand on the scale with the client, and that person's weight is subtracted from the reading. Bedridden patients are weighed supine on scales that are brought to the bedside. Many critical care units have metabolic beds with a built-in scale for monitoring weight. As weight varies throughout the day in response to dietary and elimination variables,

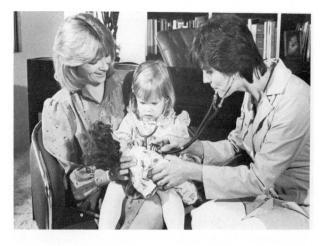

Figure 2-12. The examiner shows the toddler how she will listen to the chest of the doll.

Although some authorities recommend rectal temperature determinations for all children under age 10, most children can cooperate for oral readings earlier than this age. The pulse rate of infants is best obtained by observation of anterior fontanelle pulsations, palpation of the carotid or femoral arteries, or cardiac auscultation. Palpation of the radial artery is usually not useful until after age 3 due to the fast rate of infants and the difficulty in holding the arm of older babies still long enough. Respirations in neonates are characteristically irregular in rhythm; therefore, they are observed for at least 60 seconds. Young children also display greater excursions of the abdomen than chest; therefore, in measuring the respiratory rate the examiner views the abdomen as well as the chest.

Blood pressure determinations frequently are not obtained among children; however this is considered an omission in thorough health assessment of children over 18 months of age. As there are a variety of methods useful with young children, the method utilized is recorded. Since the same rules apply to cuff size for children, a variety of sizes ranging from 1.5 to 12 inches should be available. In young children, auscultation of the blood pressure sounds may not be possible; however, when auscultation is used, diastolic blood pressure is considered to be the point where sounds stop rather than the point where muffling of sounds begins.

In cases where auscultation is impossible, palpation of the blood pressure sometimes may be used. The systolic pressure corresponds with the level at which the radial pulse is first felt, although the palpatory pressure is generally 10 millimeters of mercury higher than that obtained by auscultation. Thigh pressures are the same as arm pressures in infants under one year of age. In infants, palpation is occasionally impossible, and the flush technique is useful. In this technique the extremity (arm or leg) is elevated to facilitate venous return, and the cuff is applied. With the limb elevated, an elastic bandage is applied, beginning distally and ending at the cuff. Then the cuff is inflated just beyond the expected systolic reading. The extremity is placed level again, and the pressure is gradually released until a flush of color returns to the pale extremity. This point corresponds to the median between the systolic and diastolic pressures.

For height determination the young baby is positioned supine with the head in contact with a bar at zero on the scale. The legs are extended, and another bar is advanced toward the child until it contacts the soles of the feet. The reading at the scale corresponds with the height. Weight is also obtained with the child supine on a baby scale until the child is willing to stand on the platform of a balance scale (usually at age two).

Measurement of the head circumference is an important aspect of the physical examination of the newborn; it is generally obtained at every visit until the child is two years of age. Head circumference is related to intracranial volume and provides a means of estimating the rate of brain growth. Normally head circumference is between 32 and 38 centimeters at birth, with an average of 34 centimeters. Head circumference in males is generally greater than in females; however, there is usually less than 1.0 centimeter mean difference in size.

Head circumference is measured with a metal or disposable paper tape. Cloth tape stretches with use and therefore provides inaccurate values over time. The examiner places the tape over the most prominent part of the occiput just above the supraorbital ridges (Figure 2-13). Individual readings are not as significant as trends in growth. Normally there is a 5.0 centimeter increase in the first four months (about 1/2 inch per month). By 12 months an additional 5.0 centimeters of growth is completed. By 18 years of age there is only another 10 centimeter increase over the head circumference at 12 months.

Frequently chest circumference is measured. However, this is not clinically significant except as an indicator of head development, as the head circumference exceeds the chest circumference until age two. For chest circumference the tape measure is applied around the chest at the nipple line.

The examiner plots the values for height, weight, and head circumference on growth curve charts. Values differ slightly for females and males (Appendix 7). Normally the individual child consistently has values on or near a given percentile curve. Values for height and weight only are plotted on growth curves for children over two years of age. Growth abnormalities

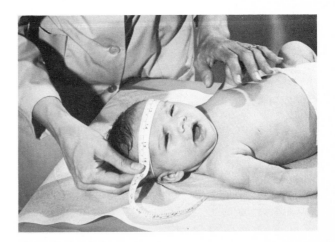

Figure 2-13. Measurement of the infant's head circumference.

are suspected in children with weight and height measurements in different percentiles, in children who shift percentile groups, and in children whose measurements are near or outside the 10th or 90th percentiles.

Adolescence

During adolescence, temperature and respiratory rates decrease, and blood pressure increases to adult values. This reflects a continuation of trends initiated at birth and existing throughout childhood. A growth spurt in body length occurs in girls from age 10 to 12 years and in boys from age 12 to 14 years.

Pregnancy

The temperature, pulse, and respiratory rates are increased slightly during pregnancy while blood pressure normally decreases. The weight increases at an approximately steady rate so that a total gain of 20 to 30 pounds occurs at the time of parturition (Appendix 8).

During pregnancy an additional measurement is taken to approximate fetal growth. This is the height of the uterine fundus; it is measured at monthly intervals until the 28th week, bimonthly until the 36th week, and then weekly. Although some agencies use a tape measure, others use calipers to measure the distance from the symphysis pubis to the fundus. Use of a tape measure includes the actual distension of the abdomen and therefore yields a larger measurement (Figure 2-14). Readings are more useful if one method is used consistently.

Late Adulthood

There are no differences in general health assessment techniques in working with older people, except that

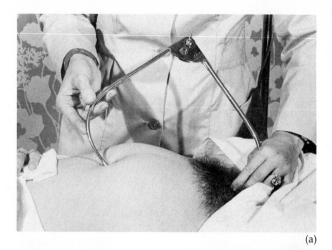

(a)

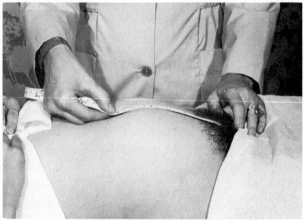

(b)

Figure 2-14. (a) Measurement of the height of the uterine fundus with calipers; (b) measurement of height of the uterine fundus with tape measure.

examiners maintain flexibility in the order of performing physical examination techniques in order to minimize fatigue. The vital signs vary with age. Temperature is generally slightly lower, while pulse and respiratory rates and blood pressure increase gradually after middle adulthood. In addition, there is a decrease in height due to a loss of collagen in the intervertebral discs.

Psychosocial assessment is an integral part of the entire health assessment process. The data obtained for the assessment come from the general history, the psychosocial history, and the mental status examination. This information provides an indication of the individual's current and past level of psychosocial functioning.

The assessment format presented in this chapter follows a developmental model encompassing the entire life cycle. The term *life cycle* refers to a concept in which an individual proceeds through a series of stages from birth to death. Changes take place in each stage, and a transition is required to progress from one stage to the next.

Within this developmental model are two major components: biological processes and environmental factors. The biological processes unfold upon a predetermined genetic and physiologic timetable. The environmental factors include the individual's interactions with the environment, that is, interactions with other people and things. The biological processes and the environmental factors interact in a reciprocal manner throughout the life cycle. These interactions lead to a sequential progression in which each new level of functioning represents a higher level of human organization and adaptation. An example is the interaction between mother and baby during early crawling. When the baby makes the first crawling attempts, the mother extends her arms toward the child and squeals with glee. The baby then crawls toward the mother. The mother's delight in a more advanced level of functioning leads the baby to repeat the activity.

With each advancement in the child's biological ability, the parent's responsiveness determines to what degree the child's biological potential will be fulfilled. In addition, each new biological advancement leads to further growth in the child's psychological abilities and social relationships. Through this process the child is able to reach higher levels of biopsychosocial development. The process described here is called developmental because it leads to a higher level of psychological organization and adaptation.

The developmental stages can be organized chronologically into infancy/toddlerhood, early childhood, adolescence, early adulthood, midlife transition, middle adulthood, and late adulthood. The ability to reach each successive stage is based upon successful completion of specific developmental tasks. The term developmental tasks refers to internal psychological processes and behaviors. A developmental task may be defined as a piece of psychological work that must be accomplished in order for a

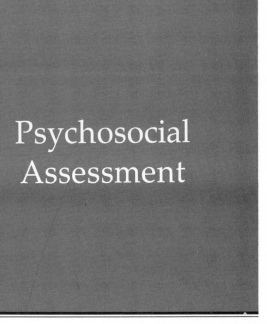

Psychosocial Assessment

_____ Objectives _____

The examiner will be able to do the following:

1. Obtain a psychosocial history including developmental stage criteria
2. Conduct a mental status examination
3. Recognize abnormalities
4. Record the information obtained

particular line of development to proceed. Tasks come about because of internal or external events. For example, the biological changes of puberty bring on adolescence, and certain social forces can bring on retirement. The individual must accept the challenge of the new task, engage in the necessary work, and create an adaptive response to the task. The concept of adaptation used here refers to the individual's ability both to accommodate to the environmental demands and to actively change the environment in keeping with personal needs.

The first developmental stage is *infancy/toddlerhood* (birth to age three). The primary task is for the infant to attach to and detach from the mother. This relationship with mother is the first significant relationship in life; its success determines to a great extent the success of future relationships. In the first few months of life bonding between mother and baby must occur; during the second six months of life the baby begins to separate physically from mother through activities such as crawling. The baby then begins to establish its own sense of self or personal identity as separate and distinct from mother. This psychological process continues to some degree throughout life.

The second stage, *early childhood* (age three to six), begins after the child solidly establishes a relationship with mother. During this stage the child continues to expand its interests to the father, siblings, other family members, and friends. During this time the child usually begins to imitate the parent of the same sex as an internal sexual identity is formed.

During *childhood* (age six to puberty) the child continues to build upon the achievement of family relationships and extends these relationships to include friends. Friends become important to the child and are valued as peers and companions.

In the latter years of early childhood and beginning years of childhood proper, the child is confronted with parental and societal rules and standards. The child must accept some of these rules, along with the accompanying frustrations. During this struggle, the child develops new outlets for expression of anger, assertiveness, and creativity. As an outcome of this process, the child forms a conscience. The development of a conscience plus the child's increased ability to express and control itself results in the formation of inner controls of behavior. These controls enable the child to expand activities to interests outside the family, such as school, hobbies, and sports.

During *adolescence* (puberty to age 20) the increased hormonal activity leads to physical changes. These changes herald the onset of the adult body. The individual is no longer a child and needs to relate to the parents as an adult. The ability for adult sexual activity and procreation is present, but open display of such activities is often uncomfortable for the adolescent and discouraged by family and societal standards. Therefore, the adolescent must find new socially acceptable outlets for these feelings. The adolescent often expresses these feelings, and the wish to become an independent adult, by rebelling against the authority of the parents, joining a peer group, and seeking relationships with the opposite sex, first on a trial basis and then on a more permanent basis.

The *young adult* (early adulthood, ages 20 to 40) has left childhood and moved into a new generation. The individual is still separating from the parents and forming an adult relationship with them. At the same time the young adult is setting goals and ideals in life, and is establishing commitments in intimate relationships and work. The individual is also confronted with decisions about having children, being in-between the younger and older generations, pursuing occupational goals, and establishing a stable marital relationship.

The *midlife transition period* (ages 35 to 45) is marked by questions and doubts about the choices that one has made in life. These questions and doubts are brought on by the awareness of personal death and the time limitations in life. The fact that life is finite means that some dreams can never be achieved. The individual must abandon unreachable goals and reorder priorities in life toward more achievable goals. This period may be a time of turmoil; life changes such as divorce and job changes may occur.

Middle adulthood (ages 40 to 60) is usually a more settled period than the midlife transition. Important career and marital decisions usually have been made by this time, and the person has the opportunity to enjoy the outcome of the decisions. Generally, realistic career goals have been reached, and the individual is part of the generation that makes the decisions in the business and social power structure. This time in life often brings personal losses (death of parents and contemporaries and loss of parental role with children) that require an adjustment in the relationship with the spouse. These changes often offer opportunities for a new and different relationship.

In *late adulthood* (age 60 and over) the individual faces the task of maintaining continuing vitality in the face of continuing losses. The losses include personal illness, threat of death, death of spouse and friends, and loss of income and social position through work. But the individual is also freed from the responsibilities of raising a family, work requirements, and other demands. Retirement offers opportunities for new activities. The individual has a perspective of the old and the new, without the necessarily intense involvement of younger years. This combination can lead to a sense of objectivity, wisdom, and serenity.

The healthy individual completes the tasks in one stage and progresses in an orderly fashion to the next stage (Table 3-1). Developmental stages do not begin and end abruptly but include a period of transition; one stage shades gradually into the next. Incomplete accomplishment of a task may lead to faulty development in future stages. The concept of completion of a task is relative; few tasks are totally resolved, and some may need to be reworked during a future stage.

An incompletely resolved task may still be sufficiently resolved to permit some progression to the next stage. With a new stage there may be new opportunities to resolve the past incompleted task and to resolve the new stage-appropriate task. For example, a woman in early adulthood becomes a parent for the first time. This new situation may revive conflicts and feelings from childhood. Therefore, parenting provides her the opportunity to have new solutions for past tasks (psychological separation from her parents) plus the opportunity to resolve cur-

Table 3-1. Developmental Tasks Throughout the Life Cycle

Stage	Task	Examples of Behavioral Indications
Infancy/toddlerhood 0-3 years	Physical and psychological separation from the mother.	Voluntarily leaves mother to play with another person or toy.
	Assumption of own individual characteristics.	Tells mother specific food preferences.
Early childhood 3-7 years	Social interaction within the family.	Engages family members in play.
	Beginning of social interaction outside family.	Plays with other children.
	Early formation of sexual identity.	Knows physical differences between sexes; recognizes and likes own sexual identity.
Childhood 6-puberty	Formation of significant peer relationships.	Has close friends.
	Development of new skills and interests.	Enjoys school, hobbies, sports.
	Internalization of parental values.	Wants to be clean and neat.
	Reinforcement of sexual identity.	Prefers to take the role of own sex in activities.
Adolescence Puberty-20 years	Completion of physical and psychological separation from parents.	Rebels against parental authority and forms new relationships.
	Beginning involvement with intimate relationships outside the family.	Becomes infatuated, dates, and experiments with falling in love.
	Completion of sexual maturity.	Develops secondary sex characteristics and experiments with sexual play.
Early adulthood 18-35 years	Achievement of intimacy.	Falls in love and marries.
	Shift in commitment from family of origin to new partner.	Moves from parents' home.
	Assumption of parental role.	Decides whether to have children.
	Establishment of occupation.	Completes education and makes career choice.
Midlife transition 35-45 years	Realization and acceptance of personal death and finiteness of life.	Prepares for economic security for spouse and children in the event of personal illness or death.
	Adjustment to aging of own body.	Accepts beginning decline in physical abilities.
	Adjustment to illness and death of parents	Mourns death of parent.
	Reordering of priorities and setting achievable goals in committed relationships and occupation.	Resolves problems in or leaves marriage; reevaluates occupational choice and decides to continue or change career.
Middle adulthood 40-60 years	Stabilization of marriage.	Maintains commitments to marriage by resolving conflicts through compromise.
	Consolidation of occupational identity.	Works toward maximum achievement in chosen occupation.
	Adjustment to adolescent children's physical and emotional independence.	Accepts children as adults.
	Commitment to children's and grandchildren's goals.	Supports children's occupational and marital choice.
Late adulthood 60 and over	Adjustment to personal illness and threat of death.	Accepts limitations of illness and adapts to altered life style.
	Adjustment to illness and death in significant others.	Mourns death of significant others and forms new attachments and interests.
	Adjustment to retirement.	Maintains active life by replacement of occupation with other interests.

rent, stage-appropriate tasks (assumption of the parental role). With the resolution of past and current tasks through parenting, the woman is able to understand her children, provide quality parenting, and relate more comfortably to her family of origin.

From a developmental perspective, emotional health can be defined as the ability of an individual to complete the previous developmental stages to a degree that enables involvement in the developmental tasks of the current stage and to derive feelings of satisfaction, happiness, and self-esteem from such development. Just as the definition of physical health is not merely the absence of physical disease, the definition of emotional health is not the absence of emotional turmoil or conflict. Conflicts and struggles are a necessary and inevitable part of life. The ability of the individual to resolve these conflicts adaptively determines the degree of emotional health.

Assessment Modalities

Preparation

The interviewer uses the same interviewing techniques to obtain the psychosocial history as for the health history (Chapter 1). Usually a transition statement is needed to inform the client of a change from physical to psychosocial questions. An example of a transition statement might be, "Now I want to talk to you about your personal life." If the client is suffering from a physical condition such as pain, the interviewer might say, "How has this pain affected your personal life?" and then continue with psychosocial questions.

The interview itself may precipitate anxiety in the client. In this situation the interviewer can assist the client by explaining that anxiety may be a normal reaction to disclosing personal information. If the anxiety interferes with the assessment process, the interviewer might say, "You seem to be getting anxious. Would you prefer to talk about this later?" If the client says yes, the interviewer then proceeds to another area and later returns to the anxiety-provoking topic. If the anxiety recurs when the subject is brought up again, the interviewer might say, "This seems to be a difficult subject for you to discuss. What do you suppose is making you anxious?" This same question is asked if the client had chosen to continue talking about the anxiety-producing subject when it first occurred.

The psychosocial assessment includes the history and the mental status examination. Aspects of the history and mental status examination are often obtained in other areas of the comprehensive health history. The mental status examination is the counterpart of the physical examination in other body systems and regions.

Psychosocial History

The psychosocial history is a collection of data giving the interviewer information about the client's life. This information is used to determine the client's current and past level of psychosocial functioning. In the developmental model the client's answers to the questions also tell the examiner to what degree the client has completed the tasks from previous stages and to what degree the client is engaged in the tasks of the present stage (Table 3-2).

The initial focus of the psychosocial history is the client's current life. The answers provide an indication of the client's thoughts, feelings, and behavior in current life situations and relationships (Table 3-3). After present circumstances are discussed, the interviewer proceeds to cover the past developmental stages in a chronological order (Tables 3-4 and 3-5).

In addition to assessing each developmental stage the interviewer looks for patterns and themes of thoughts, feelings, and behavior that have existed throughout a number of life cycle stages. These patterns help to paint a picture of the individual's personality and environment over time.

NOTE: Not all questions are asked of every client. See Tables 3-3, 3-4, and 3-5 for examples of how the developmental history may be obtained. The goal of a developmental history is to have an overall sense of whether that particular period in life was normal, or what specific problems existed.

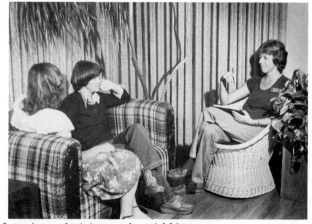

Interviewer obtaining psychosocial history.

Table 3-2. Developmental History Questions

Stage	Questions	Rationale
Infancy/ toddler-hood	Was you mother's pregnancy with you planned? What was the health of your mother during pregnancy and newborn period? What were the emotional reactions of your parents to your birth? Who was the primary caregiver?	Provides information on how parents accept and appreciate the new baby. Determines emotional climate of family into which the child was born.
	What were your mother's behavior and attitudes toward feeding you? Did you suck your thumb? for how long? What were your eating patterns? What were your sleeping patterns? What were the ages you sat, crawled, walked, talked?	Demonstrates the ability of the mother to interact in a loving and accepting manner in regard to child's feelings and dependency needs. Provides information on baby's biological maturation. Provides information of physical capacities.
	What were your parents' attitudes toward your attempts at independent behavior?	Gives information on the mother's reaction to the child's increasing independence through mobility and speech and information about the mother's ability to encourage the child's independence and self-reliance while providing protection and security.
	At what age were you toilet trained? What were your parents' methods and attitudes toward toilet training? At what age was toilet training achieved? bowel? bladder? day? night? Did you have temper tantrums? What were the attitudes of your parents toward expression of anger and defiance? What were your parents' attitudes regarding discipline? How was it provided and by whom?	Provides information on how demanding parents were in insisting on conformity from the child. Attitudes toward toilet training are often a barometer of general attitudes toward discipline and can indicate parent's ability to accept and manage child's need for power and control of own body.
	What were the attitudes of your parents toward physical illness? Were there any long separations from mother?	Provides information on parental attitudes toward physical and emotional trauma.
Early childhood	What were your parents like? How close were you with your father? mother? What was your reaction to the birth of a sibling? Your parents' reaction? What was your relationship like with your siblings? Were there any other people living in your home while you were growing up?	Provides information on family atmosphere and the quality of the relationships with both parents and siblings.
	What were your parents' attitudes toward displays of affection, both physical and verbal, toward each other? toward you and your siblings? How did your parents feel about each other? What were your parents' attitudes toward sexual curiosity and sexual play (masturbation)? How were you permitted to express anger? What forms of expressing anger were not allowed?	Provides information on the degree of strictness or permissiveness regarding sexuality and discipline, and the parent's comfort with affection, sexuality, and anger.
	Did you attend preschool? other activities? friends?	Provides evidence of beginning peer relationships.
	How did you feel about being a girl/boy?	Indicates sense of pride in sexual role.
	What were your parents' attitudes and reactions to illnesses in you, your siblings, and themselves? What were your attitudes and reactions to illness?	Provides information on parent's attitudes toward illness, which are often adopted later by the client.
	Did you ever have phobias, excessive fears, nightmares, bed wetting after completion of toilet training, nail biting?	Provides information on emotional disturbances; if mild and transient, may be phase-appropriate and without clinical significance.

Table 3-2. Developmental History Questions (*continued*)

Stage	Questions	Rationale
Childhood	What were your parents' attitudes toward school progress, friends, recreation, and other activities? Can you describe your satisfaction with progress in school, friends, recreation, and other activities? Can you describe your achievements in school? Can you describe your satisfaction with hobbies and sports?	Provides information on child's abilities and interests outside the home and to what degree these are sources of pride, self-esteem, and self-expression. Usually indicates child has sufficiently stable emotional and family life that interests can be directed to new areas.
	Can you tell me about your close friendships, not just acquaintances?	Indicates ability to establish significant and satisfying social relationships outside the home.
	What was your reaction to the birth of a sibling? Your parents' reactions? What was your relationship like with your siblings?	Describes emotional home and family life.
	What were your parents' attitudes and reactions to illnesses in you, your siblings, and themselves? What were your attitudes and reactions to this?	Provides information on parents' attitudes toward illness, which are often adopted later by the client.
	What were your reactions towards members of the same and opposite sex?	Provides information on comfort in own sexual role.
	In disagreements with family, friends, teachers, how was anger handled—expressed or inhibited? and how was it received by others?	Provides information on child's acceptance of societal standards for behavior, while maintaining opportunities for self-expression.
	Did you have any sleep disorders? habitual or ritualized behavior? Did you have any social problems—drugs, delinquency, school truancy, phobias, impaired performance in school?	Provides evidence of emotional disturbances; if mild and transient, may be phase-appropriate and without clinical significance.
Adolescence	What were your parents' attitudes toward your behavior? accepting? permissive? controlling? demanding? What were your attitudes toward your parents and parental authority? compliant? defiant? rebellious? assertive?	Provides information about emotional climate of family, how restrictive or tolerant parents were, how compliant or defiant client was.
	How shy or outgoing were you? Did you have many friends? Did you make friends easily? Did you belong to a group (crowd) of friends? Were you popular? How did you feel about yourself?	Provides information on client's self-esteem, self-confidence, ability to form social relationships outside the family; provides picture of client's personality.
	When did you first notice changes in your body? What were your emotional reactions to these changes? How did these changes make you feel? When was your first period? Did you understand what was happening? How was sexual information obtained and from whom? Do you recall masturbating? How did you feel about it? guilt? anxiety? shame? Did you have any homosexual experiences? Tell me about your sexual experience with boys/girls (heterosexual)? kissing? petting? intercourse? How did you feel about it? If yes to intercourse: Boy, did you ever get a girl pregnant? Girl, were you ever pregnant? What happened to the pregnancy? How do you feel about it?	Indicates degree of comfort and freedom client feels to permit interest and experimentation with sex. How guilty, ashamed, or inhibited? Indicates psychological reactions and consequences to sexual changes and behaviors.
	What were your parent's attitudes toward dating and sexual interests?	Provides information about family's and client's attitudes and standards regarding physical maturity and sexual relationships.
	Were you ever in love? How long did the relationship last? How and why did the relationship end?	Indicates degree of comfort and freedom in establishing an intimate relationship outside the family. Indicates fears, problems and sources of pleasure in the intimate relationship.

Table 3-2. Developmental History Questions (*continued*)

Stage	Questions	Rationale
	How did your parents feel about your being seriously involved with someone?	Indicates parents' ability to relinquish ties with child.
	What were your scholastic and other interests? How far did you go in school? How well did you do in school? If dropped out, why? What did you do next? How did you feel about it? What did you do in high school? Is this what you wanted to do? Is it what your parents wanted you to do? When you were a teenager, what did you want to be when you were an adult? (for teenager—what do you want to do when you're an adult?)	Shows initiative and sustained effort in pursuing educational or occupational goal, whether this was source of self-esteem and self-confidence, and whether child could be different from parents' expectations.
	Did you have any problems with sexual promiscuity, delinquency, or school truancy? Did you experiment with drugs? Describe (cigarettes, alcohol, marijuana, cocaine, uppers, downers, LSD, PCP, narcotics).	Provides evidence of possible emotional disturbances. If mild and transient, may be phase-appropriate and without clinical significance.
Early adulthood	When did you first move from your parents' home? What was the reason (school, military service, marriage, to live independently)?	Provides information on client's ability to function on own for the first time.
	How did you feel about living away from your parents? Did you support yourself financially? how?	
	Tell me about significant relationships. Have you ever been married? How did you meet your spouse? How long did you date prior to marriage? Who took the initiative for marriage? When did you marry? Describe spouse, satisfaction with marriage, sexual relationships with spouse. Have you had extramarital affairs?	Provides information on ability to accept responsibilities of being a marital partner and being financially independent while maintaining some ties to family of origin. Indicates ability to commit oneself to another person in a mutual relationship. Indicates capacity for trust, empathy, sincerity, and compassion. Sexual relationships are a barometer for emotional tone of a relationship. Sexual behavior can indicate the ability to assert oneself in obtaining and providing pleasure.
	Are there children? Were children planned? If no children, were they desired? How do you get along with your children? What was your reaction to pregnancy? How many children do you have? ages? sex?	Provides information on relationship to children and indicates the capacity to love and give of oneself.
	If not married, are you involved in an intimate relationship? Describe person, relationship, sex life. How committed are you to this person, person to you? Are you in love? How did previous relationships or marriages end and why?	Provides information on satisfaction in both relationships and work as sources of happiness and self-esteem.
	Describe your occupation. How do you like your work? What are your career goals and your expectations of meeting career goals? What was your highest grade completed? Did you want to go further in your education? Can you tell me more about what made you stop when you did? How did you feel about it? How do you feel now about this decision? Have you changed jobs? how often? why?	Demonstrates ability to decide upon and commit oneself to career goals. Indicates ability to have initiative and perseverance to pursue the goals.
	What is your financial situation?	Indicates ability to accept financial responsibility.
	Do you have close friends? Do you have other interests, hobbies, sports, community, and religious interests?	Indicates personal values and interests.

Table 3-2. Developmental History Questions (*continued*)

Stage	Questions	Rationale
Midlife transition	How happy are you? Do you have any problems? How close are you with your spouse? How satisfied are you with the closeness, sharing and sexual life in your marriage.	Provides information on client's current level of satisfaction in life. Indicates capacity for continued commitments toward intimacy and ability to derive pleasure from relationships.
	How old are your children? How have the sort of things that they are going through at their ages affected you? How have these affected your spouse? How close are you with your children?	Indicates quality of relationship with children. Indicates ability to understand and empathize with children passing through various developmental stages. Reflects the individual's thoughts, feelings and memories of own childhood.
	How old are your parents? How has their aging affected you and your relationship with them?	Indicates quality of continuing relationship with parents, degree to which client can relate to parents as an adult, and how parents are able to accept client as an adult.
	What experiences have you had with the death or illness of people close to you? What thoughts have you had about getting older and dying? How has the idea that life is time-limited affected you? What changes have you made in your life because of this time limitation?	Indicates recognition and acceptance of own mortality and time limitations. Indicates ability to evaluate and adapt to time limitations and set realistic goals.
	How happy are you with your work? What sort of future do you see for yourself?	Indicates to what degree work/career is a source of pleasure and self-esteem.
	What is your financial situation? How do you see it changing in the future?	Indicates to what degree client has or plans for financial security.
	What do you do for recreation? Do you have other social, community, or religious activities?	Indicates ability to engage in adult play. Indicates attitudes toward friends, civic, and spiritual matters.
Middle adulthood	How happy are you? Do you have any problems? How close are you with your spouse? How satisfied are you with the closeness, sharing, and sexual life in your marriage?	Provides information on client's current level of satisfaction in life. Indicates capacity for continued commitments toward intimacy and ability to derive pleasure from relationships.
	How old are your children? How close are you with your children? How do you feel about their growing up and leading an independent life? Do you have grandchildren? How do you get along with them? What does it mean to you to be a grandparent?	Indicates ability to relate to and accept children as independent adults. Indicates ability to allow the next generation to assume the parenting role.
	(To women—How do you feel about not being able to have children anymore?)	Indicates acceptance of loss of ability to procreate.
	How old are your parents? How has their aging affected you? How has the state of your physical health affected your lifestyle and finances? How have your spouse and children been affected? What adjustments have you made? How has the state of your spouse's health affected your life style and finances? What adjustments have you made? What has been the emotional effect of serious illness or death of friends and associates your own age?	Indicates ability to accept and adjust to aging and to chronic and limiting illnesses of self, parents, and contemporaries. Includes reactions to aging of the body and the ability to face illness and death in a realistic way.
	How happy are you in your work? Do you feel that you've achieved your career goals? How financially secure do you feel? What plans have you made for retirement?	Indicates degree of satisfaction in reaching what is probably the highest level of the client's occupation.
	What do you do for recreation? Do you have any other social, community, or religious activities?	Indicates ability to enjoy varying activities and to begin to use activities and relationships to substitute for changes in parental and occupational roles.

Table 3-2. Developmental History Questions (*continued*)

Stage	Questions	Rationale
Late adulthood	How happy are you? Do you have any problems? Is your spouse living? (If yes—How satisfied are you with the closeness, sharing, and sexual life of your marriage? If no—what was your reaction to the death of your spouse? Do you have a new partner? How satisfied are you with the relationship?)	Indicates degree of satisfaction in current intimate relationships. Indicates ability to adjust to death of spouse and to find a new and satisfying intimate relationship.
	How is your relationship with your children? grandchildren?	Indicates ability to adjust to role reversal that occurs at this time.
	What is your reaction to the death of your parents and contemporaries? How has physical illness affected you? What are your attitudes, expectations, and fears concerning your own death? What are your thoughts and plans about the future?	Indicates ability to accept the reality of one's own death as seen through the reaction to deaths of others and to increasing physical limitations, and ability to adapt to these circumstances.
	Are you retired? (If yes—How have you adjusted to retirement? What do you do for recreation? Do you have any other social, community, or religious activities? If not—What are your plans for retirement?) How do you handle your loneliness? How financially secure do you feel?	Indicates ability to adapt to a new role in life and to maintain activity and vigor despite reality of personal losses.

Table 3-3. Sample Interview: Present Psychosocial History of a 36-Year-Old Man

Dialogue	Interpretation
Interviewer: "What can you tell me about yourself—such as family and occupation?" Client: "I'm a chemist. I work for Consolidated Systems and have been there for 13 years. I like my job and someday hope to be in charge of my division. I'm married, with three kids, and live in Rockford. I met my wife in college, and we have a pretty good marriage. Our kids are 8, 5 and 3—two boys and the baby's a girl. My father died 2 years ago; it was hard for awhile but I'm okay now. My mother still lives alone in Chicago." Interviewer: "How satisfied are you with how things are going in your life? Are there any major problems" Client: "Not really, but I wish I could spend more time with my family; trying to get that promotion at work means a lot of time there." Interviewer: "What about your social life?" Client: "We go out with friends on the weekends but not during the week; I'm usually too tired. Most of our friends are from my work." Interviewer: "What about recreational and physical activity?" Client: "I play tennis but not regularly. My work often interferes."	This man has a reasonably happy and satisfying relationship with his wife and children. He seems to have adjusted to the death of his father. Although he wants to advance further in his career, the need to do more work has created pressures that limit his family, social, and recreational activities. In a developmental context, this man is in the midlife transition stage. He is engaged in and working out marital and family conflicts that will enable him to have a more stable life. Also, he is attempting to resolve the gap between his career aspirations and the realities of not having enough time in other areas of his life.

Table 3-4.   Sample Interview: Past Psychosocial History of a 23-Year-Old Single Woman
Who Lives Alone and Works as a Postal Clerk

Stage	Dialogue	Interpretation
Infancy/ toddlerhood	Interviewer: "Now I would like to learn about your background. Let's begin with your childhood and work toward the present. Many of the questions about your early childhood will involve things you don't remember. First tell me about the things you do remember or have learned about as you grew up. What do you know about the time your mother was pregnant with you; was the pregnancy planned, did your mother have any health problems?" Client: "I have no idea." Interviewer: "Okay, do you have any knowledge of what you were like as a baby?" Client: "I was told I was lazy, I wouldn't roll over or do things like that when they told me to; they even have movies showing this. But I guess I was a good baby." Interviewer: "Were there any problems with feeding; were you a good eater, picky eater, or have a history of colic?" Client: "No, I was told I was a good eater." Interviewer: "Were there major problems during the first few years of life with you or your family?" Client: "Not that I know of." Interviewer: "Were there any times when you and your mother were separated for a few days or more?" Client: "Yes. Just when my brother was born when I was 3½. My mother was in the hospital for about a week." Interviewer: "Do you remember your reactions to this separation?" Client: "I remember missing her but having a good time with my grandmother and aunt, who took care of me while she was gone." Interviewer: "Do you know when you sat up, crawled, walked, talked, or were toilet trained?" Client: "I don't know, probably the usual times." Interviewer: "What were your parents' attitudes toward you in your first few years of life: did they like having a new child, were they excited about each new thing you could do, did they find it a burden to have a small child?" Client: "Well, my mom was always excited about the things I could do, but my dad didn't pay that much attention to me till I got older."	Although the stage being discussed is infancy, it is often not possible to determine from the client what actually occurred during infancy. This interaction does demonstrate that as far as the client knows there were no major problems. Sometimes the degree of accomplishment of a developmental task in infancy may be discovered by obtaining information from the parents or it may be inferred from information obtained from later stages of development.

Table 3-4. Sample Interview: Past Psychosocial History of a 23-Year-Old Single Woman Who Lives Alone and Works as a Postal Clerk (*continued*)

Stage	Dialogue	Interpretation
Early childhood	Interviewer: "What do you recall about your brother's birth; what was your reaction?" Client: "I was really excited about it when my mom was pregnant. But after he was born, he was a real pain, he cried all the time; and besides, I wanted a sister." Interviewer: "What was it like being a little girl when you were growing up?" Client: "Oh, it was fun. I liked wearing my mom's clothes and we had several outfits that were the same! I also remember my best friend and I played dressup a lot." Interviewer: "How did you get along with your father?" Client: "My dad was pretty busy with work, but I remember playing games with him."	From this information there is evidence that as a young girl this woman's sexual identity was a source of pride and was fostered by her mother. The client had mixed feelings about her brother's birth; such mixed feelings are common. There is evidence of social interaction with her mother, father, and friend. By imitating her mother's behavior she demonstrated her wish to be an adult woman, rather than remain a small child cared for by mother. It can be inferred from this information and from her involvement with her father and friend that this little girl had begun to move toward a psychological separation from her mother. Often, when a client answers a question, she may provide information about other aspects of her life, so they do not have to be asked about directly. This client volunteered information that she had friends.
Middle childhood	Interviewer: "What can you tell me about your early school years? Was there any difficulty in leaving your mother on the first day of school?" Client: "No, I was looking forward to it because my older sister always liked school." Interviewer: "How did you like school?" Client: "I liked school. Our family moved just before I started kindergarten, and I became friends with two other girls who lived in my neighborhood. They were in my class, too. I did well in most subjects except history." Interviewer: "Were you involved in activities outside of school?" Client: "Yes. I was in the glee club and took dancing lessons. I wanted to be a ballerina." Interviewer: "Sounds like you were pretty busy. Were there ever any problems such as excessive fears, phobias, or nightmares?" Client: "Not really, but I did have nightmares after we moved and I was afraid of burglars." Interviewer: "How long did that last?" Client: "Oh, I guess about a month or so." Interviewer: "During your childhood did you ever have problems with family members?" Client: "No, my brother and I fought a lot, but we got along better as we got older." Interviewer: "Were there any major crises in the family? serious illness, death, job loss?" Client: "My father had a hernia operation but he was okay after that."	From this information there is evidence of continuing ability to separate from mother. A common indicator of problems with the task of separation is difficulty in leaving mother to attend school. The client also shows continued evidence of her identification as a girl with interest in playing with other girls and wanting to be a ballerina. Despite the move, she made friends easily. The appearance of nightmares demonstrated that the move caused some upheaval in her life. But the fact that they were transient and disappeared spontaneously indicates that she adapted to the situation. Her interests in extracurricular activities indicate a widening scope of interests in her life and suggest that her involvement in her own emotional and family problems did not interfere with her ability to direct interests elsewhere.

Stage	Dialogue	Interpretation
Adolescence	Interviewer: "Now let's turn to your adolescent years. When did you first notice changes in your body and how did you feel about it?" Client: "When I was 14 I finally got my period. I was relieved because all of my girlfriends had it before then." Interviewer: "And tell me about your dating and sexual experiences." Client: "I started going to parties in about the seventh grade, but I didn't really date until ninth grade; my parents wouldn't let me and we had big fights about it . . . what do you mean about sexual?" Interviewer: "Whatever sexual experiences you had during this time: kissing, petting, intercourse, pregnancy. And more importantly, how did you feel about it?" Client: "Well, I guess the usual, kissing and maybe a little petting; but I felt really guilty about the petting—and that's as far as I went. My parents would have really killed me." Interviewer: "And what about falling in love?" Client: "I dated a lot in high school and went steady in my senior year. But the first time I really fell in love was after I graduated." Interviewer: "What happened to that relationship?" Client: "Oh, it lasted about a year or so and we broke up. I wasn't ready to get married and settle down, and I still felt guilty about sex, and worried about what my parents would think."	This information illustrates some typical adolescent turmoil, which is age-appropriate. She had begun to sever emotional ties with her parents, to date, and to experiment sexually. She dated frequently, formed an intimate relationship, but had not felt prepared for the responsibilities of marriage. Summary of past history. The total past history illustrates that at each stage there was continuing evidence of the client's separation from her parents. In adolescence the ties with her parents were broken enough to allow her to fight with her parents, to live independently, and to fall in love. Throughout her life she has shown pride and confidence in her role as a female. Despite some minor difficulties in early life, her overall level of functioning was not restricted at any stage. Patterns of personality development emerge from the history. In following the developmental line of separation throughout these stages, it can be seen that this client fought with her parents and became independent from them. Yet, in one area this separation is incomplete: She still adopted her parents' values concerning sex. She has yet to complete this task by deciding what her own values regarding sex will be; these values may not be different from her parents' values, but they will clearly be hers and not theirs.

Mental Status Examination

The mental status examination is an evaluation tool that provides information about the client's current mental state. This information includes the client's levels of cognitive, affective, and psychomotor functioning, and is evaluated throughout the entire assessment process. The mental status examination usually requires few additional questions to the health history. The areas of examination include general appearance and behavior, sensorium and cognitive processes, thought content, thought processes, mood and affect, judgment, and insight.

General Appearance and Behavior. Observations regarding general appearance and behavior are made throughout the entire history and physical. This evaluation includes observations about the client's posture, body movements, facial expressions, speech, and attitude toward the examiner and the examination. The client's hair and clothes are normally neatly arranged and clean. Posture, body movements, facial expressions, and speech are coordinated, and the client's attitude is relaxed and cooperative.

Sensorium and Cognitive Processes. Sensorium refers to level of consciousness and orientation; the cognitive functions refer to attention and concentration, perception, memory, abstraction, and intellect. *Level of consciousness* is the degree to which an individual is alert and responsive to the surroundings. The examiner assesses both the level and consistency of the client's alertness. The level of consciousness is described in specific, objective terms. The examiner avoids the use of vague, judgmental terminology and describes exactly what is observed. The client is normally alert and responsive and maintains continuous and appropriate contact with the environment.

Table 3-5. Sample Interview: Present and Past Psychosocial History of a 72-Year-Old Widow
Who Lives Alone and Is Hospitalized for a Fractured Hip

Dialogue	Interpretation
Interviewer: "Please tell me about your current living circumstances."	From the beginning this woman communicates the central themes of her life. Her husband has died, she's lonely, and she tries to handle her loneliness partially by denying it and by involving herself with family, friends, and church activities. She is able to live within her financial means without hardship. Her attitudes toward physical illness indicate that she's a "fighter" who tries to maintain her activities despite limitations. If she doesn't overdo it, this behavior may be adaptive. In contrast, there is evidence that she has not adapted as successfully to the loss of her husband. She gets lonely, but despite offers has not allowed herself to consider a new relationship. She seems to be prepared for death and expresses a common fear: that she might have a lingering and painful illness.
Client: "What can I tell you about it? Pat died 10 years ago and it's never been the same. The children try to help but they have their own families."	
Interviewer: "And that leaves you out?"	
Client: "Well, sometimes, but I keep busy. You know, I visit the children, I'm on the advisory board for our church, and I play cards once a week with my friends."	
Interviewer: "How do you support yourself?"	
Client: "I get by. You know there's still some money from Pat's life insurance and I get Social Security."	
Interviewer: "What kind of work did you do?"	
Client: "After the kids were grown, I was a saleslady in a department store. I've been retired for 10 years."	
Interviewer: "How do you feel about your life in general?"	
Client: "I've had a good life. I just hope my hip's okay. I've never been one to just lie around."	
Interviewer: "Have you had any serious illnesses?"	
Client: "I had a mild heart attack a year after Pat died. I get a little pain once in a while, but, you know, you have to keep going."	
Interviewer: "Sounds like it was difficult for you when your husband died."	
Client: "What do you expect? After all we were married 41 years . . . . Oh, people say, 'you have to meet so-and-so,' but I never wanted any of that."	
Interviewer; "What do you do then for close companionship?"	
Client: "Well, its gets pretty bad sometimes, but you can't sit around and worry about it."	
Interviewer: "How much do you think about death?"	
Client: "I'm ready for it. I just don't want to suffer like Pat did."	
Interviewer: "How did your husband die? How did his death affect your life?"	
Client: "Pat had lung cancer and the last month or two it was pretty bad. As for me, I knew it was coming, but it was still hard. I still don't like living without him."	
Interviewer: "You must have had a good marriage."*	
Client: "We did. Oh, we had our problems like everbody, but we managed. And we had good kids."	

Here the interviewer can continue to obtain information about this developmental stage or begin to obtain information about previous developmental stages.

*Transition
(The interviewer shifts into questions about middle adulthood by selecting a convenient transition point and in this case does not point out the shift to the client in order not to interrupt the flow of the interview.

Orientation refers to awareness of the surroundings and circumstances. It includes questions about time, place, person, and situation, that is, day, date, client's name, place where the examination is being done, and the reason for the examination. Normally the client is oriented to time, place, person, and situation.

Attention and concentration refer to the ability to attend to a particular task; they are evaluated by noting whether the client is distracted and to what degree. Both attention and concentration are evaluated during the history taking by noting the client's ability to relate the history in a clear and concise manner and to answer questions directly, without drifting from the subject. If the client has difficulty in keeping to this task, attention and concentration are further tested. A common test is to ask the client to repeat a series of seven digits forward, then to repeat a different series of seven digits forward and backward. Normally, the client correctly recites at least five numbers forward and three numbers backward. Another test is to ask the client to count backwards from one hundred by sevens (serial sevens). Normally the client accomplishes this task in 90 seconds or less with no more than three errors. The results of these two tests are relative to the client's educational background.

Perception refers to the ability to receive information or to obtain knowledge through the senses. Faulty interpretation of the information received can cause perceptual distortions. Normally a perception is experienced only in the presence of a stimulus. The experience of a perception in the absence of a stimulus is called a hallucination. Most hallucinations are auditory, visual, or sometimes tactile. The examiner may evaluate the presence of hallucinations by asking the client, "Do you ever hear voices when no one is there; do you ever see things that are not there?" The misinterpretation of a stimulus is called an illusion. The examiner may evaluate the presence of illusions by asking the client, "Do you ever see a person, only to find out it was just a shadow?" Normally the client does not experience hallucinations or illusions.

Memory refers to the ability to register, retain and recall information. Long-term memory function is evaluated during the history taking when the client is asked to recall past medical history. Short-term memory is evaluated by naming three objects, telling the client to remember them, and then asking the client to recall them in five minutes and again in 30 minutes. Normally the client recalls the objects accurately and without hesitation.

Abstraction refers to the ability to explain symbolic meanings and concepts. Abstract reasoning is assessed by asking the client to describe the similarities between two things such as an apple and orange. In another technique the interviewer asks the client to explain the meaning of a familiar proverb such as, "People who live in glass houses should not throw stones." Normally the client performs these tasks accurately and easily.

Intellect refers to the client's general fund of knowledge and is evaluated by asking the client such things as the name of the president of the United States and as many preceding presidents as possible, the names of three rivers, or the materials houses are made of. The general fund of knowledge can often be inferred from noting the client's vocabulary. Normally the client's intellect is consistent with age and educational background.

Thought Content. *Thought content* refers to the subject matter of the interview; that is, what the client spontaneously says. Thought content tells the interviewer how the client understands and assigns meaning to the events in life. This information indicates how realistic, logical, and rational the individual's thinking is. Thought content is evaluated during the history by noting how the client explains what is happening in life. Normally events are explained on the basis of common logic and causality, rather than on the basis of special and unique personal attributes or powers. The interviewer also asks the client about the possession of special powers, occurrence of strange or unusual experiences, or feelings that the client is being pursued, controlled, or harmed by others (delusions). Thought content is normally rational and realistic, and the interviewer can easily follow the client's line of reasoning.

Thought Processes. *Thought processes* refer to the manner or style of thinking; that is, the way ideas are formed. Thought processes tell the interviewer how the client pursues a thought from beginning to end; whether thinking is linear, logical, and goal-directed; or whether it is interrupted, distorted, or irrelevant. Thought processes are evaluated during history taking. The client normally expresses thoughts clearly from beginning to end and can tell a series of events in a clear, sequential, and logical manner that is understandable to the interviewer.

Mood and Affect. *Mood and affect* refer to emotional states (feelings). *Mood* describes the emotional state over a period of time, whereas *affect* describes minute-to-minute fluctuations in emotional state. The interviewer evaluates mood and affect during the history. The client usually conveys mood and affect verbally and nonverbally throughout the interview. Normally the client's mood is stable and sustained, and the affect fluctuates appropriately according to the subject being discussed.

Judgment. *Judgment* refers to the ability to make decisions based upon reality and is evaluated during history taking. Judgment is indicated by how well the client manages personal, interpersonal, occupational, financial, and social aspects of life.

Insight. *Insight* refers to the ability to understand emotions, thoughts, and behavior and is evaluated during history taking. Insight is indicated by the client's spontaneous statements regarding the understanding of current and past life situations. In addition the client can be asked if there have been any changes in behavior, thoughts, or feelings. If the answer is yes, the interviewer evaluates insight by asking the client, "How do you explain these changes?" If the client states there have been no changes in behavior, thoughts, or feelings, the interviewer asks, "How do you explain your stable life circumstances?" (Table 3-6).

Recording of a Normal Psychosocial History

Identifying Data

This information is obtained at the beginning of the comprehensive health history.

Present Life Situation

A 51-year-old man has owned and operated a gas station for the past 20 years, has been married for 31 years with three children, ages 29, 27, and 24. He describes himself as reasonably happy and content with his life, except for occasional arguments with wife and children. The man is concerned with his future financial security and physical health; he admits to concerns about increased workload after having to lay off an employee due to increasing financial pressure.

The client has been in good physical health and works regularly, but business profits have declined recently due to escalating operating costs. He plans to take over work done by laid off employee but is concerned about the effects it will have on his marriage and health.

His wife is 50 years old and helps in gas station. He

feels that he loves her and describes her as a "good woman, good mother, works hard, but worries too much about our future." He states that sexual relationship is adequate.

One son, 29, is married with two children and is a draftsman for the Navy. He lives in Cherry Hill, New Jersey. A daughter, 27, is married with one child, teaches school, and lives in Philadelphia. A son, 24, is single, lives alone, and is an automobile mechanic for a car dealership in Philadelphia. The client is satisfied with children's life situation, except that he would like his younger son to work with him in the gas station, but the son wants to continue work where he is.

He likes to play baseball on weekends, goes to church occasionally, and maintains social contact with neighbors and high school friends. He feels his life situation is stable and satisfying although the economic situation may lead to increasing pressures.

Past Developmental History

He is the third of four children from a working-class family. His father was a carpenter and the mother was a housewife. A sister is six years older, brother four years older, and brother two years younger. The father is described as a hard-working, soft-spoken, kind man who "yelled a lot when angry" but was playful with the kids. The mother was described as warm, caring, and strict. The client got along well with parents and siblings.

The client believes his early development was normal and knows of no early developmental problems. He felt that he was a wanted and loved child and had a positive relationship with both parents. He fought with siblings, was particularly envious of the younger brother, "the baby," but felt close to his siblings throughout life. He recalls one playmate from early childhood. The man recalls no difficulties in separating from his mother or evidence of problems with toilet training. He had transient fears of the dark.

He started school at age six, went through 10th grade, had average grades with no major disciplinary problems. He made friends easily and "played baseball all the time." He recalls a happy childhood although he was told he had a bad temper; he got into fights, but there was no evidence of major family or school problems.

The client became interested in girls in his early teens, recalls masturbating, but was afraid of being caught. First intercourse was at age 16 with his girlfriend. He had "battles" with parents, especially with

Table 3-6. Common Abnormal Findings in History and Mental Status Examination

Condition	History	General Appearance and Behavior	Sensorium and Cognitive Processes
Mental retardation	Impairment in intellectual functioning with onset before age 18. May have impairments in social functioning.	Ranges from normal to impaired.	Impaired intellectual functioning. Other cognitive functions may be impaired.
Organic brain syndrome			
Delirium	Appearance of clinical findings over a period of hours to days. Fluctuation of symptoms over the course of a day. Disturbances in sleep-wakefulness cycle.	Motor activity usually increased, may be decreased, and often fluctuates.	Fluctuating or reduced level of consciousness, disorientation, impairment of attention and concentration, memory and abstraction, disturbances in perception (illusions, hallucinations).
Dementia	Variable, onset may be sudden, but is usually gradual, depending on causative factors and is marked by loss of intellectual functioning.	Variable; may hesitate in answering questions, may neglect personal hygiene.	Attention and concentration may be impaired, depending on severity, impaired memory, primarily short-term, and impaired abstraction.
Schizophrenia	Personality change or deterioration in functioning characterized by social withdrawal, impairment in role functioning, peculiar behavior, and impairment in ability to communicate.	Ranges from normal to impaired. May have disorder of posture, psychomotor activity, or speech; may have ritualistic or stereotyped behavior.	Auditory hallucinations, abstraction often impaired.
Affective Disorders			
Mania	Distinct period of predominantly elevated moods and associated behavior changes such as decreased sleep, increased talkativeness and activity.	Unusually cheerful, optimistic, grandiose, easily distracted, inappropriately sociable; speech may be loud, rapid, with abrupt changes from topic to topic.	Impairment of attention and concentration (distractability).
Depression	Usually gradual onset of depressed mood or loss of interest or pleasure in usual activities and relationships; usually disturbance in appetite, sleep, energy level, self-esteem, and behavior.	May appear unhappy, brooding, preoccupied with suicide. Poor personal hygiene, may have psychomotor retardation or agitation. Speech may be slow and halting.	Attention and concentration may be impaired, may have memory impairment.
Neurotic Disorders			
Depressive (dysthymic disorder)	Chronic depressed mood or loss of interest or pleasure in usual activities and relationships. Not of sufficient severity and duration to meet criteria for major depression.	May appear unhappy, sad.	Usually normal.
Anxiety (generalized anxiety disorders)	Generalized, persistent anxiety with motor tension, autonomic hyperactivity, apprehensive expectation.	Tense, anxious, apprehensive, worried.	Normal.

Thought Content	*Thought Processes*	*Mood and Affect*	*Judgment*	*Insight*
Usually normal, may be impaired.	Usually normal, may be impaired	Usually normal.	Usually impaired, depending on severity of disorder.	Usually impaired, depending on severity of disorder.
Variable, may be delusional.	Fragmented, incoherent, illogical.	Variable, may be frightened or fearful, often labile and inappropriate.	Poor.	Poor.
Ranges from normal to impaired.	Ranges from normal to impaired.	Often apathetic and withdrawn or has restricted range of affect.	Variable, generally poor.	Variable, generally poor.
Delusions.	Loosening of associations; incoherent, illogical.	Blunted, flat, or inappropriate affect.	Ranges from normal to impaired. Usually impaired.	Usually impaired.
Inflated sense of self-esteem, grandiose, may be delusional.	Flight of ideas may be present.	Elated, expansive, or irritable.	Usually impaired.	Usually impaired.
Feelings of worthlessness, self-reproach, or excessive guilt; may have suicidal thoughts; may be delusional.	Decreased or slowed thinking.	Dependent, sad, hopeless, irritable.	Usually impaired.	Usually impaired.
Feelings of inadequacy, low self-esteem.	Usually normal.	Despondent, worried, sad.	Usually normal.	Ranges from normal to impaired.
Anticipation of misfortune.	Normal.	Apprehensive, fearful, sense of dread or impending disaster.	Usually normal.	Usually normal.

Table 3-6. Common Abnormal Findings in History and Mental Status Examination (*continued*)

Condition	History	General Appearance and Behavior	Sensorium and Cognitive Processes
Phobic (phobic disorders)	Persistent, irrational fear and avoidance of a specific object, activity, or situation, leading to either significant subjective distress or impairment of occupational or social functioning.	In presence of feared object, activity, or situation, becomes frightened; otherwise normal.	Normal.
Obsessive compulsive (obsessive compulsive disorder)	Recurrent persistent ideas or thoughts experienced as involuntary, intrusive, and unwanted (obsessions). Repetitive and seemingly purposeful behaviors performed according to certain rules or in stereotyped fashion (compulsion).	Performs compulsion or becomes anxious if unable to perform compulsion; otherwise normal.	Normal.
Hysterical, conversion (conversion disorder)	Loss or alteration in physical functioning, suggesting a physical disorder. Usually sudden onset.	May appear to have relative lack of concern regarding symptoms.	Normal.

SOURCE: Adapted from American Psychiatric Association, *Diagnostic and Statistical Manual of Mental Disorders*, third edition, Washington, D.C.: A.P.A., 1980. Mental disorders are diagnosed by descriptions of the clinical features.

his father over school. He finally quit school and went to work in a gas station as did many of his friends.

He dated his wife for one year prior to marriage, later felt maybe he was too young for this long-term commitment. He had similar concerns when their first child born and had marital discord, which was accentuated by birth of second child. He was aided by emotional support from his parents and found that he could relate to his father as an adult for the first time. When the marriage improved, he and wife decided to have a third child.

He had an opportunity to buy his own gas station, and with financial help from parents, took the risk. Now he says, "Best decision I ever made in my life."

His father died of a myocardial infarction when client was 35. Client was sad, missed his father, "moped around" for a few months, and then "pulled out of it." His mother died about 1 year later from a stroke. He was again in mourning for several months. After parents' deaths, the client had some concerns about his own health but was reassured by the family doctor. He began playing baseball with high school friends for recreation and physical activity.

The client has had a good relationship with his children but feels that he may be "too strict." He wishes he had been more giving to his children when they were teenagers but feels "their generation is different from mine."

In summary, the client shows reasonably good adjustment to present and past circumstances. He grew up in a stable, loving, intact family, went through some turmoil during adolescence and early adulthood, and was able to adapt well to these challenges. He derived a great deal of support from his parents. What remains to be seen is how well he will handle the present stresses in his life without his parents; he appears to be gaining a significant degree of help from his wife. This ability to turn to others for help has been a useful resource to him at times of previous stress.

Table 3-6.   Common Abnormal Findings in History and Mental Status Examination (*continued*)

Thought Content	Thought Processes	Mood and Affect	Judgment	Insight
Normal except for irrational fears and compelling desire to avoid the specific object, activity, or situation	Normal.	Usually normal.	Usually normal.	Usually normal.
Obsessions	Normal.	Usually normal.	Usually normal.	Usually normal.
Usually normal	Normal.	Usually normal.	Usually normal.	Usually normal.

Physiology

The body meets its energy requirement from food. Energy derived from food is measured in kilocalories (KCal). A kilocalorie is the amount of heat energy required to raise the temperature of 1 kilogram of water from 15 to 16° C. A kilocalorie (KCal) is commonly called a calorie (Cal). In the metric system, joule is the unit of measurement; 1 kilocalorie equals 4.184 kilojoules.

All foods contain kilocalories. The amount of kilocalories varies due to the food's content of protein, carbohydrates, and fat. When burned for energy, protein and carbohydrates yield 4 kilocalories per gram; fat yields 9 kilocalories per gram.

Foods high in fat are high in kilocalories. These foods are butter, margarine, salad dressings, and red meat. Also, foods low in moisture content are high in kilocalories. These foods include nuts, legumes, and dried fruit. Conversely, foods high in moisture content or undigestible fiber are low in kilocalories. These foods are mainly fruits and vegetables. Poultry, fish, and starches are intermediate sources of kilocalories.

Determining Energy Requirement

An individual's kilocalorie requirement is determined by three factors: basal metabolic rate, specific dynamic action, and physical activity. Basal metabolic rate (BMR) is the minimum amount of energy required to maintain body functions in a complete mental and physical resting state. BMR is normally 40 to 65 percent of the total daily kilocalorie requirement. These kilocalories are utilized to maintain the involuntary activities of the body, including respiration, circulation, body temperature, and the functional activities of various organs. Factors influencing BMR are body size, sex, age, and climate. A heavyset person utilizes more kilocalories than a slender person; likewise males utilize more kilocalories than females. BMR decreases slowly in adulthood and drops dramatically after age 50. Climate may not play as an important role due to appropriate clothing and indoor heating and cooling systems. Average estimates of BMR are the following.

> Males—1 KCal per 1 hour per kilogram body weight per 24 hours (average = 1,600-1,800 KCal/day); Females—.9 KCal. per 1 hour per kilogram body weight per 24 hours (average = 1,250-1,450 KCal/day)

Specific dynamic action (SDA) is the kilocalories required to metabolize food. Carbohydrate and fat

Chapter 4

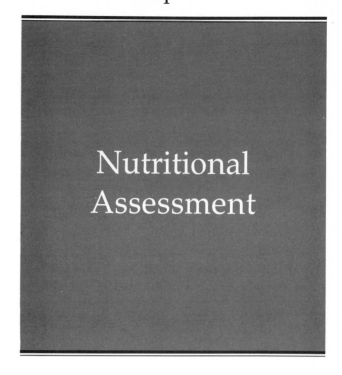

Nutritional Assessment

————— Objectives —————

The examiner will be able to do the following:

1. Obtain a nutritional history including socio-economic profile, diet history, and screening medical history

2. Obtain a food diary

3. Inspect the client for signs that reflect nutritional status

4. Obtain wrist and arm circumference measurements

5. Obtain skinfold measurements

6. Recognize abnormal physical and biochemical measurements, particularly hematocrit, hemoglobin, serum triglyceride, cholesterol, and serum glucose

7. Recognize additional abnormal biochemical measurements in clients at risk for protein-calorie malnutrition, particularly creatinine/height index, serum protein, serum albumin, lymphocyte count, nitrogen balance studies, and immune system response

8. Record the information obtained

SDA is 6 percent of the kilocalories consumed. Protein SDA is 18 to 30 percent of total protein kilocalories consumed. In a mixed diet—that is, a mixture of protein, carbohydrates, and fat—SDA is 10 percent of kilocalories consumed. Thus, for a sandwich containing 300 kilocalories, 30 kilocalories are used to metabolize the nutrients.

Physical activity increases caloric demand. The addition of two hours of walking and standing to sedentary activity such as sitting most of the day increases the caloric requirement 30 percent. A moderately active adult standing most of the day or performing light activity such as house cleaning or gardening increases the caloric requirement by 50 percent. An active person with strenuous exercise increases the caloric requirement by 75 to 100 percent.

In the office setting the examiner estimates the individual's caloric requirement by body weight. Caloric requirement for males is estimated at 35 kilocalories x kilograms of body weight. Caloric requirement for females is estimated at 35 kilocalories x kilograms of body weight x 85 percent.

When caloric intake equals caloric expenditure, body weight is maintained. When caloric intake is greater than caloric expenditure, body weight is gained. When caloric intake is less than caloric expenditure, body weight is lost. A pound equals 3,500 kilocalories.

Caloric Intake Regulation

Hunger, appetite, and satiety contribute to determining food intake. Hunger is a drive for food. After 10 to 12 hours of fasting, the stomach has rhythmic contractions that cause pain. These pains are referred to as hunger pangs. The contractions are increased with low blood sugar. Appetite is a psychic phenomenon influenced by the five senses of taste, smell, vision, hearing, and touch. Appetite is also influenced by emotions and enviroment. Appetite stimulates secretion of gastric acid, which improves digestion. Satiety is the feeling of fullness. It is a cue to stop eating. The nervous system and hypothalamus play an important role in hunger, appetite, and satiety; their interrelationships are complex and not fully understood.

Protein

Proteins are composed of amino acids. Amino acids are the structural elements of all living cells, as well as the only source of nitrogen for the body. Nitrogen is a key element for growth and maintenance of body tissues. Protein also functions to maintain fluid balance (Chapter 20 and acid-base balance (Chapter 21) and is a precursor for enzymes, antibodies, and hormones. When the body does not have enough energy from carbohydrates and fats, protein is diverted from its role in tissue synthesis and utilized for energy. However, because the body has no storage capacity for excess protein, structural tissue must be broken down (catabolized) to provide protein for energy. Therefore, protein is not an optimal energy source. In addition, protein foods are more expensive than carbohydrates and fats.

There are 22 known amino acids. Nine amino acids cannot be synthesized by the body. These 9 amino acids are known as essential animo acids (EAA). They are isoleucine, leucine, lysine, methionine, phenylalanine, threonine, tryptophane, valine, and histidine. The remaining amino acids can be synthesized by the body from the EAAs. Protein quality is determined by the composition of the amino acids. A high-quality protein, known as a complete protein, has all the essential amino acids in the correct ratio and proper quantity. Complete proteins are eggs, milk, meat, poultry, and fish. Incomplete proteins of low quality are deficient in one or more EAAs. Incomplete proteins may be complemented by a complete protein or by another protein food high in the missing EAA. For example, corn, which is deficient in methionine, may be eaten with legumes, which are a rich source of methionine; this makes the entree a complete protein. Complementing protein foods is the basis of a vegetarian diet. When incomplete proteins are consumed without being complemented, the protein is utilized as energy, and the nitrogen is excreted in the urine and not utilized for tissue building.

Protein stores are the muscle tissue, immune system, and enzyme systems. The normal adult has six to eight kilograms of protein. Protein stores are not normally used as an energy source since depletion of protein stores compromises health. The body preferentially uses carbohydrates and fats as energy sources in order to spare structural protein. This is known as protein-sparing.

The requirement for complete protein is estimated at 0.8 gram per kilogram of body weight. This requirement averages 12% of the diet, and is an average of 56 grams per day for a 70 kilogram man and 44 grams per day for a 55 kilogram woman. The average intake of protein in the American diet is 70 to 100 grams or 20 percent of the total diet.

Carbohydrates

Carbohydrates are the major source of energy for the body and have a protein-sparing effect. That is, carbo-

Table 4-1. Classification of Carbohydrates

Simple Sugars	Complex Carbohydrates

Monosaccharides
  Glucose
  Fructose
  Galactose
Disaccharides
  Sucrose (table sugar)
    Glucose and fructose
  Lactose (milk sugar)
    Glucose and galactose
  Maltose
    2 glucose molecules
	All are composed of long-chain glucose molecules
	Starch
	Cellulose (fiber)
	Glycogen

hydrates are burned for energy, which allows utilization of proteins for tissue building. Carbohydrates are classified into simple or complex carbohydrates (Table 4-1). Once ingested, all forms of carbohydrates are converted to glucose for utilization by cells; excess carbohydrate is stored as glycogen or metabolized into triglycerides for fat deposition.

There is no established minimum or maximum of carbohydrate requirement. On a carbohydrate-free diet, fat catabolism, breakdown of body protein stores, loss of energy, and fatigue occur. Carbohydrate intake of 50 to 100 grams per day prevents these symptoms. In the American diet an average of 40 to 50 percent of calories are carbohydrates; therefore, a 2,000 kilocalorie diet contains 200 to 250 grams of carbohydrates.

Fat

Fat serves as the body's major reserve of energy. Dietary fat also supplies linoleic acid, an essential fatty acid that cannot be synthesized in the body. Dietary fat serves as a carrier for fat-soluble vitamins A, D, E, and K. Fat also serves as an insulator, protecting vital organs.

The major portion of dietary fat occurs as triglyceride. Triglyceride is composed of a glycerol molecule and three fatty acids.

Fatty acids vary in the number of carbon molecules. Medium-chain fatty acids contain 6 to 10 carbon units.

Long-chain fatty acids contain 16 to 20 carbon units. Most of the naturally occurring fatty acids have 16 to 18 carbon molecules.

Fatty acids are classified as unsaturated or saturated. Saturation depends on the number of hydrogens attached to the carbon molecule. A saturated fatty acid has two hydrogens for each carbon. An unsaturated fatty acid has two hydrogens between two carbons, which forms a double bond between the carbon molecules. Monounsaturated fats have one double bond and no nutritional significance. Polyunsaturated fats have multiple double bonds (Table 4-2).

Polyunsaturates play a vital role in maintaining the function and integrity of the cell membranes. They are found naturally in plant oils (like corn, safflower, and cotton seed) and are liquid at room temperature. Saturated fats occur naturally in animal sources and are solid at room temperature.

Other forms of fat are phospholipids and sterols. Phospholipids are the structural component of all cell membranes. Lecithin is the most common phospholipid and serves as an emulsifying agent. The most common sterol is cholesterol. It is an important constituent in the myelin sheath around the nerve fibers and is a precursor of steroids and sex hormones.

Excess dietary fat and carbohydrate are transported from the liver to fat stores in the form of lipoproteins. Lipoproteins are classified as very-low-density (VLDL), low density (LDL), and high-density (HDL) lipoproteins. VLDLs are primarily triglycerides and a small percentage of cholesterol. LDLs are primarily cholesterol. HDLs are primarily phospholipids with a small percentage of cholesterol. Because phospholipids are water soluble, it is theorized that HDLs prevent precipitation of cholesterol in the blood stream.

Excess fat is stored in adipose tissues. Common areas of fat deposition are the thighs, upper arms, and midabdomen. Although research suggests that 25 to 30 percent of calories be ingested as dietary fat, most Americans consume more than 30 to 40 percent.

Table 4-2. Classification of Fatty Acids

Saturated Fatty Acids		Unsaturated Fatty Acids		
Name	Number of Carbons	Name	Number of Bonds	Number of Carbons
Myristic	14	Palmitoleic	1	16
Palmitic	16	Oleic	1	18
Stearic	18	Linoleic	2	18
		Linolenic	3	18
		Arachidonic	4	20

Table 4-3. Recommended Dietary Allowances, Revised 1980*
Designed for the maintenance of good nutrition of practically all healthy people in the U.S.A.
FOOD AND NUTRITION BOARD, NATIONAL ACADEMY OF SCIENCES-NATIONAL RESEARCH COUNCIL.

Age and Sex Group	Weight		Height		Protein	Fat-soluble Vitamins			Water-soluble Vitamins	
	kg.	lb.	cm.	in.		Vitamin A	Vitamin D	Vitamin E$_P$	Vitamin C	Thiamin
					gm.	μg.R.E.[†]	μg[‡]	mg.αT.F.[#]	$\longleftarrow$	mg. $\longrightarrow$
Infants										
0.0-0.5 yr.	6	13	60	24	kg. × 2.2	420	10	3	35	0.3
0.5-1.0 yr.	9	20	71	28	kg. × 2.0	400	10	4	35	0.5
Children										
1-3 yr.	13	29	90	35	23	400	10	5	45	0.7
4-6 yr.	20	44	112	44	30	500	10	6	45	0.9
7-10 yr.	28	62	132	52	34	700	10	7	45	1.2
Males										
11-14 yr.	45	99	157	62	45	1,000	10	8	50	1.4
15-18 yr.	66	145	176	69	56	1,000	10	10	60	1.4
19-22 yr.	70	154	177	70	56	1,000	7.5	10	60	1.5
23-50 yr.	70	154	178	70	56	1,000	5	10	60	1.4
51+ yr.	70	154	178	70	56	1,000	5	10	60	1.2
Females										
11-14 yr.	46	101	157	62	46	800	10	8	50	1.1
15-18 yr.	55	120	163	64	46	800	10	8	60	1.1
19-22 yr.	55	120	163	64	44	800	7.5	8	60	1.1
23-50 yr.	55	120	163	64	44	800	5	8	60	1.0
51+ yr.	55	120	163	64	44	800	5	8	60	1.0
Pregnancy					+30	+200	+5	+2	+20	+0.4
Lactation					+20	+400	+5	+3	+40	+0.5

Reproduced from *Recommended Dietary Allowances*, Ninth Revised Edition, 1980, with the permission of the National Academy of Sciences, Washington, D.C.

*The allowances are intended to provide for individual variations among most normal persons as they live in the United States under usual environmental stresses. Diets should be based on a variety of common foods in order to provide other nutrients for which human requirements have been less well defined.

Recommended Dietary Allowances

Recommended dietary allowances (RDAs) have been established by the Food and Nutrition Board of the National Academy of Sciences. The RDAs are guidelines for specific nutrients for the normal, healthy population. The nutrient allowances are based on current scientific data. Determinations are based on balance studies, biochemical measurements, and clinical evaluations. The RDAs have a 20 to 30 percent margin of safety, because it is recognized that individual variation exists. Certain conditions such as surgery, chronic drug ingestion, and stress vary the need for specific nutrients. Scientists believe that an individual who consistently ingests less than two-thirds of the RDA for a specific nutrient is at risk for a clinical deficiency. Not all nutrients essential for life are included in the RDAs due to lack of scientific data. (Tables 4-3 and 4-4).

Vitamins

Vitamins are organic compounds required in minute amounts by the body. Vitamins perform specific and vital functions in the metabolic processes of the body and cannot be synthesized by humans. Inadequate intake or improper absorption of vitamins causes specific deficiency states.

Vitamins differ from each other in physiologic function and chemical structures. They are classified as fat-soluble or water-soluble. Vitamins A, D, E, and K are fat-soluble, are stored in the body, and are not lost from foods during cooking or processing. Because fat-soluble vitamins are stored in the body, excessive intake can result in toxicity. The water-soluble vitamins are vitamin C and the B complex. B complex vitamins are thiamine, riboflavin, niacin, pyridoxine, biotin, choline, folic acid and pantothenic acid. Because they are water-soluble, concentration of vi-

Table 4-3. (continued)

	Water-soluble Vitamins				Minerals					
Ribo-flavin	Niacin	Vitamin B₂	Folacin‡	Vitamin B₁₂	Calcium	Phosphorus	Magnesium	Iron	Zinc	Iodine
mg.	mg.N.E.¶	mg.	←— µg. —→		←——————— mg. ———————→					µg.
Infants										
0.4	6	0.3	30	0.5**	360	240	30	10	3	40
0.6	8	0.6	45	1.5	540	360	70	15	5	50
Children										
0.8	9	0.9	100	2.0	800	800	150	15	10	70
1.0	11	1.3	200	2.5	800	800	200	10	10	90
1.4	16	1.6	300	3.0	800	800	250	10	10	120
Males										
1.6	18	1.8	400	3.0	1,200	1,200	350	18	15	150
1.7	18	2.0	400	3.0	1,200	1,200	400	18	15	150
1.7	19	2.2	400	3.0	800	800	350	10	15	150
1.6	18	2.2	400	3.0	800	800	350	10	15	150
1.4	16	2.2	400	3.0	800	800	350	10	15	150
Females										
1.3	15	1.8	400	3.0	1,200	1,200	300	18	15	150
1.3	14	2.0	400	3.0	1,200	1,200	300	18	15	150
1.3	14	2.0	400	3.0	800	800	300	18	15	150
1.2	13	2.0	400	3.0	800	800	300	18	15	150
1.2	13	2.0	400	3.0	800	800	300	10	15	150
+0.3	+ 2	+0.6	+400	+1.0	+400	+400	+150	††	+ 5	+ 25
+0.5	+ 5	+0.5	+100	+1.0	+400	+400	+150	††	+10	+ 50

†Retinol equivalents; 1 retinol equivalent = 1 ug. retinol or 6 ug. B-carotene. See text for calculation of vitamin activity of diets as retinol equivalents.

‡As cholecalciferol: 10 ug. cholecalciferol = 400 I.U. vitamin D.

#Octocopherol equivalents; 1 mg. d-x-tocopherol = 1 T.E.

¶1N.E. (niacin equivalent) = 1 mg. niacin or 60 mg. dietary tryptophan.

tamin C and the B complex is decreased during cooking, processing, and aging. Unlike the fat-soluble vitamins, excessive intake of the water-soluble vitamins results in increased excretion by the kidneys.

Individual foods vary in their content of vitamins. Therefore, a diet with a variety of fresh, under-processed foods is essential to ensure adequate intake (Table 4-5). Vitamin preparations may be deficient for three reasons: the metabolic demand requires absorption of vitamins throughout the day; not all vitamins are known, nor do many vitamins have an established daily requirement.

Minerals

Minerals are inorganic elements. Like vitamins, the diversity of functions of the individual minerals is great. Minerals have vital roles in hormonal regulation, metabolism, heme formation, water balance, muscle contractions, and bone formation. Deficiency syndromes occur if the body's mineral stores are depleted or if food intake or absorption is inadequate.

Minerals are classified by daily requirements. Macrominerals are required in amounts of 100 milligrams or above per day. Examples are calcium, phosphorous, magnesium, sodium, potassium, chloride, and sulfur. Microminerals, also known as trace elements, are required in amounts less than 100 milligrams per day and are stored in the body. Examples are iron, iodine, fluorine, zinc, copper, chromium, selenium, cobalt, and manganese. Many trace elements are still being studied as to their function in the body and possible requirements. There is considerable controversy whether certain trace elements are contaminants or whether they have an essential role in the body. The trace elements in question are molybdenum, vanadium, tin, silicone, and cadmium.

Mineral requirements have been established by the Food and Nutrition Board of the National Academy of Sciences (Table 4-4). It had been believed that if an individual consumed adequate amounts of calcium, iron, and iodine, other minerals would be present in adequate amounts. However, food-processing methods and increasing reliance on processed foods may result in loss of essential nutrients. To ensure adequate intake, eating a wide variety of fresh, under-processed foods is essential (Tables 4-5 and 4-6).

Table 4-4. Estimated safe and adequate daily dietary intakes of additional selected vitamins and minerals*

Age Group	Vitamins			Trace elements[+]						Electrolytes		
	Vitamin K	Biotin	Pantothenic acid	Copper	Manganese	Fluoride	Chromium	Selenium	Molybdenum	Sodium	Potassium	Chloride
	μg		mg									
Infants												
0.0-0.5 yr.	12	35	2	0.5-0.7	0.5-0.7	0.1-0.5	0.01-0.04	0.01-0.04	0.03-0.06	115- 350	350- 925	275- 700
0.5-1.0 yr.	10- 20	50	3	0.7-1.0	0.7-1.0	0.2-1.0	0.02-0.06	0.02-0.06	0.04-0.08	250- 750	425-1,275	400-1,200
Children and adolescents												
1-3 yr.	15- 30	65	3	1.0-1.5	1.0-1.5	0.5-1.5	0.02-0.08	0.02-0.08	0.05-0.1	325- 975	550-1,650	500-1,500
4-6 yr.	20- 40	85	3-4	1.5-2.0	1.5-2.0	1.0-2.5	0.03-0.12	0.03-0.12	0.06-0.15	450-1,350	775-2,325	700-2,100
7-10 yr.	30- 60	120	4-5	2.0-2.5	2.0-3.0	1.5-2.5	0.05-0.2	0.05-0.2	0.1 -0.3	600-1,800	1,000-3,000	925-2,775
11+ yr.	50-100	100-200	4-7	2.0-3.0	2.5-5.0	1.5-2.5	0.05-0.2	0.05-0.2	0.15-0.5	900-2,700	1,525-4,575	1,400-4,200
Adults	70-140	100-200	4-7	2.0-3.0	2.5-5.0	1.5-4.0	0.05-0.2	0.05-0.2	0.15-0.5	1,100-3,300	1,875-5,625	1,700-5,100

Reproduced from: *Recommended Dietary Allowances*, Ninth Revised Edition, 1980, with the permission of the National Academy of Sciences, Washington, D.C.

*From *Recommended Dietary Allowances*, Revised 1980, Food and Nutrition Board, National Academy of Sciences—National Research Council. Because there is less information on which to base allowances, these figures are not given in the main table of the RDAs and are provided here in the form of ranges of recommended intakes.

[+]Since the toxic levels for many trace elements may be only several times usual intakes, the upper levels for the trace elements given in this table should not be habitually exceeded.

Table 4-5. Food Sources and Functions of Vitamins and Related Deficiency Syndromes

Vitamins	Food Source	Function	Deficiency Syndromes
Ascorbic acid C	Citrus fruit Green peppers Broccoli	Collagen formation Wound healing Neurotransmitter synthesis Enhancement of iron absorption	Scurvey Weakness Lassitude Bleeding gums
Thiamine B_1	Whole grains Brown rice Brewer's yeast Fish Meat Nuts Organ meats	Energy metabolism Protein, fat, and carbohydrate metabolism Muscle tone maintenance	Beriberi Irritability Disorderly thinking Nausea
Riboflavin B_2	Black strap molasses Nuts Organ meats Whole grains	Energy release from carbohydrate, fat, and protein metabolism Oxidation/reduction reactions Red blood cell formation	Deficiency usually in conjunction with other B vitamin deficiency Growth retardation Cheilosis Glossitis Dry, scaly skin Dermatitis
Pyridoxine B_6	Black strap molasses Brewer's yeast Green leafy vegetables Meat Organ meats Wheat germ Whole grains	Coenzyme in protein and amino acid metabolism Fatty acid utilization	Nausea Depression Neuritis Dermatitis
Cobalamine B_{12}	Cheese Milk and milk products Fish Organ meats	Coenzymes in synthesis of nucleic acids Red blood cell formation	Pernicious anemia General weakness Nervousness
Niacin	Brewer's yeast Seafood Lean meats Milk and milk products Poultry	Energy released from carbohydrate, fat, and protein	Pellagra Dermatitis Diarrhea Dementia
Pantothenic acid	Brewer's yeast Legumes Organ meats Wheat germ Whole grains	Factor in coenzyme A metabolism of carbohydrate, fat, protein, fatty acid, and sterol synthesis	No known deficiency
Biotin	Legumes Whole grains Organ meats	Coenzyme in amino acid metabolism, and protein synthesis Carbohydrate metabolism Formation of antibodies	Dermatitis Anorexia Lassitude Nausea *Consumption of raw egg whites may cause biotin deficiency
Folic acid	Green leafy vegetables Milk and milk products Organ meats Whole grains	Coenzyme in protein metabolism Heme synthesis Red blood cell formation and maturation	Megaloblastic anemia Diarrhea Glossitis Growth retardation

Table 4-5. Food Sources and Functions of Vitamins and Related Deficiency Syndromes (*continued*)

Vitamins	Food Source	Function	Deficiency Syndromes
A	Green and yellow vegetables and fruits (carotene) Milk and milk products Oil	Functions in visual cycle from bright light to dim light Maintaining growth and maintenance of epithelial cells	Night blindness Growth retardation Increased susceptibility to infection *Toxicity-nausea Headaches Peeling and flaky skin Dizziness Pain of long bones
D	Egg yolks Organ meat Sunlight Enriched milk	Increased absorption of dietary calcium Affects bone mineralization	Rickets Osteomalacia *Toxicity-nausea Weight loss Anorexia Calcification of bones and soft tissue
E	Dark green vegetables Eggs Organ meats Vegetable oils	Postulated role in heme synthesis Increased stability of cellular and intracellular structures Antioxident "Protects" polyunsaturated fats	Deficiency found only in premature infants Symptoms of irritability Edema Hemolytic anemia No known toxicity
K	Green leafy vegetables Vegatable oil	Blood-clotting mechanism	Decreased blood coagulation Deficiency unlikely unless interference with fat absorption or presence of liver disease No known toxicity

Table 4-6. Food Sources and Functions of Minerals and Related Deficiency Syndromes

Minerals	Food Source	Function	Deficiency Syndromes
Calcium	Milk and milk products	Bone formation Transmission of nerve impulses Muscle contractions Blood coagulation Cell membrane permeability	Osteoporosis Rickets Muscle cramps Nervousness
Phosphorus	Eggs Meats Whole grains Milk	Component of RNA and DNA Component of cellular membranes Component of high-energy phosphate complex ATP Component of vitamin B coenzymes	Depletion by taking high doses of antacids Weakness Anorexia Malaise Bone pain Bone demineralization
Sulfur	Bran Cheese Eggs Nuts	Structure of amino acids Composition of thiamine and biotin Required for many oxidation-reduction reactions Active in detoxification mechanism	No specific deficiency syndrome
Magnesium	Green vegetables Nuts Milk and milk products	Mobilization of calcium from bone Component of many enzyme systems Role in protein synthesis	Tremors Tetany Seizures Mental disorientation

Minerals	Food Source	Function	Deficiency Syndromes
Iron	Red meat Black strap molasses Eggs Wheat germ Organ meats	Oxidation mechanism of all cells Vital component of hemoglobin	Microcytic, hypochromic anemia Weakness Fatigue Lassitude
Iodine	Seafood Iodized salt	Component of thyroid hormones	Goiter
Fluoride	Fluoridated enriched water sources Bone meal	Protects against dental caries	Dental caries Possible osteoporosis *Toxicity-mottling of tooth enamel
Copper	Legumes Nuts Organ meats	Constituent of several enzymes Synthesis of hemoglobin	Hypoproteinemia Hypocupremia Anemia Poor growth
Zinc	Brewer's yeast Liver Soybeans	Constituent for activity of a number of metalloenzymes Component of insulin Role in taste and olfactory acuity Normal growth Wound healing	Hypogeusia Anorexia Weight loss Poor growth *Toxicity-fever Vomiting Diarrhea
Manganese	Bananas Celery Cereals Egg yolks Green leafy vegetables Legumes Nuts	Bone formation Brain function Reproduction	No known deficiency syndrome
Cobalt	Meats Legumes Nuts	Component of B-12	No known deficiency syndrome
Selenium	Whole grains Brewer's yeast Meats	Component of enzyme glutathione perioxidase	No known deficiency syndrome
Chromium	Brewer's yeast Vegetable oils Whole grains	Cofactor in insulin	No known deficiency syndrome

Essentials of an Adequate Diet

The basic four food groups were developed by the Dairy Council. The food groups include meat, milk, grains, and fruits and vegetables. Foods high in fat or sugar with low nutrient density are classed outside the four food groups. The basic four food groups can be utilized as a crude evaluation guide or as an educational tool to select an adequate diet. Following the basic four guidelines usually ensures meeting the basic nutrition requirments for the general population (Table 4-7).

Table 4-7. Basic Four Food Requirements for Adults

Food Group	Serving Size	Servings per Day—Adult
Milk	8 ounces milk or yogurt 1-½ ounces of cheese 1-½ cups of cottage cheese	2
Meat	2 ounces meat, poultry, fish, cheese 2 eggs 4 tablespoons peanut butter ½ cup lentils	2
Vegetable and fruit	½ cup vegetable or fruit 4 ounces fruit juice	4 or more
Grains	1 slice of bread ½ cup of cereal, pasta	4 or more

Assessment Modalities

Preparation

For nutritional assessment the examiner obtains a nutritional history; inspects physical size and the condition of the skin, hair, eyes, and mouth; and obtains anthropometric and biochemical measurements when indicated.

The examining room requires a table, two chairs, and a beam balance weight and height scale. The tools required are a flexible, nonstretch measuring tape; skinfold calipers; food models; and forms to plot data. Skinfold calipers have two pincers that exert a constant pressure over the entire operating range.

Food models are usually plastic replicas of food. They are used to evaluate portion sizes that the client consumes. Measuring cups and spoons and various sizes of drinking glasses are also helpful (Figure 4-1).

Nutritional History

The nutritional history includes a socioeconomic profile, a diet history, and a screening medical history. The socioeconomic profile provides information

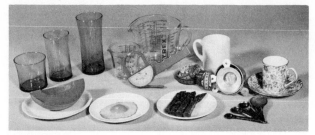

Figure 4-1. Equipment used for nutritional assessment.

on the client's ability to procure and prepare food and gives insight into the client's caloric demands by answering questions concerning his occupation, recreation, and exercise habits (Table 4-9). The diet history gives information on actual food intake, approximate calories ingested, meal and snacking pattern, food beliefs, and supplements taken (Table 4-8). The medical history is important in identifying risk factors that indicate a need for diet manipulation. The medical history also gives information on conditions that interfere with adequate food intake, such as shortness of breath, arthritis, diabetes, or colostomy (Table 4-10).

Table 4-8.   Diet History

Food	Frequency (amount per day or week)
Dairy	
Milk Fat—whole/reduced	
Cheese	
Yogurt	
Fruit	
Canned	
Whole	
Juice	
Vegetable	
Fresh/frozen	
Canned	
Breads	
Whole	
Refined	
Sweetened (doughnuts, etc.)	
Meats	
Red	
Luncheon	
Fish/fowl	
Eggs	
Beans	
Fats	
Saturated	
Unsaturated	
Caffeine	

Food	Frequency (amount per day or week)
Soda	
Sweets	
Alcohol	
Favorite foods	
Dislikes	
Food beliefs	
Vegetarian	
Vitamin supplements	
Ovo-lacto-vegetarian	
Frequent fasting	
Source of nutritional information	
Magazines	
T.V.	
Radio	
School	
Other	
Have you ever been on a specific diet or counseled on a diet restriction?	
Type of diet	
Place of instruction	
Personalized	
Printed information	
Length of adherence to diet	
Problems with adherence	

Table 4-9. Socioeconomic Profile

1. Occupation
2. Recreation/hobbies/exercise—time spent in each per week
3. Number of people in household
4. Who is responsible for major procurement of food? Who is responsible for major preparation of food?
5. Kitchen facilities in home: Community kitchen facility
   Refrigerator
   Stove
   Oven
   Hot plate
6. Participation in federal food programs: WIC(Women, Infants, Children)
   Food stamps   Meals on Wheels   Other
7. Dollars per week spent on food
8. Number of meals per week eaten away from home
   Fast food restaurants   Work/school cafeteria
   Chain restaurants   Ethnic   Exclusive restaurants
   Number of meals eaten away from home per week less than $2   Less than $5
   Less than $10   Greater than $10
9. Religion   Ethnic group
10. Is any produce grown in a home garden or orchard?
11. Is there participation in a food cooperative plan?
12. Where is food purchased?
13. What proportion of diet comes from prepared foods?
14. What proportion of diet comes from "start from scratch" foods?

Table 4-10.   Screening Medical History

Medical Condition	Past History	Current History	Family History
Allergy			
Arthritis			
Cancer			
Cardiovascular			
Colostomy			
Diabetes			
Gastrointestinal			
Hypertension			
Lung disease			
Neurological			
Renal			
Dental			
Other			
Ingestion of drugs			
Over-the-counter preparations			
Prescribed			
Illicit			
Recent Complaints	*Yes*		*No*
Frequent fevers/infections			
Headaches			
Nausea			
Vomiting			
Early fatigue			
Malaise			
Indigestion			
Heartburn			
Diarrhea			
Constipation/hemorrhoids			
Slow wound healing			
Shortness of breath			

To evaluate nutrient intake further, a written food daily is sometimes requested. Advantages of a written diary are the following:

1. The dairy is kept over several days covering variations of food intake due to changes in schedule.

2. Portions of food may be weighed or measured.

3. Behavioral influences may be recorded.

4. As compared to a dietary recall, the problem of forgotten food is eliminated.

The client is instructed to record all food and beverages consumed for three to seven days and is encouraged to record food immediately after ingestion in order to avoid omissions. Food and beverages are weighed or measured to clarify portion sizes (Table 4-11).

The diary is analyzed using the basic four food groups, food composition tables, or nutrient-computerized programs. Food composition tables and nutrient computer programs give approximate nutrient content of foods. The values are usually given for 100-gram portions or portions commonly used. The diet is evaluated for one or all of the following: calories, protein, fats, carbohydrates (refined, complex), and specific minerals or vitamins. The information gathered provides a data base for dietary counseling.

Inspection

The examiner inspects for physical signs that reflect nutritional status. Abnormal physical signs or lesions are a clue to nutrient deficiencies and excesses, and are documented with diet and laboratory evaluation. Many other diseases have clinical manifestations similar to nutrient lesions (Table 4-12).

With the client standing, the examiner evaluates physical size and distribution of body tissues. Physical size is judged subjectively in terms of cachectic, small-petite, slender, medium, stout, large, or athletic (Figure 4-2). Physical size aids in assessing caloric demand. Distribution of body tissues is an estimate of excessive fat deposits, extreme bony protrusions, or muscle atrophy. Excessive fat deposits are a risk factor in diseases of aging including heart disease, hyper-

Table 4-11. Sample of a Food Diary from Awakening to Lunchtime

Time	Food/Preparation	Amount	Location	Position	With Whom
7:00	Whole wheat toast	1 slice	Kitchen	Standing	Alone
	Margarine	1 tsp.			
7:30	Coffee with sugar	10 oz.	Car	Sitting	Alone
	Sugar	3 tsp.			
10:00	Glazed doughnut	1	Office break room	Sitting	3 co-workers
11:30	Cottage cheese	$\frac{1}{2}$ cup	Cafeteria	Sitting	2 co-workers
	Diet cola	12 oz.	Cafeteria	Sitting	2 co-workers
	Apple	1	Cafeteria	Sitting	2 co-workers
	Jello	1 cup	Cafeteria	Sitting	2 co-workers

Table 4-12. Abnormal Physical Signs Related to Nutritional Deficiencies

Finding	Condition	Description
Hair		
Lackluster hair	Protein-calorie deficiency	Dull, dry, wirelike
Thin and sparse hair	Protein-calorie deficiency	Wide gaps between hair
Face		
Diffuse pigmentation	Protein-calorie deficiency	General lightness of skin color
Nasolabial seborrhea	Riboflavin, niacin, or pyridoxine deficiency	Scaly with dry, grey-yellowish threadlike material around nostrils, bridge of nose, eyebrows
Eyes		
Bitot's spots	Vitamin A deficiency	Dry, grayish, or yellow foamy spots on whites of eyes.
Conjunctival xerosis	Vitamin A deficiency	Whites appear dull, rough, and pigmented.
Lips		
Angular stomatitis	Riboflavin, niacin deficiency	Bilateral cracks, redness, flaking at corners of mouth.
Cheilosis	Niacin deficiency	Vertical cracks of lips, usually at center of lips.
Tongue		
Magenta tongue	Riboflavin deficiency	Purplish-red color.
Atrophic papillae	Folate, niacin, riboflavin deficiency	Tongue appears smooth, pale, and slick.
Glossitis	Niacin, folate deficiency	Tongue appears swollen, red; taste buds atrophied, painful.
Gums		
Spongy, bleeding	Vitamin C deficiency	Purplish-red spongy, swollen gums that bleed easily.
Skin		
Petechiae, ecchymoses	Vitamin C, K deficiency	Small black-blue hemorrhagic spots on skin.
Pellegrous dermatosis	Niacin deficiency	Hyperpigmented areas. Acute: red, swollen with itchy and cracking skin. Chronic: dry, rough thickened and scaly skin.
Follicular hyperkeratosis	Essential fatty acid deficiency	Skin feels like sandpaper, looks like gooseflesh, flaky, and dry.
Nails		
Koilonychia	Iron deficiency	Bilateral thin, concave spoon-shaped nails.
Legs		
Knock-knee	Calcium deficiency	Knees turned inward, ankles cannot touch.
Bowlegged	Calcium deficiency	Legs curved outward, ankles cannot touch.

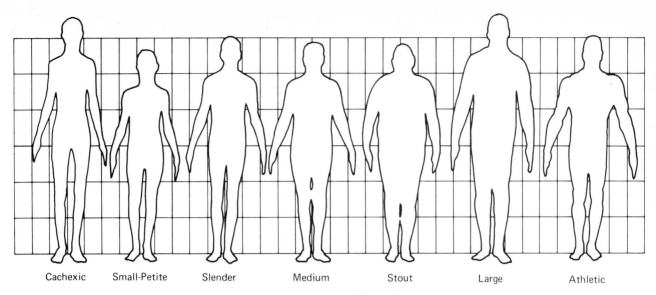

Cachexic   Small-Petite   Slender   Medium   Stout   Large   Athletic

Figure 4-2. Examples of physical size.

tension, and diabetes mellitus. Bony protrusion or muscle atrophy reflects weight loss, commonly the first clinical sign of a chronic disease process such as cancer, obstructive lung disease, or hyperthyroidism. With the client seated, the examiner inspects the skin, hair, eyes, and mouth (Chapters 5, 7, and 9).

Measurement

Measurement includes two areas: anthropometric and biochemical. Anthropometric measurements evaluate the size, weight, and proportions of the body. Biochemical measurements determine levels of various nutrients in the blood and urine or examine metabolic functions that depend on adequate nutrient intake.

Anthropometric measurements. Anthropometrics for the adult client include weight and height (Chapter 2), wrist circumference, skinfold measurements and arm circumference.

Wrist circumference reflects an estimate in body frame size (Table 4-13). It is taken with a flexible non-stretch tape, at the smallest part of the wrist, proximal to the styloid process of the ulnar bone (Figure 4-3). When the body frame size is determined, ideal weight for height is determined by use of Appendix 5 or 6. The percentage of standard is calculated by the following equation:

$$\frac{\text{Actual weight}}{\text{Standard weight}} \times 100$$

Less than 70 percent is a significant weight deficit; greater than 120 percent, a significant weight excess (Table 4-14). Quick guides for determining appropriate weight for height are the following equations:

For women: Height of 5'1" equals 100 lbs. For every 1" of height above 5'1", 5 lbs. are added.

For men: Height of 5' equals 110 lbs. For every 1" of height above 5', 6 to 7 lbs. are added.

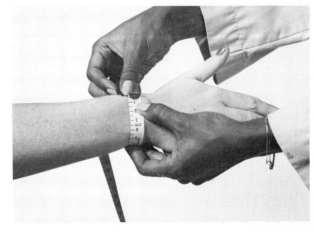

Figure 4-3. Measurement of wrist circumference.

Table 4-13. Determination of Body Frame Size

Body Frame Type

Small	Medium	Large

Height (vertical axis, top to bottom): 6'0", 5'11", 5'10", 5'9", 5'8", 5'7", 5'6", 5'5", 5'4", 5'3", 5'2", 5'1", 5'0", 4'11", 4'10", 4'9", 4'8"

Arm circumference (horizontal axis): 5", 5¼", 5½", 5¾", 6", 6¼", 6½", 6¾"

Skinfold thickness measurements reflect fat stores. The two most clinically useful skinfolds are the triceps and subscapular. The triceps skinfold is measured on the nondominant arm at the midpoint of the upper arm. To locate the midpoint, marks are made at the acromion and olecranon processes. A measuring tape is placed at the posterior portion of the arm between the two marked points, and the midpoint is marked. The client's arm hangs relaxed at the side. A pinch of skin and fat is taken between the thumb and forefinger to assure that no muscle tissue is included with the fold. The examiner notes that when the client flexes his arm, no pulling occurs. If pulling occurs, the examiner regrasps the skin and fat until no muscle tissue is present. Skinfold calipers are placed at the midpoint and are read to the nearest 0.5 millimeter (Figure 4-5).

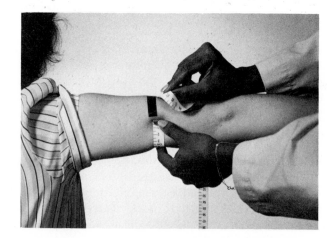

Figure 4-4. Measurement of arm circumference.

Table 4-14. Nutritional Disorders: Abnormal Weight

Finding	Condition	Description
Excessive caloric intake or inactivity without decrease in caloric intake	Obesity More than 20% over ideal weight	Excessive fat deposition.
Edema Obesity of face and trunk Muscle wasting Skin atrophy	Cushing syndrome	Hyperactivity of the adrenal cortex.
Goiter, large tongue, puffiness of hands and face	Hypothyroidism	Iodine deficiency, thyroid hypertrophy.
Overeating, gradual weight gain of 1 to 3 pounds over multiple years	Overweight Less than 20% over ideal body weight	Excessive fatty deposits.
Severe underweight	Anorexia nervosa	Distorted body image leading to compulsive under-eating and strenuous exercise. Weight 10 to 20% below ideal body weight. Most common in teenage girls.
Severe muscle wasting with severe weight loss	Cachexia	10% below ideal body weight accompanied by taste changes, early satiation. Frequently occurs in chronic disease processes, especially cancer and chronic obstructive lung disease
Nervousness, weakness, weight loss with increased appetite	Hyperthyroidism	Excessive thyroid hormone secretion with elevated BMR, increased serum protein bound iodine (greater than 8 mcg/100 ml).

The subscapular skinfold is measured at the inferior angle of the scapula with the fold running parallel to the axillary border.

The triceps and subscapular skinfold measurements are plotted on the nomogram in Table 4-15, and the percentage of body fat is determined. The normal for men is less than 16 percent; for women, less than 19 percent. Body fat is excessive when it is greater than 20 percent for men and greater than 25 percent for women. People at or below the fifth percentile for standard are at risk for protein-calorie malnutrition (Table 4-16).

Persons at risk for marasmus (post trauma such as burns or major surgery) are further assessed for protein stores. Arm circumference is used in the calculation of arm muscle circumference, a sensitive index of muscle protein stores (Table 4-17). Arm circumference is taken on the nondominant arm, at the midpoint of the upper arm. It is measured with a flexible, nonstretch tape and read to the nearest 0.1 centimeter (Figure 4-4). People at or below the fifteenth percentile for standard are at risk for protein calorie malnutrition (Table 4-18).

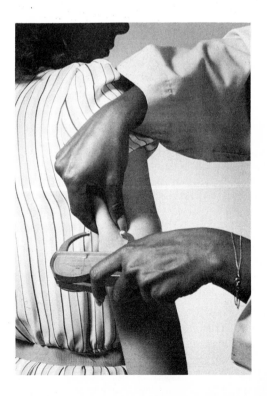

Figure 4-5. Measurement of triceps skinfold thickness.

Table 4-15. Determination of Percentage of Body Fat

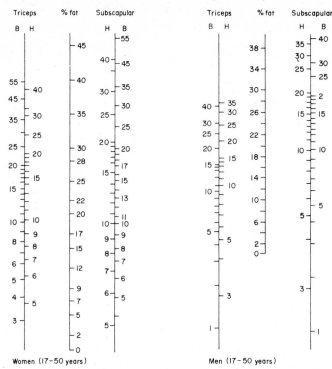

Women (17–50 years)   Men (17–50 years)

Reproduced by permission from Parizkova et al., *Body Fat and Physical Fitness,* Hingham, MA: Martinus Nijhoff, 1977.

Table 4.16. Standards for Triceps Fatfold

Triceps Skinfold Percentiles (millimeters)

	Male					Female				
Age	5th	15th	50th	85th	95th	5th	15th	50th	85th	95th
0–5 mo.	4	5	8	12	15	4	5	8	12	13
6–17 mo.	5	7	9	13	15	6	7	9	12	15
1½–2½ yr.	5	7	10	13	14	6	7	10	13	15
2½–3½	6	7	9	12	14	6	7	10	12	14
3½–4½	5	6	9	12	14	5	7	10	12	14
4½–5½	5	6	8	12	16	6	7	10	13	16
5½–6½	5	6	8	11	15	6	7	10	12	15
6½–7½	4	6	8	11	14	6	7	10	13	17
7½–8½	5	6	8	12	17	6	7	10	15	19
8½–9½	5	6	9	14	19	6	7	11	17	24
9½–10½	5	6	10	16	22	6	8	12	19	24
10½–11½	6	7	10	17	25	7	8	12	20	29
11½–12½	5	7	11	19	26	6	9	13	20	25
12½–13½	5	6	10	18	25	7	9	14	23	30
13½–14½	5	6	10	17	22	8	10	15	22	28
14½–15½	4	6	9	19	26	8	11	16	24	30
15½–16½	4	5	9	20	27	8	10	15	23	27
16½–17½	4	5	8	14	20	9	12	16	26	31
17½–24½	4	5	10	18	25	9	12	17	25	31
24½–34½	4	6	11	21	28	9	12	19	29	36
34½–44½	4	6	12	22	28	10	14	22	32	39

Adapted from: Frisancho, A.: "Triceps Skin Fold and Upper Arm Muscle Size Norms for Assessment of Nutritional Status," *Journal of Clinical Nutrition,* 27:1052, 1974.

These percentiles were derived from data obtained on all white subjects in the United States Ten-State Nutritional Survey of 1968–1970. In this survey, obesity in adults was defined as a fatfold greater than the 85th percentile.

Table 4-17. Calculation of Muscle Circumference and Cross-Sectional Muscle and Fat Areas

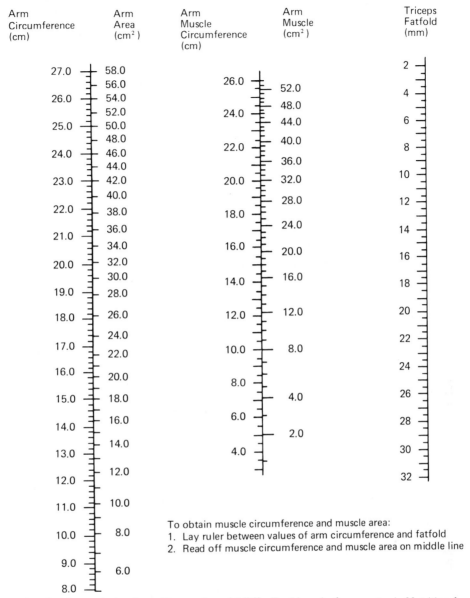

Arm Circumference (cm)	Arm Area (cm²)	Arm Muscle Circumference (cm)	Arm Muscle (cm²)	Triceps Fatfold (mm)

To obtain muscle circumference and muscle area:
1. Lay ruler between values of arm circumference and fatfold
2. Read off muscle circumference and muscle area on middle line

Reproduced with permission from: Gurney, J. and Jelliffe, D.: "Arm Anthropometry in Nutritional Assessment; Nomogram for Rapid Calculation of Muscle Circumference and Cross-Sectional Muscle and Fat Areas," *American Journal of Clinical Nutrition* 26:912, 1973.

Biochemical Measurements. The purposes of biochemical measurements are to screen for subclinical deficiencies or excesses before overt clinical signs occur and to quantify existing clinical abnormalities. The most common tests are hematocrit, hemoglobin, serum triglyceride, cholesterol, and serum glucose. Normal values are listed in Appendix 9.

Hematocrit and hemoglobin reflect iron stores. Cholesterol and triglycerides are drawn to assess risk of heart disease, particularly atherosclerosis. A fasting glucose or urine dipstick for glucose is performed to rule out glucose metabolism abnormalities. In addi-

tion an electrophoresis pattern quantitates LDLs, VLDLs, and HDLs.

The hospitalized patient undergoing major surgery or under metabolic or psychological stress is at risk for protein-calorie malnutrition. Futher evaluation of protein stores is performed to assess adequate nutritional status. This includes creatinine/height index (CHI), serum protein, serum albumin, lymphocyte count, nitrogen balance studies, and immune system response. Normal values are presented in Appendix 9.

Table 4.18. Standards for Arm Muscle Circumference

Arm Muscle Circumference Percentiles (centimeters)

	Male					Female				
Age	5th	15th	50th	85th	95th	5th	15th	50th	85th	95th
0–5 mo.	8.1	9.4	10.6	12.5	13.3	8.6	9.2	10.4	11.5	12.6
6–17 mo.	10.0	10.8	12.3	13.7	14.6	9.7	10.2	11.7	12.8	13.5
1½–2½	11.1	11.7	12.7	13.8	14.6	10.5	11.2	12.5	14.0	14.6
2½–3½	11.4	12.1	13.2	14.5	15.2	10.8	11.6	12.8	13.8	14.3
3½–4½	11.8	12.4	13.5	15.1	15.7	11.4	12.0	13.2	14.6	15.2
4½–5½	12.1	13.0	14.1	15.6	16.6	11.9	12.4	13.8	15.1	16.0
5½–6½	12.7	13.4	14.6	15.9	16.7	12.1	12.9	14.0	15.5	16.5
6½–7½	13.0	13.7	15.1	16.4	17.3	12.3	13.2	14.6	16.2	17.5
7½–8½	13.8	14.4	15.8	17.4	18.5	12.9	13.8	15.1	16.8	18.6
8½–9½	13.8	14.3	16.1	18.2	20.0	13.6	14.3	15.7	17.6	19.3
9½–10½	14.2	15.2	16.8	18.6	20.2	13.9	14.7	16.3	18.2	19.6
10½–11½	15.0	15.8	17.4	19.4	21.1	14.0	15.2	17.1	19.5	20.9
11½–12½	15.3	16.3	18.1	20.7	22.1	15.0	16.1	17.9	20.0	21.2
12½–13½	15.9	16.9	19.5	22.4	24.2	15.5	16.5	18.5	20.6	22.5
13½–14½	16.7	18.2	21.1	23.4	26.5	16.6	17.5	19.3	22.1	23.4
14½–15½	17.3	18.5	22.0	25.2	27.1	16.3	17.3	19.5	22.0	23.2
15½–16½	18.6	20.5	22.9	26.0	28.1	17.1	17.8	20.0	22.7	26.0
16½–17½	20.6	21.7	24.5	27.1	29.0	17.1	17.7	19.6	22.3	24.1
17½–24½	21.7	23.2	25.8	28.6	30.5	17.0	18.3	20.5	22.9	25.3
24½–34½	22.0	24.1	27.0	29.5	31.5	17.7	18.9	21.3	24.5	27.2
34½–44½	22.2	23.9	27.0	30.0	31.8	18.0	19.2	21.6	25.0	27.9

Adapted from: Frisancho, A.: "Triceps Skin Fold and Upper Arm Muscle Size Norms for Assessment of Nutritional Status." *American Journal of Clinical Nutrition,* 27:1052, 1974.

These percentiles were derived from data obtained on all white subjects in the United States Ten-State Nutritional Survey of 1968–1970.

The creatinine/height index allows a comparison between muscle mass per height and actual body cell mass. Height is unaltered in the malnourished state and under normal conditions creatinine excretion is constant. During tissue breakdown, creatinine excretion is decreased. A 24-hour urine creatinine is compared to expected excretion for height. Normal creatinine excretion for height is listed in Table 4-19. The formula is:

$$CHI = \frac{urinary\ creatinine\ excretion}{ideal\ urinary\ creatinine\ excretion \times 100}$$

Values of 90 to 100 percent are considered normal. With a value less than 90 percent the client is considered at risk for protein/calorie malnutrition.

During malnutrition the visceral protein stores are the first protein stores to be broken down for energy. Visceral protein includes serum protein and albumin, hemoglobin, lymphocytes, and the immune system. Low levels of visceral protein may reflect inadequate protein and calorie intake. Many other diseases cause low levels of serum protein, albumin, and lymphocytes. If they are low, further evaluation for protein intake by a written diet history or oral recall is indicated.

Nitrogen balance studies are performed to determine anabolism, catabolism, or equilibrium state. That is, nitrogen balance studies reflect tissue building (anabolism), tissue breakdown (catabolism), or a homeostatic state. Protein contains 16 percent nitrogen, or 1 gram of nitrogen equals 6.25 grams of protein. Nitrogen balance is determined by the following equation:

$$Nitrogen\ balance = \frac{protein\ intake}{6.25}$$
$$- (urea\ nitrogen + 3)$$

The number 3 is a constant factor for daily nitrogen lost in the feces, hair, and skin. The balance study is performed over a 24-hour period. A 24-hour urine collection is analyzed for urea nitrogen since urea is the major excretion route of nitrogen. Using the equation, a positive value means nitrogen is retained, or the body is building tissue (anabolism). A negative value means protein tissues are broken down for energy (catabolism). A value of zero means that protein breakdown equals protein tissue building or the body is in an equilibrium state. Most healthy adults are in zero nitrogen balance.

Table 4-19. Expected 24-hour Urinary Creatinine Excretion

Women

Height		Small Frame		Medium Frame		Large Frame	
in.	cm.	Ideal Weight	mg Creatinine per 24°	Ideal Weight	mg Creatinine per 24°	Ideal Weight	mg Creatinine per 24°
56	142.2	43.2	778	46.1	830	50.7	913
57	144.8	44.3	797	47.3	851	51.8	932
58	147.3	45.4	817	48.6	875	53.2	958
59	149.8	46.8	842	50.0	900	54.5	981
60	152.4	48.2	868	51.4	925	55.9	1006
61	154.9	49.5	891	52.7	949	57.3	1031
62	157.5	50.9	916	54.3	977	58.9	1060
63	160.0	52.3	941	55.9	1006	60.6	1091
64	162.5	53.9	970	57.9	1042	62.5	1125
65	165.1	55.7	1003	59.8	1076	64.3	1157
66	167.6	57.5	1035	61.6	1109	66.1	1190
67	170.2	59.3	1067	63.4	1141	67.9	1222
68	172.7	61.4	1105	65.2	1174	70.0	1260
69	175.2	63.2	1138	67.0	1206	72.0	1296
70	177.8	65.0	1170	68.9	1240	74.1	1334

Men

in.	cm.	Ideal Weight	mg Creatinine per 24°	Ideal Weight	mg Creatinine per 24°	Ideal Weight	mg Creatinine per 24°
61	154.9	52.7	1212	56.1	1290	60.7	1396
62	157.5	54.1	1244	57.7	1327	62.0	1426
63	160	55.4	1274	59.1	1359	63.6	1463
64	162.5	56.8	1306	60.4	1389	65.2	1500
65	165.1	58.4	1343	62.0	1426	66.8	1536
66	167.6	60.2	1385	63.9	1470	68.9	1585
67	170.2	62.0	14.26	65.9	1516	71.1	1635
68	172.7	63.9	1470	67.7	1557	72.9	1677
69	175.3	65.9	1516	69.5	1598	74.8	1720
70	177.8	67.7	1557	71.6	1647	76.8	1766
71	180.3	69.5	1599	73.6	1693	79.1	1819
72	182.9	71.4	1642	75.7	1741	81.1	1865
73	185.4	73.4	1688	77.7	1787	83.4	1918
74	187.9	75.2	1730	80.0	1846	85.7	1971
75	190.5	77.0	1771	82.3	1893	87.7	2017

Reprinted with permission from: Anne Grant, *Nutritional Assessment*, Box 25057, Northgate Station, Wa, 1979.

Table 4-20. Sample Worksheet for Hospitalized Patients

Measurement	Value Obtained	At Risk for Protein-Calorie Malnutrition
1. Fat stores % body fat % triceps skinfold		At or below the fifth percentile for standard (Table 4-16).
2. Somatic protein Actual body weight Ideal body weight		Less than 20% ideal body weight
Midarm circumference Arm muscle circumference Arm muscle %		At or below the fifteenth percentile for standard (Table 4-18).
Creatinine/height index		85% or less
3. Visceral protein Serum albumin		Less than 3.0 grams
Total lymphocyte count		Less than 800
Immune system response		Negative

Table 4-21. Selected Carbohydrate Abnormalities

Condition	Finding	Explanation
Tooth enamel decalcified; decaying teeth	Dental caries	Sugar is fermented on the teeth, which forms a weak acid. Frequency and duration of carbohydrates ingested are important factors
Polyuria, thirst, hunger, weakness, weight loss	Diabetes mellitus	Elevated fasting blood sugar greater than 100 mg/100 ml. Urine positive for glucose. Elevated two hour postprandial blood sugar greater than 160 mg./100 ml. Insulin secretion is insufficient for adequate transportation of glucose across cell membranes.
Two to three hours after eating, onset of sweating, flushing, hunger, headaches, or dizziness	Hypoglycemia	Oversecretion of insulin. Postprandial blood glucose less than 50 mg./100 ml. Possible inappropriate eating habits.
Diarrhea, gas, abdominal cramping after ingestion of milk products	Lactose intolerance	Lactase deficient, cannot digest lactose.
Risk factors in chronic heart disease	Hypertriglyceridemia	Diets high in refined sugars cause elevated triglycerides. Elevated levels of serum triglyceride greater than 120 mg/100 ml. Elevated levels of VLDL.
Infrequent bowel movements with straining or pain occuring during bowel movement. Feces are hard and small	Constipation	Lack of fiber and liquid in diet.
Pouches protruding from colon lumen	Diverticulosis	Lack of fiber in diet causes increased lumen pressure.

Table 4-22. Selected Protein Abnormalities

Condition	Finding	Explanation
Edema Poor growth in children Skin lesions Hair color changes	Kwashiorkor	Inadequate protein intake.
Muscle wasting Similar to Kwashiorkor except no edema	Marasmus	Inadequate protein and calorie intake.
Mental deficiency Inability to metabolize amino acid phenylalanine	Phenylketonuria	Urine phenylalanine 0.3 to 1 gms. per day. Serum phenylalanine 5 to 60 mg/100 ml.
Swelling around eyes Fluid retention in feet and hands	Edema	Low intake of high-quality protein over a period of time.

Table 4-23. Selected Fat Abnormalities

Condition	Finding	Explanation
Dry, scaly skin	Linoleic acid deficiency	Less than 1% of calories contain linoleic acid over a protracted period of time.
Creamy appearance of blood; eruptive xanthomas. Bouts of abdominal pain.	Hyperlipoproteinemia I	Hereditary inability to clear chylomicrons in the plasma.
Premature vascular disease. Tendon and tuberous xanthomas.	Hyperlipoproteinemia IIa	Elevated LDL with elevated serum cholesterol greater than 300 mg./100 ml. Cholesterol plaque formation in arteries.
Premature vascular disease, tuberoeruptive or planer xanthomas. Commonly occurs with glucose intolerance or obesity.	Hyperlipoproteinemia IIb	Elevated LDL and elevated VLDL. Serum cholesterol greater than 300 mg./100 ml. Serum triglycerides greater than 150 mg./100 ml. Low serum HDL.
Tuberoeruptive or planer xanthomas, premature vascular disease.	Hyperlipoproteinemia III	VLDL and LDL of abnormal composition.
Premature vascular disease, commonly overweight.	Hyperlipoproteinemia IV	Elevated VLDL, triglycerides greater than 120 mg./100 ml.
Eruptive xanthomas, bouts of abdominal pain, pancreatitis, hepatosplenomegaly.	Hyperlipoproteinemia V	Elevated VLDL, chylomicrons present.

Immune System Response. Intradermal skin tests for the recall of antigens may be applied to assess immune deficiencies. Common antigens are Candida, Streptokinase/Streptodormase, or PPD (purified protein derivative). A normal reaction is a red, irritated induration at the site of the antigen injection. The spot is measured in centimeters; normal reaction is an induration greater than 5 centimeters. A negative response is no irritant reaction within 48 hours. This is interpreted as anergy, one cause of which is protein deficiency.

Collection of Data. A worksheet for collection of data is tabulated, and the nutritional status is assessed. Appropriate recommendations are made based on the collected data (Tables 4-20, 4-21, 4-22 and 4-23).

Life Cycle Variations

Childhood

Modifications to the socioeconomic profile and diet history for infants include questions about the following: breast-feeding, formula feeding (how formula is prepared), use of prepared baby foods, time and order of introduction of foods, kind and amount of food taken at each feeding, vitamin and mineral supplementation, and stool pattern (Table 4-24).

Parents of older children are asked about snack foods and patterns, attitudes toward food and eating, the atmosphere in the home during meals, and meal patterns.

Table 4-24. Normal Stool Pattern for Infants

Feeding	Frequency per Day	Description
Breast-feeding	4 to 5	Yellow, mushy
"Regular" formula Milk-based or soy	2 to 4	Pale, brown, mushy to soft form
"Predigested" formula i.e., Pregentimal Nutramigen	4 to 5	Green, liquid to pasty

Table 4-25. Abnormal Findings in Childhood

Finding	Condition	Description
Inadequate subcutaneous fat Lassitude or excessive irritability	Failure to thrive	Inadequate weight gain or growth. Possible maternal deprivation.
Pale, weak, sleeps excessively	Iron-deficient anemia	Microcytic-hypochromic red blood cells. Hemoglobin less than 9 g./100 ml. Hematocrit less than 30%.
Very pale Excessive fat deposits Obese infant up to 2 yrs. of age	Milk baby	Baby's major source of calories is milk, causing too many calories, leading to obesity and also iron-deficient anemia.
Weakness Anorexia Nausea Vomiting Incoordination Hypertonicity History of vegan mother (eats only fruits, vegetables, grains, and legumes) who is breast-feeding; or history of child, infant on nonenriched soy milk as major source of calories	Pernicious anemia	Lack of intrinsic factor or positive Schillings test. CO-labeled B-12 excretion less than 2%.
Infant on goat's milk with no supplements Pale Weakness	B-6 deficient anemia	Megablastic macrocytic anemia. Serum folic acid less than 5 mcg./ml.
Diarrhea Abdominal cramping	Lactose intolerance	Lactase, the enzyme to digest milk sugar, is deficient.
Steatorrhea Voracious appetite No weight gain	Cystic fibrosis	Fibrosis of endocrine glands, particularly lungs and pancreas, causing deficiency of pancreatic enzymes.
Straining or crying on elimination Stools hard, small pellets	Constipation	Inadequate fluid or fiber intake.
High incidence of dental caries	Fluorine deficiency or high sugar intake	Multiple fillings or decaying teeth.

Measurements include height and weight for all children with the addition of head circumference for infants (Table 4-25 and Appendix 7). The values for hemoglobin and hematocrit are age-specific and reflect iron stores (Appendix 9).

Adolescence

The nutritional requirements are dictated by the physiological state rather than chronological age. Puberty increases the demands for calories, protein, calcium, and iron. The presence of orthodontic braces frequently necessitates changes in the diet eaten by the family and peer groups.

Inspection for appropriate height-to-weight, excessive fat deposition, or depletion of fat stores is important. The normal physiologic fat deposition that occurs in females during puberty may raise concern regarding weight among some adolescents. Adolescents are vulnerable to radical weight loss programs at a time when protein and calorie requirements are high. Evaluation of the client's own body image is important so the examiner may deter harmful dieting. Teenage girls taking oral contraceptives require increased vitamin B-6. Adolescents who abuse over-the-counter drugs such as aspirin and alcohol increase the metabolic demands for protein, calcium, and vitamins C and B-6.

Pregnancy

Adequate nutrition is vital to optimize the growth and development of the fetus and to minimize obstetric complications. Inadequate food intake is associated with difficult deliveries, stillbirths, prematurity, and congenital defects. Pregnancy increases the demand for most nutrients (Table 4-3). Supplements of iron and folic acid are required. If the diet provides for these added requirements, vitamin and mineral supplements are not necessary. Supplements cannot compensate for poor food habits.

Nutritional assessment is performed on every client during the first prenatal visit and at each trimester. If the client falls into one or more risk categories or if disparity is observed during the initial assessment, more frequent follow-up is indicated. The risk categories include the following: adolescence, high parity, obesity, dietary fadism, low-income status, alcoholism, drug addiction, history of rapid weight gain, previous obstetric complications, and excessive smoking.

The most important measurement is weight. Adequate weight gain ensures the fetus of sufficient kilocalories and nutrients for growth. *Pregnancy is not the time for weight reduction.* Recommended weight gain is 11 kilograms (24 pounds) for most American women. Normal weight gain pattern is 3 to 4 pounds the first trimester, $\frac{1}{2}$ pound per week for the second trimester, and one pound per week for the third trimester (Appendix 8).

Late Adulthood

During the aging process, multiple physiological changes directly affect the nutrient intake of the geriatric client. The decrease in hearing, vision, taste, and smell take away some of the social aspects and ability to eat. Decreased muscle tone, decreased peristalsis, and delayed esophageal emptying can make eating meals an uncomfortable experience. This leads to complaints of "heartburn," early satiety, or "gas." Loss of teeth or ill-fitting dentures also influences nutrient intake. Fifty percent of Americans have lost all their teeth by age 65, 65 percent by age 75. The accumulative effect of these physiological changes places the geriatric client at risk for nutritional disease.

Various sociologic changes during the later years of the life cycle place older people at risk for nutritional disorders. These include a fixed income during an inflationary economy, living alone, and the decreased ability to shop for foods. Careful review and evaluation of the diet history are the basis of nutritional assessment of the older adult. Manifestation of overt lesions or symptoms of dietary indiscretion occur gradually. By evaluation of the dietary history early intervention is possible (Table 4-26).

Table 4-26. Abnormal Findings in Late Adulthood

Finding	Condition	Explanation
Chest pain Elevated cholesterol	Atherosclerosis	Intimal thickening of the arteries by local accumulation of lipids
Fatigue Headaches Diastolic blood pressure greater than 90 mm./Hg.	Hypertension	Cardiac hypertroply accentuated with obesity and high sodium intake
Bone pain, bone decalcification on X-ray	Osteomalacia	Deficient calcium intake; inappropriate Ca:P ratio
Fatigue	Muscle wasting	Insufficient intake of proteins

Anatomy and Physiology

The skin is the outermost covering of the body and has numerous functions: protection of the internal environment from the external environment; regulation of body temperature; and sensory reception for touch, temperature and pain. Anatomically the skin is divided into three layers; epidermis, dermis, and subcutaneous. Appendages to the epidermis include the nails, hair, sebaceous glands, apocrine glands, and eccrine glands (Figure 5-1).

The epidermis is the most superficial layer of the skin. This paper-thin cellular membrane is devoid of blood vessels, connective tissue, and lymphatics. It performs several important functions. It protects the body from the surrounding environment by preventing the entry of microorganisms, chemicals, other foreign substances, and ultraviolet radiation. In addition the epidermis prevents the egress of water and electrolytes and aids in heat regulation by conduction, radiation, and convection.

There are several strata within the epidermal layer. The outermost stratum, the horny layer or stratum corneum, consists of dead keratinized cells. These dead cells shed constantly but are quickly replaced by keratinocytes from the deeper layers. By this process the epidermis continually renews itself. Thickness of this epidermal layer varies, depending on body region. It is extremely thin over the eyelids, scrotum, and penis and attains its greatest thickness over the palms of the hands and soles of the feet.

The innermost stratum, the basal layer, is where melanin is formed. Production of this pigment is stimulated by the melanocyte-stimulating hormone (MSH) of the anterior pituitary gland and by exposure to sunlight. Melanin protects the body against ultraviolet radiation and determines skin color characteristics of different races. This skin color differentiation is based upon the size and activity level of melanocytes rather than the number of melanocytes present. Thus, a person with darkly pigmented skin has larger and more active melanocytes than a person with lighter skin color.

The dermis, the corium or true skin, is the layer of skin directly beneath the epidermis and is the major portion of the skin. The dermis has the property of being tough, flexible, and elastic because of its fibrous components collagen and elastin. This dense connective tissue layer also contains sensory nerve endings, lymphatics, and blood vessels; it stores water and electrolytes. Functionally the dermis has a protective function by shielding the body from gross physical trauma.

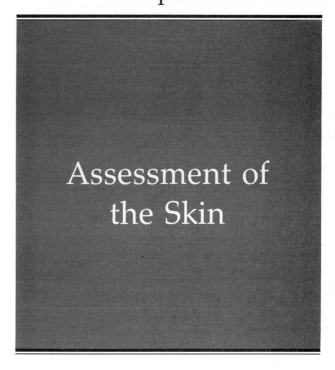

Assessment of the Skin

Objectives

The examiner will be able to do the following:

1. Inspect the skin
2. Palpate the skin for temperature, moisture, texture, and turgor
3. Observe the appearance, color, and texture of the hair and nails
4. Recognize abnormalities of the skin and its appendages
5. Record the information obtained

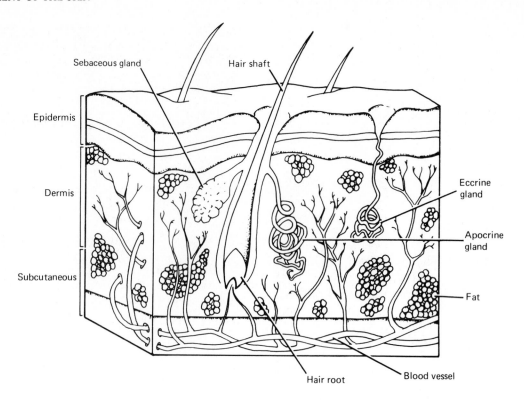

Figure 5-1. The skin and its appendages.

The subcutaneous layer of the skin is where fat is manufactured and stored. This tissue is a depot for fat storage; it also insulates and cushions the body.

The nails are appendages to the skin, and each consists of a nail plate, matrix, bed, and root (Figure 5-2). The nail plates are made of hard keratin material that grows at the rate of 0.1 millimeter per day. At the base of each nail is a white semilunar region, the lunula. The lunula corresponds to the nail matrix. It is often hidden by the skin but is especially noticeable in the thumb. The matrix is the area of the nail responsible for growth. The nail bed is an area of epithelial tissue found directly beneath the nail plate. Although the nail plate rests on and adheres to the nail bed, the nail bed does not contribute to the formation or growth of the plate. The nail plate is inserted into the skin laterally and posteriorly. The nail edges are inserted into shallow grooves called nail folds. The root is the proximal portion of the nail and is inserted deeply into the posterior groove.

Hair is another appendage of the skin. Each hair consists of a shaft and a root (Figure 5-1). The shaft is the portion of the hair that projects above the skin's surface. The root is located beneath the skin and is surrounded by a hair follicle. The follicle is a tubular invagination of the epidermal layer that extends inferiorly and obliquely into the dermal layer. When hair is exceedingly long, the follicle penetrates the subcutaneous tissue. An enlarged bulbous area at the end of the follicle contains the cellular material that determines hair structure and pigmentation. Similar to the skin, hair color is dependent on the activity of melanocytes.

Hair is composed of tightly woven keratinized cells. Growth of hair is cyclical with periods of activity gen-

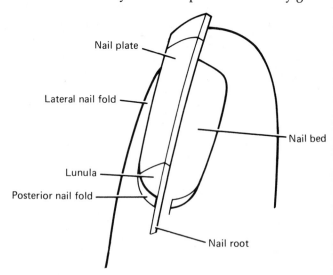

Figure 5-2. Components of the nail.

erally followed by shorter periods of rest. Each hair follicle functions independently of adjacent follicles; while one hair is in a period of growth, another may be resting. Hair in different regions of the body has different cycles. Hair on the scalp has long growing periods interspersed with short periods of rest. Hair on the trunk, eyebrows, and extremities has brief growing periods followed by longer resting phases.

The entire body, except for the soles of the feet, palms of the hands, and a few other areas, is covered with vellus, a fine, barely visible, lightly colored hair. Terminal hair is the longer, thicker, coarser and darker hair found on the rest of the body. Terminal hair assumes different characteristics depending on location and hormonal stimulation.

The sebaceous glands are epidermal appendages that provide constant, imperceptible lubrication for the skin (Figure 5-1). They are widely distributed throughout the body. Sebaceous glands are most numerous on the scalp, face, and scrotum; appear in lesser numbers on the upper trunk and extremities; and are absent on the palms of the hands and soles of the feet. They secrete sebum, a complex fatty substance that passes to the skin through the hair follicles. Sebum secretion is influenced by hormonal activity. For instance, estrogen and androgen activity increases sebum production.

The apocrine glands are vestigial appendages that are not widely distributed (Figure 5-1). The apocrine glands are found in greatest numbers in the axillae, but are also located in the areolae of the nipples and the periumbilical, perianal, and genital regions. Other apocrine glands are found in the ear canal, where their secretions contribute to the formation of ear wax. The apocrine glands are simple, coiled, tubular glands attached to the hair follicles. They secrete a milkish, white fluid onto the skin in response to emotional stress. This secretion initially is odorless but assumes an unpleasant odor in the presence of normal skin bacteria. Functionally the apocrine gland's secretions are of no benefit to the body. The apocrine glands are inactive in childhood, become productive during puberty when stimulated by sex hormones, and decrease their production as a normal consequence of aging.

The eccrine glands are epidermal appendages that control body temperature (Figure 5-1). This thermoregulatory activity is governed by the heat regulatory mechanism of the hypothalamus. Stimulation of cholinergic fibers activates the glands and eccrine sweat immediately appears on the skin. While the prime stimulus for sweating is heat, sweating may also occur as a result of emotional stress. Sweat is a dilute saline solution; the quantity of sweat produced may vary from a few drops to several thousand milliliters per hour. Eccrine glands are widely distributed but are most numerous on the forehead, palms of the hands, and soles of the feet. The pores of the eccrine glands open directly onto the skin.

Assessment Modalities

Preparation

Examination of the skin is best achieved with adequate exposure and proper positioning. In most situations the client wears a gown and is appropriately draped. The only equipment necessary is a transparent ruler for measuring lesions.

There are two different methods for examining the skin; both utilize a systematic approach that compares symmetrical parts. In one method the examiner assesses the entire skin by starting with the head and proceeding to the rest of the body. In the other method the examiner assesses the skin with the body parts and regions being examined. For example, the skin of the abdomen is assessed during assessment of the abdomen.

Inspection

Inspection is used to determine color, vascularity, and lesions. Normal skin color is determined by the presence of hemoglobin, carotenoids, and melanin in the skin and their ability to absorb and reflect light. The range of skin color is great and reflects genetic background as well as exposure to sun and weather. Thus, skin color varies among people and in different areas of the same person. The face, ears, and back of the neck, hands, and arms are usually the areas that receive greatest sun exposure; therefore they are normally darker in color than other areas (Table 5-1). Although the skin is a highly vascular organ, normally it is free of vascular markings (Table 5-2).

Erythema (diffuse redness) may be a normal finding from blushing on the part of an embarrassed client or from an overly warm examining room. It results from capillary dilatation in response to nervous stimuli. This vascular flush is most commonly seen on the cheeks, bridge of the nose, neck, and upper chest.

Striations, or stretch marks, are frequently observed on the abdomen. They occur when elastic fibers are ruptured from prolonged stretching. Pregnancy and obesity are common predisposing factors. Recent striae appear pink while those of long duration assume a silvery-white discoloration.

Table 5-1. Selected Color Abnormalities of the Skin

Finding	Condition	Explanation
Brown	Addison's disease	Increased pigmentation that appears as a diffuse tanning in both exposed and unexposed portions of the body. Areas where hyperpigmentation most likely occurs include pressure points (sacrum, elbows), skinfolds, scars, and extensor surfaces.
	Exposure to sunlight	Hyperpigmentation occurs only in those areas of the body exposed to sunlight.
Grayish-brown	Hemochromatosis	Increased pigmentation and deposition of iron in skin due to defect in iron metabolism.
Pallor (decreased color)	Albinism	Generalized hypopigmentation of skin, hair, and eyes due to congenital inability to produce melanin.
	Vitiligo	Localized patchy areas of hypopigmentation that have sharply demarcated borders. Size varies. Commonly seen on backs of hands, sides of neck, axillae, genitalia, and trunk.
	Anemia	Nail beds, mucous membranes, and skin appear pale due to decrease in the amount of oxyhemoglobin.
	Shock	Nail beds, mucous membranes, and skin appear pale due to decrease in the amount of blood available to superficial vessels.
Yellow	Liver disease	Generalized yellow appearance to skin, sclerae and mucous membranes. Results from red blood cell hemolysis with increase in cutaneous bilirubin.
	Carotenemia	Discoloration occurs on palms, soles, and face, although it may be generalized and is due to increased presence of carotene pigments in skin. May result from increased consumption of vegetables and fruits containing carotene pigment. (Sclerae unaffected.) Also seen in myxedema and diabetes.
Red	Fever Drug eruptions Infections (streptococcal)	Due to vascular dilatation. Erythema due to inflammatory response.
	Sunburn	Erythema on exposed parts of body due to prolonged exposure to sun.
Blue	Central cyanosis Congenital heart defect Congestive heart failure Chronic lung disease	Nailbeds, lips, and oral mucosa appear cyanotic due to presence of increased amounts of deoxygenated hemoglobin.
	Peripheral cyanosis Anxiety Cold	Appearance of cyanotic nailbeds and lips results from peripheral vasoconstriction.

Because most people have at least a few clinically insignificant lesions, it is imperative that the examiner be familiar with their distinctive characteristics. These include the following; distribution, configuration, and morphology. Distribution refers to where the lesions occur. Terms used to describe distribution are as follows: localized, generalized, involving the exposed surfaces, and involving the intertriginous (skinfold) areas. Configuration refers to the pattern of distribution and includes the following: annular (circle), arciform (arc), serpiginous (wavy line), linear (straight line), and irregular (no definite pattern). Morphology refers to structural characteristics (Tables 5-3 and 5-4).

Table 5-2. Selected Abnormalities of the Dermal Vascular System

Finding	Condition	Description	Illustration
Small, bright, red, slightly raised lesion	Cherry angioma (de Morgan's spot)	Found primarily on thorax and arms. Appears more frequently with increasing age. Has no pathological significance. Pressure induces only partial blanching.	
Red, small central body with radiating legs	Spider angioma (arterial spider)	Most lesions found above the waist. Seen most frequently in liver disease, vitamin B deficiencies, and pregnancy. May be seen in healthy person. Pressure on central portion produces blanching of spider. After pressure is released, blood returns to central portion and then fills branches.	
Bluish central body of variable size and shape with radiating branches (shapes include flare, cascade, comet, rocket, and tangle)	Venous star	Found on dorsum of foot, leg, medial aspect of thigh and back of neck. Most often lies above vein. More common in women. Associated with the aging process or venous obstruction. Pressure on central body produces blanching of body but not of branches.	
Small, thin-walled bluish papule	Venous lake	Most frequently seen on ears and face, especially lips. Uncommon other than on head and neck. Appears after age 35 and numbers increase with age. Pressure produces emptying of papule. No pathological significance.	
Small, dark red to purple discrete round lesions	Petechia	May be found anywhere on body. Present when there is extravasation of blood outside the vessel. May be associated with bleeding tendency. Pressure does not produce blanching.	
Purplish-blue variable sized and shaped areas	Ecchymoses	Location varies. Caused by extravasation of blood into skin. May be secondary to trauma or evidence in bleeding disorders. Pressure does not product blanching. Larger than petechiae.	

Table 5-3. Primary Lesions of the Skin (Lesions that develop on normal skin in response to external or internal stimuli. Except for the macule, they are palpable lesions.)

Finding	Condition	Description	Illustration
Macule	Freckle Vitiligo Rubella	Circumscribed change in skin color generally less than 1 cm. in diameter. Shape varies.	
Papule	Wart Insect bite	Solid, elevated area of varying colors less than 0.5 cm. in diameter.	
Plaque	Psoriasis	Solid, elevated area greater than 0.5 cm. in diameter.	
Nodule	Xanthomas Gouty tophi	Elevated solid area that extends into dermal layer. Diameter ranges from 0.5 cm in 1–2 cm.	
Tumor	Dermatofibroma	Elevated solid lesion of greater size than nodule extending into dermal and subcutaneous layer. Usually larger than 2 cm. in diameter.	
Wheal	Insect bite Urticaria	Circumscribed, elevated irregular, relatively transient. Varies in color from pale to red.	
Vesicle	Herpes simplex Chicken pox	Circumscribed fluid-filled elevation up to 0.5 cm. in diameter.	
Bulla	Second-degree burn	Similar to vesicle but larger in size. Diameter greater than 0.5 cm.	
Pustule	Acne Furuncle Impetigo	Pus-filled vesicle or bulla. Appearance depends on infecting organism.	

Table 5-4.   Secondary Lesions of the Skin (Lesions that develop from alterations in primary lesions.)

Finding	Condition	Description	Illustration
Scales	Psoriasis Dry skin	Flaking due to exfoliated epidermis	
Crusts	Impetigo	Dried exudate of pus, serum, or blood	
Fissure	Angular chelitis Chapped skin	Linear crack extending into dermis	
Erosion	Superficial scratches	Loss of superficial epidermis	
Ulcer	Stasis ulcer	Loss of epidermal layer with extension into dermal layer	
Scar	Healed surgical incision or trauma	Smooth, fibrotic area of dermis; color indicates age: red—of recent origin; pink—after 6 weeks color of surrounding skin or hyperpigmented after 6 months; pale—after long period of time	
Keloid	Hypertrophic scar	Formation of dense hyperplastic fibrous tissue over scar; occurs in black and yellow-skinned persons	

Palpation

Palpation assesses temperature, moisture, texture, and turgor. The examiner uses the back of the hand or fingers to palpate the skin for temperature. Since skin temperature is dependent on the amount of blood circulating through the dermal vessels, slight variations in temperature normally occur. This is especially true of the digits, which are usually somewhat cooler than the hands and feet.

Moisture on the skin varies among different body regions. It is not unusual for the palms of the hands, soles of the feet, forehead, axillae, and groin to be moist since sweat glands are most numerous in these areas. Localized sweating is more likely to occur in response to emotional stimuli while a generalized moist feeling to the skin occurs in response to thermal stimuli, for example, fever or an overly warm examining room. Dry skin may be a normal finding in winter when temperatures and humidity are lower.

Skin texture refers to the characteristic "feel" of the skin's surface. Texture is assessed by gently palpating the skin's surface with the fingertips, and is influenced by body region, age, and sex. The texture of normal skin varies from delicately fine (nipples) to extremely rough (soles of the feet, and palms of the hands). It is finest in infancy, and becomes coarser with aging, and is finer in women than men.

Skin turgor is a measure of the elasticity of the skin. It is assessed by gently pinching the skin over the sternum or forearm between the thumb and forefinger and releasing it. Turgid skin immediately resumes its original shape (Figure 5-3, Table 5-5).

Appendages to the Skin

The hair is assessed for distribution, quantity, and quality. Normal distribution of hair is dependent upon age, sex, the influence of sexual hormones, and genetic background. Terminal hair distribution in women includes the head, axillae, pubis, and legs. In males terminal hair distribution also includes the face, chest, hypogastric region, back, buttocks, and extremities. People of Asian and African ancestry often have sparser distribution of terminal hair.

The quality of hair refers to color and texture, which are genetically determined. Color and texture may be altered by the use of chemical agents, such as dyes, permanent solutions, and straighteners. Texture ranges from very fine in persons of light complexion to quite coarse in darkly pigmented people (Table 5-6).

The normal fingernail is thin, smooth, firm, translucent, and convexly shaped. The dorsal or free edges of the nail plates have a whitish appearance due to the presence of free air. White spots or streaks on the nails (leukonychia) result from incomplete keratinization and are a variation of normal. Fine longitudinal ridges are also sometimes seen in the normal nail plate. The skin surrounding the nail is intact, and

Table 5-5. Selected Abnormalities of Palpation of the Skin

Finding	Condition	Description
Generalized hyperthermia	Systemic infection	Skin feels warmer than usual. Accompanied by generalized flushed appearance.
Generalized hypothermia	Shock	Skin feels cold.
Localized hyperthermia	Sunburn Cutaneous inflammation	Skin feels warmer in certain areas, for example, sun-exposed areas.
Localized hypothermia	Peripheral vascular disease	Skin feels cooler in areas of vascular insufficiency.
"Tenting" (Poor turgor)	Fluid volume deficit Senile cutaneous atrophy—loss of elasticity Sunlight damage	Persistence of the skinfold following pinching with a slower return to the original shape.
Edema	Local trauma Cardiovascular disease	Depression formed in skin by examiner's finger pressing firmly. Recorded as one of the following: 1+ Barely detectable 2+ Indentation less than 5 mm. 3+ Indentation less than 1 cm. 4+ Indentation greater than 1 cm.

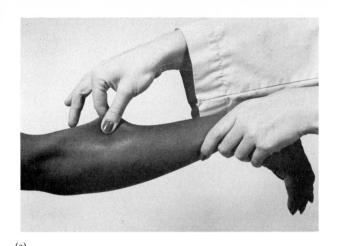

(a)

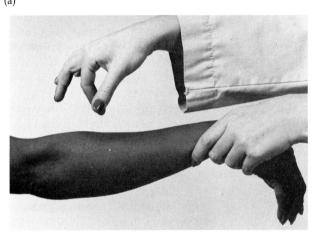

(b)

Figure 5-3. *Assessment of skin turgor: (a) the examiner pinches the skin; (b) the examiner releases the skin.*

the angle between the nail and proximal portion of the finger is approximately 160 degrees (Figure 5-4). This unguophalangeal angle is firm to palpation (Table 5-7).

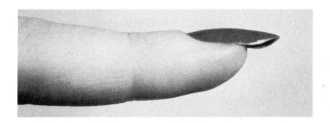

Figure 5-4. *Normal unguophalangeal angle.*

Life Cycle Variations

Childhood

The skin of the neonate has unique characteristics. An erythematous flush appears in the first 8 to 24 hours but gradually disappears and is replaced by a pinkish skin color. This pinkish color predominates except in the hands and feet, which may appear cyanotic. Acrocyanosis is cyanosis of the extremities and may occur throughout early infancy due to vasoconstriction with exposure to cold.

The appearance of jaundice in the second or third day of life is a frequent occurrence. Jaundice is best detected in natural daylight. The examiner observes a yellow discoloration, which is most obvious on the nose when pressure is applied. "Physiologic jaundice" represents a normal phenomenon because it results from the immature liver's inability to conjugate bilirubin. Accumulation of unconjugated bilirubin in the blood imparts a characteristic yellow color to the skin and sclerae. Physiologic jaundice appears gradually and disappears slowly during the first few

Table 5-6. Selected Abnormalities in Hair Quantity

Finding	Condition	Description
Hirsutism	Cushing's disease Acromegaly	Increase in the growth and distribution of hair in males. Growth of hair in unusual places in females (on face and chest). Due to congenital or acquired conditions.
Alopecia (Partial or complete loss of hair)	Alopecia areata	Loss of hair in patches.
	Fever Hypopituitarism Hypothyroidism	Patterns vary but usually begin as overall thinning.
	Physiologic baldness in males	Inherited variation from normal, which begins over frontal regions of scalp and extends posteriorly. Sometimes begins over occiput and extends anteriorly.

Table 5-7. Selected Abnormal Conditions of the Nail

Finding	Condition	Description
Transverse furrow across nail	Beau's line	A white line appears across the nail usually following an acute illness or injury. As the nail grows, the line moves distally until it eventually reaches the free margin where it is filed or cut off.
Concave nails	Spoon nails	Nail plate loses its convexity and assumes a more concave shape. Associated with hypochromic and iron deficiency anemia. Can be congenital.
Unguophalangeal angle > 160°	Hippocratic nails Clubbing of the nails	A painless, bilateral occurrence seen in pulmonary and cardiovascular disease. On palpation nails feel resilient and spongy.

weeks of life. However, jaundice can result from serious pathology (infection, hemolytic disease of the newborn, or biliary atresia) and cause rapid and sustained elevations in serum bilirubin. Serum bilirubin greater than 17-23 mg./100 ml. can result in kernicterous, a condition of irreversible brain damage due to cerebral accumulation of bilirubin. Because of this serious complication of hyperbilirubinemia, the presence of jaundice necessitates daily serum bilirubin determinations.

In older infants a yellowish skin hue may be a normal finding when large quantities of yellow vegetables and fruits containing carotene are consumed. The discoloration of carotenemia normally concentrates on the palms of the hands, soles of the feet, and nasolabial folds. While the entire skin may be involved, the scleare are not affected.

The skin of the black newborn appears dusky pink except in the fingernails and genitalia, which are highly pigmented. Gradually pigmentation develops and the infant becomes darker in color. A normal finding in many black, Asian, and Indian infants is the appearance of an undefined bluish area in the lumbosacral region, a Mongolian spot. This coloration occurs when there is an overgrowth of pigmented cells in the dermis. The spot becomes less noticeable as the infant grows and usually disappears in early childhood as the surrounding areas of pigmentation become more evident.

Harlequin color changes are a normal finding in the infant turned on the side. The side on which the infant is lying appears red while the other side becomes pale; a line of demarcation appears to divide the body into two halves. Harlequin color changes are transient, result from vascular instability, and have no pathological significance. Mottling is the appearance of alternating patches of rubor and pallor; it is normal on the extremities of babies under one month of age

who are cold. It is abnormal when it occurs over the entire body. This generalized mottling is seen predominantly in premature infants and those with Down's syndrome.

The skin of the newborn may normally appear to be shedding. This may vary from a slight flakiness to large patches of desquamation.

On palpation, the skin of the newborn normally feels smooth, soft, and warm. A slight moisture in the axillae and on the palms of the hands may be palpable. Varying quantities of vernix, a cheeselike, greasy substance are found on the skin of newborns. This substance protects the infant's skin in utero and often accumulates in the skinfolds and vaginal folds and under the fingernails.

Slight edema may be a normal finding shortly after birth due to the presence of retained fluids. It normally appears in the hands, feet, lower legs, sacrum, and pubis and disappears in the first few days of life.

The newborn is often covered with fine downy hair called lanugo. It is commonly seen on the back and shoulders and gradually disappears during the first few weeks of life. The amount of scalp hair present at birth varies from a scanty covering to hair in great abundance. The original hair, shed during the first several months, is replaced with new hair, which sometimes differs in color from the original.

A common finding in babies is a macular rash in the diaper area, "diaper dermatitis." It may result from an allergy to the diapers or to the detergents or soaps used in laundering them. Another cause is prolonged exposure to urine and feces.

The skin of children frequently provides the first manifestations of systemic viral infections. These skin changes are known as exanthems (Table 5-9). Children frequently contract bacterial skin infections and skin infestations from close physical contact with other children (Table 5-10).

Table 5-8. Selected Skin Lesions of the Newborn

Finding	Condition	Description
Whitish pinhead-sized papules on nose, forehead, and cheeks	Milia	May be present at birth but can also appear during first few weeks of life due to the collection of secretions from sebaceous glands.
Large red spots with white centers scattered diffusely	Erythema neonatorum toxicum	Usually appear during first few days. May be due to irritation (for example), rubbing against nursery cribsheet). Disappear spontaneously.
Smooth flat red to purplish area	Nevus flammeus (port wine stain)	Present at birth and commonly located on face or neck. Can vary in size from a few mm. to being so large that it covers face and neck. Due to proliferation of skin's capillary bed. Rarely disappear.
Slightly raised bright red lesion	Nevus vasculosus (strawberry mark)	May be present at birth but usually appears shortly thereafter. Commonly located on face or neck. May vary in size from a few mm. to several cm. Does not blanch on pressure. Usually disappears spontaneously by age 5, although residual scarring, brown pigmentation, or wrinkling may be seen.
Small brown macule	Freckle	Commonly appears in areas exposed to sunlight.
Circumscribed light brown to black macule or papule	Nevi (moles)	May be present at birth but usually develop later. Formed by clustering of specialized epithelial cells containing melanin. Vary in size, shape, texture, and degree of hair present. Very small precentage undergo changes and become malignant melanomas later in life.

Table 5-9. Viral Exanthems

Finding	Description	Condition
Red maculopapular confluent rash	Rash begins at hairline, spreads inferiorly over the face and body within 3 days, and lasts 7 to 10 days. Follows 3-day prodrome of cough, rhinitis, conjunctivitis. Accompanied by Koplick spots (Table 9-6).	Measles (rubeola)
Pinkish discrete maculopapular rash	First appears on face, spreads to the trunk and arms, and in 2 days disappears from the upper body, and appears on legs where it lasts 2 to 3 days. Usually accompanied or preceded by lymphadenopathy (Chapter 19) and mild fever.	German measles (rubella)
Discrete rosy-pink macular rash with general distribution	Rash may be barely discernible and transient and usually occurs after 3 days of sustained high fever in a child who appears well.	Roseola
Red punctate sandpaper feelings rash on body and red confluent rash on face with circumoral pallor	Rash begins on neck and chest, spreads to extremities, and disappears in 2 to 3 days. Follows 1 to 2 days prodrome of fever, vomiting, and sore throat. Accompanied by strawberry tongue initially and raspberry tongue later (Table 9-6).	Scarlet fever
Erythematous, slightly raised rash on cheeks giving them a "slapped cheek" appearance.	About 1 day after facial rash appears, maculopapular rash appears on extremities. Rash intensifies during warm baths and assumes a lacy appearance after several days.	Fifth disease (erythema infectiosum)
Crops of maculo-papular and vesicular lesions	Lesions begin as erythematous macules, which develop rapidly into papules and vesicles. Greatest concentration of lesions is on the trunk.	Chicken pox (varicella)

Table 5-10. Infections and Infestations Common among Children

Finding	Condition	Explanation
Pruritus accompanied by inflammation and secondary bacterial infection resulting in papules, pustules and crusting, and nits (eggs) of lice adherent to hair shafts of scalp, eyelashes, or pubic hair. Lice may not be visible on body but found in seams of underwear.	Pediculosis capitus	Infestation by pediculosis humanus. Lice acquired by physical contact or use of infested brushes, combs, head garments, or bed linen.
	Pediculosis corporis	Infestation by pediculosis humanus corporis; lice acquired by physical contact or use of infested clothing or bed linen.
	Pediculosis pubis	Infestation by phthirus pubis; lice acquired by sexual contact, use of infested clothing, toilet seats, or bed linen.
Intense itching of hands (especially between fingers), wrists, areolae, axillae, genitalia, or face (in infants) from eggs and feces of mites in burrows beneath skin; may be accompanied by papules, vesicles or pustules from secondary infection.	Scabies	Infestation by sarcoptes scabeii; acquired by physical contact or use of infested clothing or bed linen. Pregnant females burrow under the skin and deposit eggs in channels several mm. to cm. long. Examiner uses a number 15 blade to scrape unscratched burrow or papule and smear glass slide. Slide is treated with 1 drop of 10% potassium hydroxide and inspected microscopically.
Vesicles, bullae and honey-colored crusted pustules.	Impetigo	Infection by Group A Streptococci.
Groups of erythematous papules surrounded by urticaria (papular urticaria) on the shoulders, upper arms, and buttocks of infants.	Delayed hypersensitivity to insect bites	Delayed transient hypersensitivity response to insect bites (usually fleas, but also mosquitoes, lices and scabies); sensitivity lasts 4-5 months.

Adolescence

During adolescence the child begins to assume some of the physical attributes of the adult. Noticeable skin changes include an increase in pigmentation in the mammary areaolae of the female and the genitalia in both sexes. In males the skin of the scrotum appears more reddish. The skin thickens in both sexes but to a greater degree in males.

The sebaceous glands become larger and begin their secretory activity. Unfortunately for many adolescents, this also heralds the appearance of acne. Because acne vulgaris occurs with such frequency, a mild involvement could almost be considered a normal physiologic process. Acne develops when the ducts of the sebaceous glands become blocked with a keratin plug that blackens; the surrounding area also becomes inflamed. Commonly affected areas include the face, neck, chest, and back. While both sexes are equally affected, males seem to have the more serious cases. It is also not unusual for females to have premenstrual flare-ups that last for several days beyond the menstrual flow.

Hair distribution also begins to show the typical adult and sex-related distribution. An increase in hair in the pubis, axillae, and other parts of the body occurs. Pubic hair growth begins as a sparse, downy hair and becomes more heavily pigmented, dense and curly over a one- to two-year time span. In males pubic hair growth occurs between ages 10 and 14 and assumes a diamond shape. In females pubic hair growth occurs between ages 8 and 13 and assumes a triangular shape. Axillary hair growth begins one to two years after pubic hair growth. It also begins as sparse down that becomes more heavily pigmented and dense. In males facial hair changes from vellus to sparse down to more heavily pigmented and finally to dense hair. This change in facial hair begins at approximately the same time or after axillary hair growth.

Pregnancy

During the second trimester of pregnancy, noticeable skin changes occur. There is an increase in pigmentation on the areolae, vulva, linea alba, and face. Primary areas of melanin deposition may occur on the face, including the cheeks, nose, and forehead and are referred to as the "mask of pregnancy." Upon termination of the pregnancy, a marked decrease in the amount of pigmentation occurs, although a slight residue may remain permanently.

Other skin changes that normally develop in pregnancy include the appearance of striae gravidarum or stretch marks of pregnancy. The causative factors are hyperactivity of the adrenal cortex and stretching of the skin. Striae appear most frequently on the breasts, thighs, abdomen, and buttocks; they vary in color from pinkish red to purple. Following delivery these striae fade and take on the silvery-white appearance of scar tissue.

Vascular spiders (spider angiomata) on the face, neck, upper chest and arms may be seen. These usually disappear after childbirth. In addition it is not unusual for the palms of the hands to appear erythematous.

Late Adulthood

Pigmentation changes appear with greater frequency in late adulthood. Blotchy, irregularly pigmented areas (mottling) develop in older persons of lighter skin and hair color. Blacks, Asians, and Indians do not demonstrate the same mottling tendency due to their more permanent pigmentation. Increased pigmentation may normally occur on the backs of the hands, face, and genitoanal region. Yellowish papules and plaques may also appear due to fat deposition. The skin appears pale as a result of changes in the blood vessels and decreased blood supply.

Lesions appear more frequently as skin growths seem to increase with aging. Although many of these lesions appear as a normal consequence of aging, their presence is noted (Table 5-11).

Thinning of the epidermis causes the veins to appear more prominent. Senile purpura may occur due to the degeneration of the supportive connective tissue surrounding the dermal vasculature and the increased fragility of the vessels themselves. These areas of reddish-purplish discoloration are most often located on the backs of the hands and forearms.

On palpation the skin of the older person may feel cool. This decrease in temperature is due to a decrease in the ability to regulate body temperature. The texture is drier as a result of the reduced activity of the sebaceous glands and reduced number of sweat glands. In addition, the loss of elasticity and subcutaneous fat gives the extremities and face a more wrinkled appearance. Loss of elasticity also causes decreased skin turgor.

Epidermal appendages also show age-related changes. A generalized thinning of hair occurs due to a reduction in the numbers of hair follicles. This thinning is apparent not only on the scalp but also on the extremities, axillae, and pubis. The hair becomes gray due to decreased melanocyte activity. Other changes that normally occur include a decrease in facial hair on males, an increase in facial hair on women, and a coarsening and thickening of hair in the nasal orifice and ear. Nails tend to grow more slowly, and the nail plate becomes thicker, tougher, more brittle, and less lustrous.

Table 5-11. Selected Skin Lesions of the Elderly

Finding	Condition	Description
Slightly raised, yellowish-brown wavy areas with greasy appearance.	Seborrheic keratoses	Found at hair margin on neck, face, trunk, and arms.
Flat or raised red, brown or grayish appearing lesions which may or may not be well-defined. (May be palpable only and feel as roughened skin texture.)	Actinic keratoses	Found on sun-exposed areas such as face, back of hands, lips, and helix of ear. Should be distinguished from seborrheic keratoses. Premalignant lesions.
Small, flat brown pigmented areas.	Lentigo senilis	Benign condition that results from an increase in deposition of melanin. Located on back of hands, wrist, face.
Small, bright red areas.	Senile telangiectasia	Dilatation of dermal capillaries frequently appearing on trunk and face.
Soft, flesh-colored cutaneous tags.	Acrochordons ("Skin tags")	Vary in size. Appear most commonly on neck, axillae, and eyelid. Have no pathological significance. Increase with age.

Anatomy and Physiology

This chapter focuses on assessment of the structural components of the head (the skull and the face) and of two neck structures (the thyroid gland and trachea). The head also contains the brain, lymph nodes, and four of the sensory receptor organs: eyes, ears, nose, and tongue. The neck also contains the jugular veins, carotid arteries, sternocleidomastoid and trapezius muscles, lymph nodes, spinal cord, and esophagus. Assessment of these head and neck structures is presented in other chapters.

The Skull and the Face

The skull consists of the cranial bones (cranium) and facial bones. The cranium encompasses the brain and consists of the frontal, temporal, parietal, and occipital bones. The facial bones include the orbits, nasal bones, zygomatic bones, maxilla, and mandible, the only movable facial bone. The other bones of the skull do not move and are joined by immovable joints known as sutures (Figure 6-1).

The mandible is the only bone of the lower face; the other facial bones are the bones of the midface. The bones of the midface are the origins for the muscles of facial expression. The insertions of the facial muscles are in the soft tissues of the eyelids, nose, and cheeks.

The mandible is the insertion for the muscles of mastication. They originate in the cranium (the temporalis muscle) and the facial bones (the masseter muscle) and are innervated by cranial nerve V (the trigeminal nerve).

The skull is covered by the scalp, a five-layer, thick, tough, and vascular protective covering. The outermost layer is the skin that covers the second layer, the subcutaneous tissue. Beneath these layers is the epicranius. The epicranius consists of the occipitofrontalis muscle. These first three layers are tightly bound to one another by numerous fibrous bands. The fourth layer contains loose fatty tissue; the fifth layer is the pericranium, a fibrous membrane surrounding the cranium that extends down into the suture lines.

The head contains the salivary glandular system, which secretes saliva into the mouth. Saliva contains enzymes that initiate carbohydrate digestion. The largest salivary glands are the parotids, located in the lateral cheeks. Two other glands are located in the lower face: the sublingual (under the tongue) and the submandibular glands (under the mandible). The submandibular glands are also known as the submaxillary glands and lie inferior and anterior to the

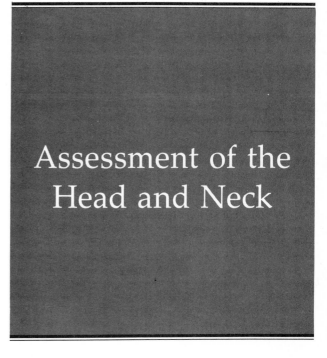

Chapter 6

Assessment of the Head and Neck

Objectives

The examiner will be able to do the following:

1. Inspect and palpate the head
2. Auscultate the head
3. Inspect the neck
4. Palpate the trachea and thyroid gland
5. Auscultate the thyroid
6. Palpate the cranial sutures of the newborn
7. Palpate and measure the anterior fontonalle of babies under 18 months of age
8. Transilluminate the head of newborns
9. Recognize abnormalities of the head and neck
10. Record the information obtained

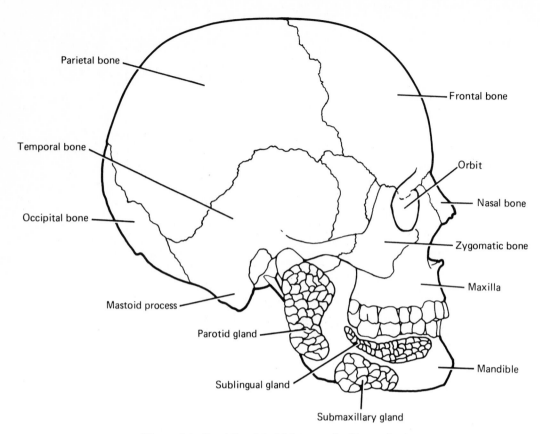

Parietal bone

Temporal bone

Occipital bone

Mastoid process

Parotid gland

Sublingual gland

Submaxillary gland

Frontal bone

Orbit

Nasal bone

Zygomatic bone

Maxilla

Mandible

Figure 6-1. Cranial and facial bones and salivary glands.

sublingual gland. The parotids and submandibular glands are assessed during examination of the head while the openings of their ducts and the sublingual glands are assessed during examination of the mouth (Chapter 9).

The Neck

The topographical anatomy of the neck includes two pairs of muscles and the larynx. The trapeziae and sternocleidomastoids (Chapter 17) are muscles that divide the neck into an anterior triangle and two posterior triangles. The anterior triangle is between the right and left sternocleidomastoids. The posterior triangles are between each of the respective sternocleidomastoid muscles and the trapezius on the same side (Figure 6-2). The larynx or voice box contains the thyroid cartilage (Adam's apple) and the cricoid cartilage (Figure 6-3). The thyroid cartilage is the main cartilage of the larynx. It is notched in the midline and is visible during swallowing. The cricoid cartilage is the lowermost laryngeal cartilage or uppermost tracheal ring.

The Trachea. The trachea is the section of the respiratory tract that transports inspired and expired air between the larynx and the bronchi. It is a segmented tube of cartilaginous rings about 10 to 12 centimeters long, extending from the sixth cervical vertebra to the fifth thoracic vertebra in the anterior midline.

The Thyroid Gland. The thyroid gland is located in the anterior neck and consists of two lateral lobes and a connecting bridge, the isthmus. The isthmus overlies the trachea at about the third tracheal ring; the lobes are located on either side of the trachea and extend from the inferior border of the thyroid cartilage to the sixth tracheal ring. The thyroid is an endocrine gland with widespread metabolic and somatic functions. It secretes three hormones: thyroxine, triiodothyronine, and calcitonin. Since thyroxine and triiodothyronine have similar effects, they are discussed together as thyroid hormone. Thyroid hormone affects secretion of other endocrine glands and affects four general body functions: metabolism, growth, and nervous and cardiac activity. Calcitonin is important in the regulation of serum calcium, since it decreases bone resorption of calcium (Chapter 20).

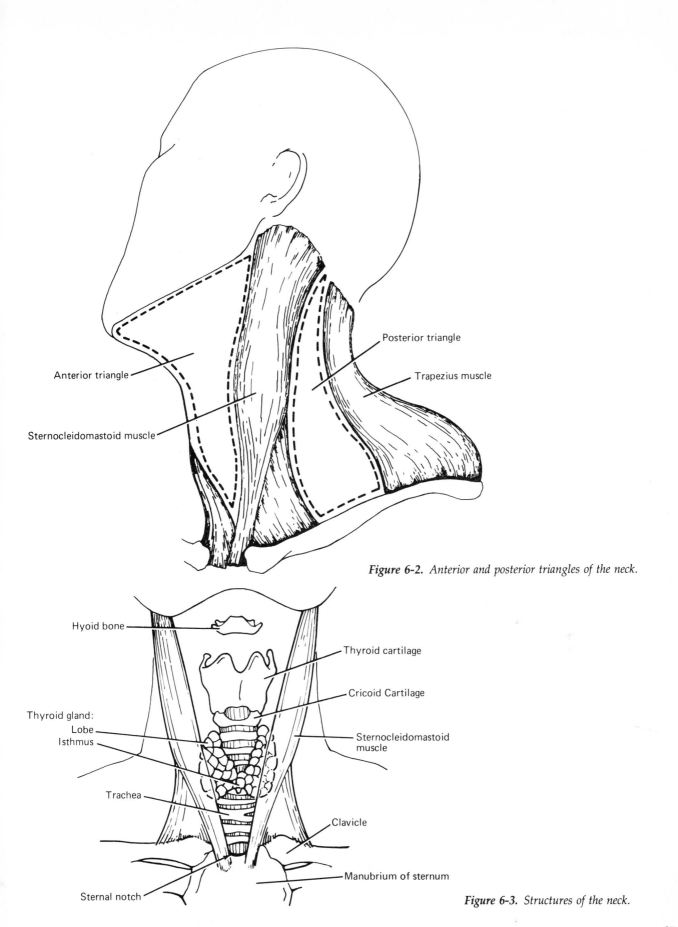

Figure 6-2. Anterior and posterior triangles of the neck.

Posterior triangle

Trapezius muscle

Anterior triangle

Sternocleidomastoid muscle

Hyoid bone

Thyroid cartilage

Cricoid Cartilage

Thyroid gland:
Lobe
Isthmus

Sternocleidomastoid
muscle

Trachea

Clavicle

Manubrium of sternum

Sternal notch

Figure 6-3. Structures of the neck.

Assessment Modalities

Preparation

Clients are asked to remove wigs, hairpieces, or toupees prior to the examination. The client usually sits for examination of the head and neck but can be supine or standing. In assessing the head and neck, inspection and palpation are the most important modalities. Since auscultation is sometimes performed, a stethoscope is generally the only instrument necessary. In addition, a cup of water often helps the client swallow, an important maneuver in the examination of the thyroid gland.

Inspection and Palpation of the Head

The head is inspected for size, contour, position, and consistency. Estimation of head size is generally subjective in the adult. Size is proportional to overall body size. The head is normally symmetrical and rounded with prominent frontal areas anteriorly and prominent occipital areas posteriorly. The position of the head is straight and midline. The examiner's hands are placed firmly on the client's head, and consistency is assessed. It is normally bony hard with no areas of fluctuance or compressibility. The term that describes normal findings is normocephalic.

The scalp is inspected for color and texture. Color is usually consistent with the color of the unexposed skin areas. Clients with hair loss have varying degrees of tanning from sun exposure. The texture is smooth.

The face reflects mood and emotion. It is inspected for symmetry, expression, mobility, color, and texture. It is normally symmetrical; the expression is alert and interested. It is normally animated; that is, facial movements correspond with conversation and are smooth in character. The color is consistent with the remainder of the body, and the texture is smooth. There is normally no bulging in the lateral cheeks, the areas over the parotid glands. The examiner palpates the face at the temporomandibular joints, which are normally nontender (Figure 6-4).

Auscultation of the Head

The examiner auscultates the head to detect the presence of any abnormal sounds (bruits). Bruits are soft rushing sounds produced by abnormal blood flow. The examiner usually listens over both temporal arteries by placing the bell of the stethoscope lightly

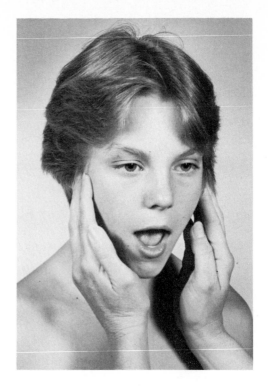

Figure 6-4. *Palpation of the temporomandibular joints.*

on the scalp. Normally there are no sounds audible (Figure 6-5, Table 6-1).

The Neck

The examiner assesses the neck for general appearance and for the characteristics of the trachea and the thyroid gland. In general appearance the neck is symmetrical; that is, the angles of the jaw are equidistant from the shoulders. It is flexed slightly at an angle less than 20 degrees, with cervical concavity.

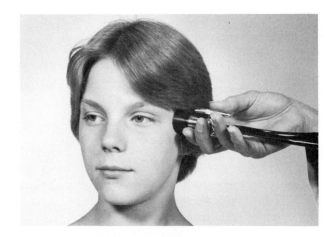

Figure 6-5. *Auscultation of the head.*

Table 6-1. Selected Abnormalities of the Skull, Scalp, and Face

Finding	Condition	Explanation
Enlarged cranium in comparison to the facial bones.	Paget's disease (osteitis deformans)	Bones of the skull thickened by the replacement of normal osseous tissue with porous vascular osseous tissue. A bruit may be audible. The client may relate that hat size has changed.
Prominent frontal bone, enlargement of nose, prognathism (growth of mandible resulting in overbite).	Acromegaly	Overproduction of growth hormone after epiphyseal closure results in growth of membranous bone (occurs in the extremities also). The client may relate that hat size has changed.
Bruit over the skull.	A-V fistula, arterial constriction	Interference with normal blood flow results in vibrations of arterial wall, causing production of abnormal sounds.
Single or multiple firm, nontender masses on the scalp.	Sebaceous cyst (wen)	Arises from skin and subcutaneous tissue; moves easily over the skull.
Sharply localized fluctuant mass, which slides over the skull.	Hematoma Abscess	Blood or pus in skin or subcutaneous layer of scalp is localized because of the numerous fibrous bands that join them to the epicranium.
Fluctuant mass bounded by the suture lines of a skull bone.	Depressed skull fracture; blood or pus under the pericranium	Hematoma or abscess is limited by suture lines because the pericranium extends into the suture lines.
Dry or greasy scales or flakes on the scalp.	Seborrheic dermatitis (dandruff)	Hereditary condition that accompanies oily skin.
Unilateral swelling below and in front of the ear (also may be behind the ear).	Neoplasm Infection	Abnormal formation of tissue in the parotid gland. Swelling from the inflammatory process.
Swelling and pallor; edema most marked in periorbital areas.	Nephrotic syndrome	During glomerular disease proteins are lost in the urine as well as extravasated into the interstitial tissue, which draws water and results in edema.
Dull, puffy facies (edema is nonpitting, is most marked in periorbital areas). Skin is dry; hair and eyebrows are dry, coarse and sparse.	Myxedema	Hypothyroidism due to inadequate secretion of thyroid hormone.
Round or moon face with red cheeks.	Cushing's syndrome	Usually accompanied by hirsutism in females (increased facial hair in mustache and sideburn areas).
Distorted facial expression; unilateral paralysis of muscles controlling facial expression (rarely bilateral); unilateral ptosis, and when talking cannot move affected side of mouth.	Bell's palsy Cerebrovascular accident	Acute inflammation in or near cranial nerve VII (facial nerve). Diminished blood supply to cranial nerve VII (the facial nerve) causes unilateral facial muscle paralysis.

The Trachea. The examiner inspects the neck and, in the healthy client, observes that the trachea does not deviate to the right or left. The examiner palpates the trachea by placing the forefinger in the suprasternal notch. It normally is palpable several centimeters posterior to the sternum (Figure 6-6, Table 6-2).

Thyroid Gland. The thyroid is assessed for size, symmetry, shape, and consistency. The thyroid isthmus overlies the trachea inferior to the cricoid cartilage. The thyroid lobes extend laterally from the isthmus and curve posteriorly around the cartilages and the upper tracheal rings. (Figure 6-3).

Table 6-2   Selected Abnormalities of the Neck

Finding	Condition	Explanation
Bulge in the anterior neck (may be unilateral or bilateral)	Goiter	Enlarged thyroid gland. May be due to dietary iodine deficiency, hypo- or hyperthyroidism or thyroiditis. Abnormal growth of tissue.
Soft rushing sound over a thyroid lobe (bruit over thyroid coincident with arterial pulsation persists when pressure is applied on the stethoscope)	Tumor Thyrotoxicosis	Accelerated blood flow through the thyroid arteries causes the production of abnormal sounds synchronous with the heart rate.

Lateral deviation of the trachea at the level of the clavicles	Goiter
	Cervical lymphadenopathy (Chapter 19)
	Chest pathology:
	  Pleural effusion
	  Tension pneumothorax
	  Pulmonary atelectasis
	  Spontaneous pneumothorax
		Neck masses can exert pressure resulting in tracheal compression and displacement.
		Displacement of the trachea to the contralateral side.
		
		Displacement of the trachea to the ipsilateral side.

The thyroid is a soft, small gland that is usually not visible. Each of the lobes are approximately 5.0 centimeters in length, 3.0 centimeters in width, and 2.0 centimeters in thickness. In thin clients the isthmus is frequently palpable, but in obese clients the thyroid is sometimes not palpable even when enlarged.

During inspection the neck is observed with the head erect, in slight extension, and while the client swallows a sip of water (Figure 6-7). Normally no bulges or masses are seen, and the only motion visible during swallowing is ascent of the thyroid cartilage.

There are four principles the examiner observes during palpation:

1. The thyroid is more apparent when the neck muscles are relaxed as in neck flexion.

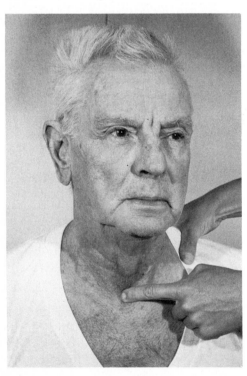

Figure 6-6. *Palpation of the trachea.*

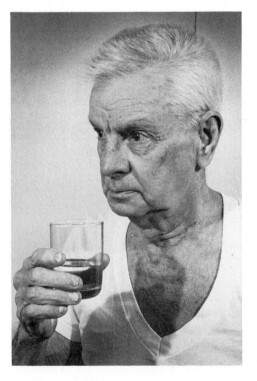

Figure 6-7. *Inspection of the neck.*

2. Palpatation is a bimanual technique; while one hand displaces neck structures medially, the other hand palpates the opposite lobe.

3. One lobe of the gland is compared with the other.

4 The thyroid ascends during swallowing.

There are two techniques for palpation of the thyroid: examination from the front and examination from the back. During examination from the front, the examiner faces the client. The examiner places the palmar aspects of the second and third fingers on the neck below the cricoid cartilage. As the client swallows some water, the neck is palpated for motion of the isthmus under the examining fingers (Figure 6-8). To palpate the right anterior lobe, the examiner asks the client to flex the neck (drop the chin) slightly and tilt the head slightly to the right. The left thyroid lobe is displaced toward the right by exerting pressure with the right hand in a medial direction. The left hand palpates for the anterior right lobe while the client swallows a sip of water. (Figure 6-9). The examiner palpates for the posterior portion of the right lobe by grasping the right sternocleidomastoid muscle between the thumb and fingers of the left hand and sliding them in superior and inferior directions (Figure 6-10). The procedure is reversed for the left lobe.

During the examination from the back, the examiner stands behind the client and asks that the neck be flexed slightly. The fingertips of both hands are

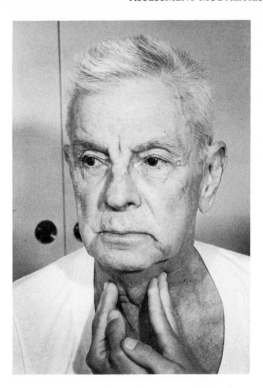

Figure 6-9. Anterior approach to palpation of the anterior right lobe of the thyroid.

placed over the trachea below the cricoid cartilage. The isthmus is palpated while the client swallows a

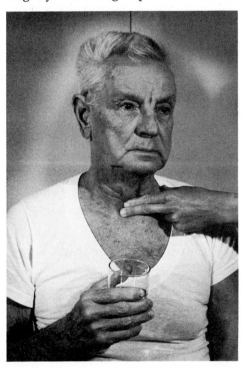

Figure 6-8. Anterior approach to palpation of the thyroid isthmus.

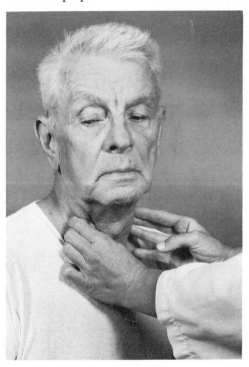

Figure 6-10. Anterior approach to palpation of the posterior right lobe of the thyroid.

sip of water. (Figure 6-11). Similar to the anterior approach, the examiner requests the client to tilt the head slightly toward the side being examined. In assessing the anterior left lobe, the examiner displaces the right thyroid lobe medially (toward the left) with the right hand and palpates for the left lobe with the fingers of the left hand while the client swallows a sip of water. (Figure 6-12). The examiner then palpates for the posterior left lobe by hooking the thumb and fingers around the left sternocleidomastoid and moving the hand in superior and inferior directions while the client swallows a sip of water (Figure 6-13).

The examiner auscultates the neck over both lobes of the thyroid gland with the bell of the stethoscope. Normally there are no sounds (Figure 6-14, Table 6-2).

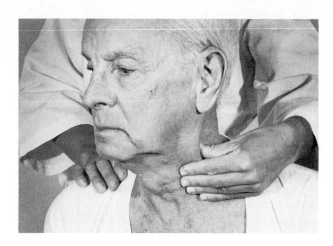

Figure 6-13. Posterior approach to palpation of the posterior left lobe.

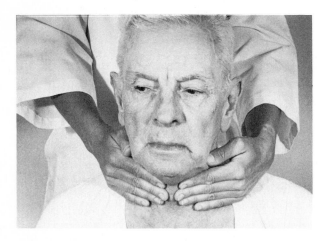

Figure 6-11. Posterior approach to palpation of the thyroid isthmus.

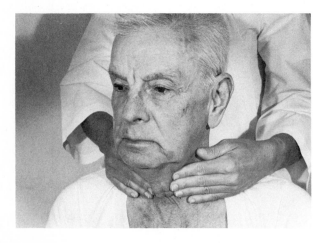

Figure 6-12. Posterior approach to palpation of the anterior left lobe.

Life Cycle Variations

Childhood

The examiner assesses the same characteristics of the head of the newborn—that is, size, shape, symmetry, and consistency—although there are considerable variations in findings. Additional necessary equipment includes a measuring tape and flashlight.

Head size is proportionately larger in early development. At birth the head is almost one-quarter the

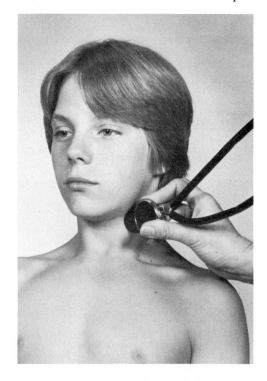

Figure 6-14. Auscultation of the neck.

length of the body while at adulthood it is approximately one-eighth of the length of the body. (Figure 6-15). Head size is an indicator of brain growth, and is measured at each visit in babies up to age 2 years (Chapter 2, Appendix 7).

The cranial sutures are movable and the fontanelles are open at birth. This enables temporary overlapping of the cranial bones during birth, which decreases the skull's diameter. The result is molding of the head, a temporary deformity in shape due to pressure against the presenting part of the vertex (head) during labor and delivery, which lasts up to several days (Figure 6-16).

At birth the sutures may be palpable as ridges due to overriding of bones. The sutures most frequently palpable are the coronal, sagittal, and lambdoidal. Others that may be palpable are the petrosquamal and metopic. In American Indians an additional suture may be palpable, the mendosal (Figure 6-17). By six months the sutures are no longer palpable, al-

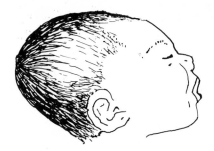

Figure 6-16. *Molding of the head of the newborn.*

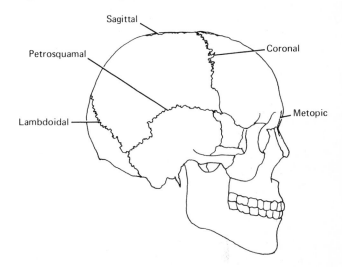

Figure 6-17. *Cranial sutures that may be palpable at birth.*

though they do not become firmly closed until just prior to puberty when synostosis (bony union) occurs. Until this time, increases in intracranial pressure can cause reopening of the sutures.

Besides molding, two additional head deformities that result from pressure against the head during parturition are caput succedaneum and cephalhematoma. Caput succedaneum is an area of edema over the presenting part of the head, which crosses the suture lines. It rarely lasts beyond several days after delivery (Figure 6-18).

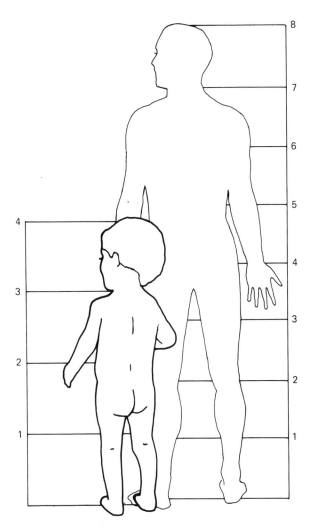

Figure 6-15. *Comparison of head-to-body-size ratio between the infant and the adult.*

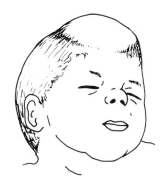

Figure 6-18. *Caput succedaneum.*

Cephalhematoma results from bleeding into the subperiosteal space on a skull bone and is confined to the borders of that individual bone (most frequently the parietal bone). It can last up to several months if calcification occurs but usually subsides in several days (Figure 6-19).

Another normal variation in appearance and palpation of the head among newborns is the presence of the anterior fontanelle. When the baby is upright, it appears as a slight depression, which pulsates with the heart rate. It is soft, as it represents a space between the bones, and feels compressible against the fingertips in the well-hydrated infant. In fact, at birth there are six fontanelles, although usually only two are palpable: the anterior and posterior fontanelles (Table 6-3, Figure 6-20). The anterior fontanelle is routinely measured at each visit until closure, varies from 1.0 cm. to 4.0 cm. in any direction and decreases in size over time. (Figure 6-21). The head is usually symmetrical after the neonatal period.

Transillumination. Transillumination is a technique used to assess the absence of cranial tissue in infants. In a dark room the examiner places a

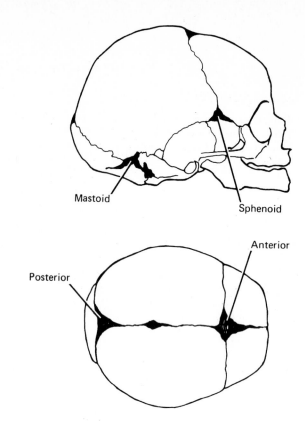

Figure 6-20. Fontanelles.

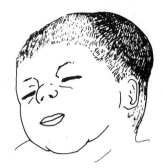

Figure 6-19. Cephalhematoma.

flashlight against the head and shines it into the cranium. Normally the circle of light extends no more than 1.5 centimeters in fullterm babies and 2.0 centimeters in preterm babies. The circle of light gives evidence of fluid rather than brain tissue. Extension of the circle of light greater than 2.0 centimeters gives evidence of decreased brain tissue or increased fluid. (Figure 6-22).

There are normally no other age-related structural changes in the head, skull, scalp, face, and neck (Table 6-4).

Table 6-3. Fontanelles

Name	Location	Palpable Until Which Month
Anterior	Junction of frontals and parietals	10-16 months
Posterior	Junction of parietals with occipitals	May be palpable at birth and up to 1-2 months
Right sphenoid	Junction of right parietal with right sphenoid	Usually not palpable
Left sphenoid	Junction of left parietal with left sphenoid	Usually not palpable
Right mastoid	Junction of right parietal with right temporal	Usually not palpable
Left mastoid	Junction of left parietal with left temporal	Usually not palpable

Table 6-4   Abnormalities of the Head, Skull, Scalp, Face, and Neck during Childhood

Finding	Condition	Description
Small head size in comparison with overall body size (microcephaly).	Mental retardation	Small head size is frequently associated with delayed brain growth.
Large head size for body size and age (macrocephaly).	Most frequently is hereditary when present at birth but may be due to abnormal growth of tissue within the cranium or excessive fluid in cranial vault (hydrocephaly)	Prior to closure of the sutures the cranial vault is capable of enlarging to accommodate increased tissue or fluid.
Pointed, conelike, or dome-shaped head.	Oxycephaly	Results from premature closure of the coronal sutures.
Boat-shaped head (narrow, long cranium)	Scaphcephaly	Results from premature closure of the sagittal sutures. Common in premature babies.
Palpation of temporoparietal or parieto-occipital areas results in momentary yielding similar to how a ping-pong ball would respond to similar pressure ("Ping-pong head").	Craniotabes	Results from osteoporosis of bone due to increased intracranial pressure, rickets, congenital syphilis, hypervitaminosis A, or hydrocephalus.
Increased circle of light during transillumination.	Hydrocephaly	Light shines through fluid, which displaces cranial tissue.
	Anencephaly	Light shines through head because of absence of brain tissue.
Excoriated papules and pustules on scalp; matted hair with gnats adherent to hair shafts and numerous small wingless insects.	Pediculosis capitus infestation (lice)	Usually occurs in other members of the child's household and among playmates, particularly at day care centers and in the classroom.
Facial distortion—unaffected side of the mouth moves normally during crying while affected side does not.	Facial nerve palsy	Results from birth pressures or use of forceps.
Swelling below and in front of the ears, usually bilateral although one side swells first.	Mumps	Acute viral inflammation of the parotid glands.
Asymmetry of neck muscles, which causes tilting of the head to one side.	Torticollis	Results from bleeding into the sternocleidomastoid muscle or spasm due to fibrosis in the muscle body.

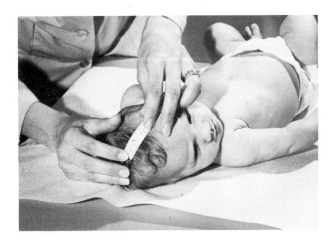

Figure 6-21. The pediatric nurse practitioner measures the anterior fontanelle at the six-month well-baby check-up.

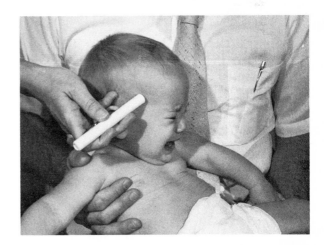

Figure 6-22. The head of the normal infant does not transilluminate.

Anatomy and Physiology

The structures of the eye can be viewed as having three types of functions: protection, support, and vision. The facial bones and accessory structures provide protection and support, while most of the structures of the globes contribute toward the function of vision.

Ocular Orbits

The ocular orbits are bony sockets cushioned with fat which provide protection on all but the front portions of the eyes (Figure 7-1). Portions of the frontal, sphenoid, maxillary, lacrimal, zygomatic, and palatine bones compose the ocular orbits.

Accessory Structures

The accessory structures are the eyelids, eyebrows, and lacrimal apparatus. Anteriorly the eyelids shield the eyes (Figure 7-2), and have a dual protective role. They protect by creating a mechanical barrier to foreign objects during blinking; they also protect the eyes against drying by spreading the lubricating fluid of tears across the ocular surface. The muscles of lid closure, orbicularis oculi, are innervated by cranial nerve VII (the facial nerve). The inner strength of the lids derives from the tarsus, a platelike fibrous structure.

The upper and lower eyelids join to form two angles. Laterally the angle is called the external canthus; medially, the internal canthus. In the internal canthus

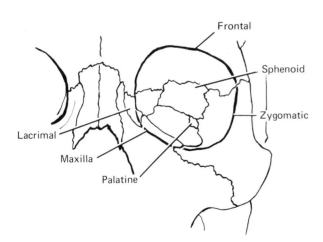

Figure 7-1. Ocular orbits.

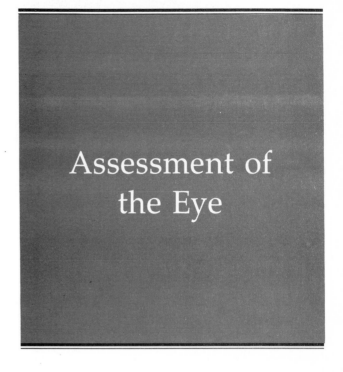

Chapter 7

Assessment of the Eye

Objectives

The examiner will be able to do the following:

1. Inspect the eyes and accessory structures
2. Palpate and auscultate the eyes
3. Measure visual acuity
4. Test visual fields
5. Observe extraocular movements
6. Check pupillary responses
7. Perform an ophthalmoscopic examination
8. Perform tonometry
9. Perform the cover-uncover and alternate cover tests
10. Recognize abnormalities of the eyes
11. Record the information obtained

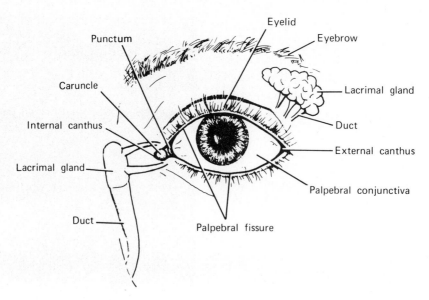

Figure 7-2. Accessory structures of the eyes.

there· is a small projection of mucous membrane known as the caruncle.

The conjunctiva lines the eyelids. The conjunctiva is divided into two parts, the palpebral portion and the bulbar portion. The palpebral portion lines the lids; it is a shiny pink transparent membrane that joins the bulbar conjunctiva. The bulbar portion covers the anterior eye surface and is presented with the other anterior eye structures.

The lacrimal apparatus consists of the lacrimal glands and ducts and the puncta. The glands are located superiorly and temporally to the eyes. Innervated by cranial nerve VII (the facial nerve), they produce tears, which are washed across the eyeball surface by the lids. The ducts transport tears to the puncta, small openings on the nasal portions of the upper and lower lids through which the tears drain. Tears then flow via the nasolacrimal duct into the nose.

Anterior Structures of the Eye

The structures of the anterior eye are the following: bulbar conjunctiva, cornea, anterior chamber, iris, pupil, lens, and posterior chamber (Figure 7-3).

The bulbar conjunctiva is a clear transparent membrane continuous with the palpebral conjunctiva. It overlies the sclera up to the limbus. The sclera, a protective, opaque, white, fibrous covering over the entire eyeball, with the exception of the iris and pupil, is the only visible anterior structure that extends beyond the anterior globe. The limbus is the circular margin where the sclera joins the cornea. The cornea is a convex, avascular, transparent covering over the iris and pupil. The cornea is protective in that it is an extension of the sclera; it is directly involved with vision because of its transparency and refractive ability.

The anterior chamber, iris, pupil, and lens are also directly involved with vision. Together they serve to regulate lighting conditions and focus light rays on the retina. Behind the cornea and anterior to the iris and lens is the anterior chamber. It contains aqueous humor, a transparent fluid. Behind the iris and lateral to the lens is the posterior chamber. Aqueous humor is secreted into the posterior chamber by the ciliary body and passes through the pupil to the anterior chamber. The aqueous humor drains from the anterior chamber via the canal of Schlemm, which is located in the angle of the anterior chamber.

The iris is a circular colored structure that contains two pairs of muscles: the sphincter pupillae and dilator pupillae. These muscles regulate the size of the pupil dependent upon two factors: available light and the distance from the object viewed. The sphincter is innervated by cranial nerve III (the oculomotor nerve) and constricts the pupil in the presence of bright light or when the object viewed is close to the eyes. The dilator, by sympathetic stimulation, increases the size of the pupil when there is decreased lighting or when the object in view is at a distance.

The pupil is a circular aperture surrounded by the iris. It dilates and constricts in response to the muscles of the iris.

The lens, a biconcave disc located behind the anterior chamber, contains many transparent fibers within a strong elastic capsule. Arrangement of the

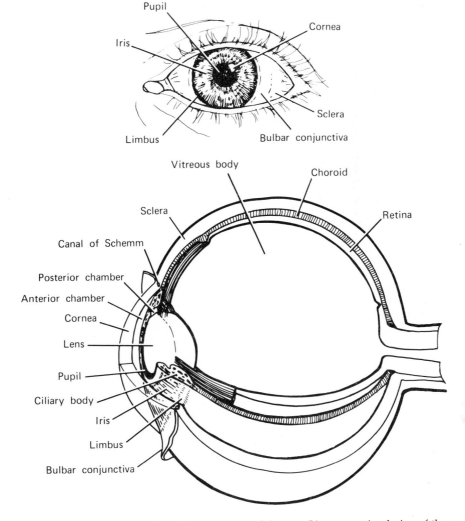

Figure 7-3. *(a) Anterior view of the structures of the eye; (b) cross-sectional view of the eye.*

fibers in a normal lens causes parallel light rays from an object in view to bend upon entering the pupil. This refraction normally results in convergence of light rays on the retina.

The lens capsule is suspended radially from the ciliary body. The ciliary body consists of two sets of small muscles that control the shape of the lens, depending on the distance an object in view is from the eyes. Cranial nerve III (the oculomotor nerve) innervates the muscles of the ciliary body. Further discussion of the mechanics of vision follows this section.

For optimal vision the transparent anterior structures enable light rays to enter the eye; and the iris and its muscles function to assure that the pupil admits appropriate light; and the ciliary body causes the lens to refract light rays which focuses them on the retina.

Interior Structures of the Eye

Behind the lens are the vitreous body, retina, choroid, and sclera. The vitreous is a transparent, semigelatinous substance that provides inner support. It also affects refraction of light similar to the aqueous humor.

After passing through the vitreous, light finally reaches the neurosensitive retina, where visual images are projected. The retina is the only place in the body where blood vessels and a nerve (cranial nerve II—the optic nerve) are visible. The retina has characteristic features called landmarks identifying the normal placement of its structures. These structures, visible during ophthalmoscopic examination, are the arteries, veins, optic disc, and macula (Figure 7-26). The retinal arteries and veins course peripherally after emerging from the optic disc. The optic disc is the nerve head of the optic nerve. The macula contains the highest concentration of cones; therefore, it is the area of central vision and most acute color vision. The rods and cones are the neurosensitive cells of the retina. They synapse with other cells within the retina, which in turn synapse with cells whose axons converge toward the optic disc to form the optic nerve. Light rays stimulate image formation on the retina, which results in transmission of electrical impulses via the optic nerve to the visual center in the cerebral cortex.

Immediately posterior to the retina are the vascular choroid and the sclera. The choroid provides the eye with its blood supply, while the sclera has a protective function.

Mechanics of Vision

Refraction and Accommodation

Refraction is the property of bending light rays. Accommodation refers to the ability of the lens to change shape in order to focus light rays on the retina. The cornea refracts light rays slightly because of its convexity. The lens of the eye changes shape by the action of the muscles of the ciliary body in order to bend light rays to focus them on the retina. Since not all objects in the field of vision are equidistant from the globes, refraction enables convergence of light rays on the retina. Without refraction, convergence of light rays would occur in a variety of locations anterior and posterior to the retina and fuzzy vision would result. The refractive power of the lens is many more times powerful than necessary. Its refraction of light rays is decreased by the aqueous humor and vitreous body.

Although the lens of the eye is convex and varies in its degree of convexity only, there are basically two types of refractive lenses. These are convex and concave lenses. A convex lens increases convergence of light rays, while a concave lens diverges light rays (Figure 7-4).

When the two sets of muscles of the ciliary body contract, the lens thickens or assumes a move convex spherical shape. This increased anteroposterior diameter causes increased bending of light rays and enables focus on near objects. When focusing on distant objects, the relaxation of the muscles of the ciliary body causes the lens to assume a more flattened or less convex shape and decreases refraction. Thus, the lens accommodates by increasing its convexity when

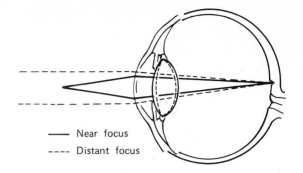

— Near focus
---- Distant focus

Figure 7-4. *Refraction of the light rays by the lens: (a) focus on a near object results in more convexity and more refraction; (b) focus on a distant object, in less convexity and less refraction.*

focusing on near objects and by decreasing its convexity when focusing on distant objects.

Fusion

Fusion refers to the property of combining the two images formed during binocular vision. Since the eyes are approximately 5 centimeters (2 inches) apart, images from near objects form on different locations on the retinae. The more distant an object is from the eyes, the more closely images are formed on corresponding locations of the retinae. The visual center of the cerebral cortex fuses and interprets the images from the two retinae; this phenomenon results in depth perception.

The Visual Pathway

The visual pathways of each eye contain six essential components: the visual field, retina, optic nerve, optic chiasm, optic tract, and visual center. (Figure 7-5). The visual field refers to the area in view. It is divided into two sections: the nasal (medial) and temporal (lateral) aspects. The retina receives light rays and converts light energy into the chemical energy necessary for image formation. This chemical energy is converted into electrical energy for transmission along the optic nerve. The optic nerve conducts impulses to the optic chiasm, an X-shaped area in the brain where some of the optic nerve fibers cross. Fibers that originate in the nasal half of each retina cross; those from the temporal halves do not cross. Beyond the chiasm the optic pathway is called the optic tract. Impulses continue along the optic tract to the cerebral cortex. The occipital region of the cerebral cortex is the area where vision is interpreted.

In summary, the eyes operate similarly to a camera. Reflected rays of light from an object in the field of vision first pass through the pupil, which is adjusted

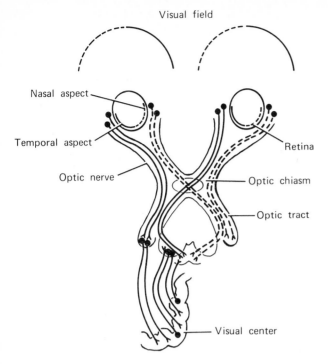

Figure 7-5. *Visual pathway.*

asm prior to continuing along the optic tracts. Nerve fibers from the temporal aspect of the retina (nasal field of vision) continue to travel along the lateral sides of the optic nerve. Therefore, the optic tracts beyond the chiasm contain fibers from one-half of the field of vision. In other words, the right optic tract contains only fibers from the right half of each retina, which are actually stimulated by objects in the left half of each field of vision. Consequently the shape and form of the visual field of each eye provides information regarding proper functioning of six separate areas in the visual pathway.

Extraocular Muscles

Six pairs of muscles work together to cause the full range of ocular movement. These are the lateral rectus, medial rectus, superior rectus, inferior rectus, inferior oblique, and superior oblique muscles. The four rectus muscles move the eyes in the direction implied by their names. However, due to the insertion of the oblique muscles in a pulley fashion, they cause movement in the direction opposite their names (Figure 7-6).

The eyes move in the same direction because each muscle of one eye acts synergistically with a corresponding muscle of the other eye. For instance, the right lateral rectus and left medial rectus act together in turning the eyes to the right along the horizontal plane.

Three of the cranial nerves innervate the six pairs of extraocular muscles: cranial nerve III (the oculomotor nerve) innervates the medial, superior, and inferior rectus and inferior oblique muscles; cranial nerve IV (the trochlear nerve), the superior oblique muscle; and cranial nerve VI (the abducens nerve), the lateral rectus muscle.

by the autonomic nervous system for varying light conditions and distances. Then light rays are refracted by the lens and projected as a reversed and inverted image on the retina, the analogue of photographic film. Therefore, an object in the lower temporal field of vision forms an inverted image on the upper nasal quadrant of the retina.

While traveling along the optic nerve, fibers from the nasal aspect of the retina (temporal aspect of the field of vision) "decussate" or cross at the optic chi-

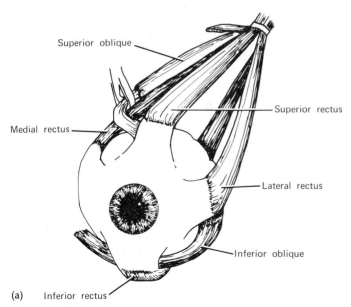

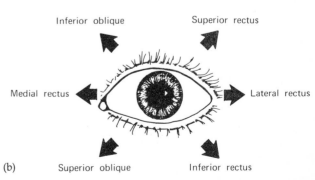

Figure 7-6. *Extraocular muscles: (a) insertions on the eyeball; (b) direction of action in the left eye.*

The eyes move in the same direction simultaneously when observing distant objects (conjugate movements) and inward symmetrically when viewing near objects (convergence). Both of these types of movements result from the proper functioning of the extraocular muscles. Conjugate movements maintain the vertical axes of the eyeballs in a parallel relationship, which prevents diplopia (double vision). On the other hand convergence is necessary for the eyes to focus simultaneously on near objects.

Assessment Modalities

Preparation

Routine assessment of the eyes includes the techniques of inspection, palpation, and sometimes auscultation. In addition, there are various other specialized techniques: measurement of visual acuity, visual field testing, examination of extraocular movements, pupillary response checks, ophthalmoscopy, and tonometry.

The client sits for most of the assessment, unless bedridden or uncooperative, but usually stands for testing visual acuity of distant objects. Acuity testing is frequently performed with the collection of general data such as height and weight measurements.

The equipment necessary includes a light source (penlight), ophthalmoscope, two opaque cards, cotton-tipped applicator, visual testing charts, wisp of cotton, and tonometer (Figure 7-7). The area for examination should provide variable light conditions since a well-lit area enhances inspection of the external structures, and a darkened area is necessary for ophthalmoscopy.

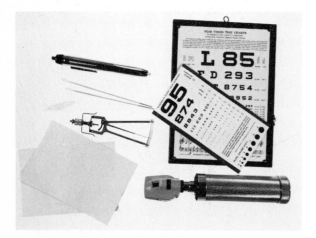

Figure 7-7. Equipment necessary for assessment of the eyes.

Visual Acuity

Visual acuity is a measurement of a person's ability to see clearly. It reflects the transparency of the cornea, anterior chamber, lens, and vitreous body; the functioning of the macula or central vision area; and the integrity of the visual pathway.

Distant vision is most frequently tested by means of one of several Snellen eye charts and should be performed prior to instillation of drops for pupillary dilation. The charts enable standardization of measurement; they consist of 11 lines of characters arranged with the largest at the top in the middle column. Scores range from 20/200 to 20/10 and are found in the left column. Distances of 200 feet (61 meters) to 10 feet (3.05 meters) are placed in the right column beside the line designations (1-11) (Figure 7-8).

The client stands 20 feet (6 meters) from the chart; each eye is tested while the other eye is covered with a card (Figure 7-9). If the scores differ between the eyes, both eyes are tested together. If corrective lenses are used for distant vision, the client is tested with and without them to verify that they are effective in correcting the particular refractive error.

A visual acuity score reflects the smallest line of print read correctly by the client. The score is expressed in fraction form; the numerator represents the distance from the chart (20 feet), and the denominator designates the distance a person with normal

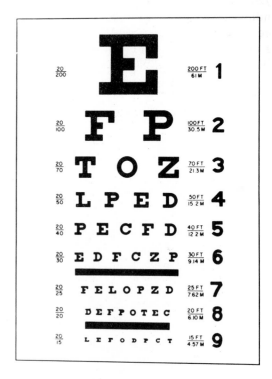

Figure 7-8. Snellen eye chart.

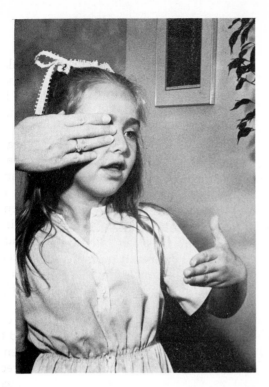

Figure 7-9. The school nurse tests visual acuity with the Snellen eye chart. The 5-year-old indicates the direction of the E with her hand.

right eye alone can see at 20 feet what a person with normal vision (20/20) sees at 40 feet; the left eye alone can see at 20 feet what a person with normal vision sees at 100 feet; together both eyes can see at 20 feet what a person with normal vision can see at 70 feet.

If the client is unable to read the largest letters or line one of the Snellen eye chart, the examiner holds up several fingers three feet away and asks the client to tell how many fingers are seen. This represents a test of grosser visual acuity deficit. If the client is unable to count the fingers correctly, the examiner attempts to ascertain whether the client can see any hand movements and screens for even more pronounced visual difficulties. If the client fails to detect movement, the examiner shines a flashlight beam into the client's eyes and asks from which direction the light originated. This maneuver differentiates near blindness from functional blindness, the inability to perceive light.

If standard Snellen eye charts are not available, a rough estimate of visual acuity can be made by asking the client to read various sizes of newspaper print. This is a test of near vision only. People over 40 years of age and those who report blurred near vision, for example, while reading, should have near vision tested also. The smallest size of the letters differentiated from a given distance is recorded. For example, O.S. 1.5 millimeters characters at 5.0 centimeters, O.D. 1.5 millimeters characters at 5.0 centimeters. A variety of Snellen eye charts can be used with illiterate people as well as with children and others unfamiliar with the names of the letters of the alphabet (Figure 7-10).

vision can see clearly what the client sees clearly at 20 feet from the chart. A person with normal vision (20/20) clearly sees the figures on line nine when standing 20 feet from the chart. If the client misses more than 2 figures on line nine, the ability to read line eight is tested. The results "O.D. 20/40, O.S. 20/100, O.U. 20/70" are interpreted as follows: The

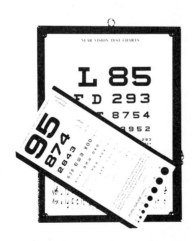

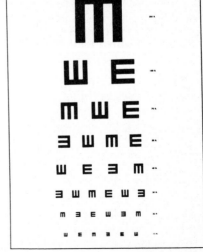

Figure 7-10. Other Snellen eye charts.

Screening for the most common variety of color vision abnormality, red-green blindness, can be performed with a Snellen eye chart by asking the client to read the line of characters above the red line (line nine) or below the green line (line six). For more precise testing, a book of Isihara plates is necessary. These consist of patterns of colored circles arranged to make certain numbers apparent to individuals with normal color vision and other numerical configurations apparent to persons with various forms of color blindness (Figure 7-11).

Inspection

General Characteristics and the Corneal Reflex. Inspection begins with a general look at the eyes as they relate to each other and their position on the face. The eyes are symmetrical; the space between them varies but is approximately 5 centimeters (2 inches). There is normally no deviation, that is, medial or lateral turning of the eyes with respect to each other (Table 7-1).

One way to ascertain if a deviation exists is to elicit the corneal light reflex (Hirschberg test). In this tech-

nique a penlight is shown on both corneas while the client stares straight ahead. The reflection is in the same area on both corneas if the eyes are parallel (Figure 7-12). This test provides an initial screening for cranial nerves III, IV, and VI (the oculomotor, trochlear, and abducens nerves) and the extraocular muscles that they innervate. Further discussion of testing for deviation follows in the life cycle variations section of this chapter (cover tests).

Accessory Structures. The supraorbital ridges are smoothly arched and covered with the eyebrows, moderate to dense arrangements of hair. The color and amount of hair are consistent with age and genetic heritage. The eyelashes or cilia are evenly distributed and curve outwardly from the skin surface of the lid margins in a double row configuration. The hairs of the brows and lashes are shiny, unbroken, and flexible.

The eyelids are normally the same color as the rest of the skin, smooth in contour and freely movable and blink about 6 to 12 times per minute. The upper eyelid extends beyond the superior limbus to approximately

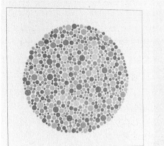 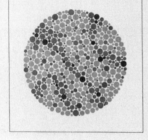

Figure 7-11. Isihara plates.

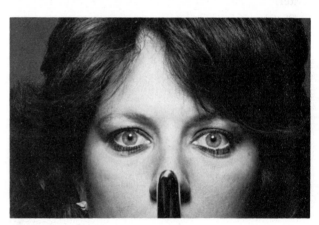

Figure 7-12. Corneal light reflex test.

Table 7-1.   Selected Abnormalities of General Appearance of the Eyes

Finding	Description	Condition
Hypotelorism	Abnormally closely set eyes	May be variation of normal or it may indicate trigonocephaly (triangle-shaped head or absence of nasal bridge).
Hypertelorism	Abnormally widely spaced eyes	May be variation of normal but is frequently associated with retardation.
Microphthalmia	Abnormally small eyes	May be variation of normal or may be associated with toxoplasmosis or retrolental fibroplasia.
Macrophthalmia	Abnormally large eyes	May be variation of normal or indicate genetic disorder.
Enopthalmos	Abnormally recessed eyes	When bilateral, may be variation of normal. When unilateral, may indicate blow out fracture of orbit.
Exophthalmos	Abnormally protruding eyes	Graves' disease.
Esotropia	Medial deviation	Weakness of one or several of the extraocular muscles.
Exotropia	Lateral deviation	Weakness of one or several of the extraocular muscles.

2 to 3 millimeters over the iris. The lower lid extends about 2 millimeters below the inferior limbus. The space between the lids is known as the palpebral fissure.

It is important to note any widening of the palpebral fissure which is known as lid spasm. Lid spasm is evident when the white sclera is exposed superiorly. This may represent a variation of normal; however, it deserves further investigation if it is a recent or unilateral finding.

Two other normal variations of lid configurations are epicanthal folds and mongolian folds. These are discussed in the life cycle variations section. Inspection of the palpebral conjunctiva is usually combined with inspection of the bulbar conjunctiva.

Although the puncta are the only visible features of the lacrimal apparatus, inspection of the skin overlying the lacrimal glands provides insight into the condition of this system. The skin overlying the glands has the same color as the remainder of the body and is smooth in contour, that is, without bulging or swelling (Table 7-2).

Anterior Structures of the Eye. The anterior structures are inspected for color and clarity. Normally there is no evidence of irritation or opacities. The bulbar conjunctiva is moist and transparent. The eyelids are gently retracted with the thumb and forefinger in order to maximize visualization of the bulbar conjunctiva (Figure 7-13). The palpebral conjunctiva is moist and pink. To inspect the inferior palpebral conjunctiva, the lower lid is everted by gently placing the thumb on the loose skin overlying the infraorbital margin and pushing downward (Figure 7-14).

Inspection of the superior bulbar and superior palpebral conjunctivae necessitates eversion of the upper lid. Lid eversion also uncovers any lacrimal gland enlargement. After explaining the procedure and assuring the client that the sensation of examination will be unusual, although not painful, the examiner requests that the client keep the eyes open while looking downward. The examiner holds some medial eyelashes with the thumb and forefinger and gently pulls downward and outward. Lid eversion is accomplished when the examiner presses against the lid above the upper edges of the tarsal plate with a cotton-tipped applicator and flips the lid upward (Figure 7-15). The examiner maintains lid eversion with the thumb. The lid easily returns to normal when the examiner releases it and the client glances upward.

The sclera underlies the bulbar conjunctiva and is white or pigmented. Pigment in the sclera is characteristic in members of darker-skinned racial groups. Usually a few superficial scleral blood vessels are visible branching from the periphery toward the limbus. The deeper vessels are not normally visible; when apparent, they radiate near the limbus since they originate in the iris.

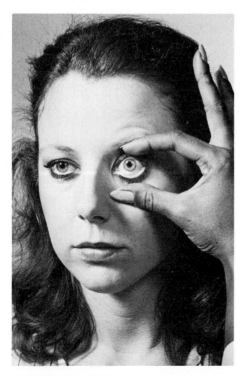

Figure 7-13. *Retraction of the eyelids.*

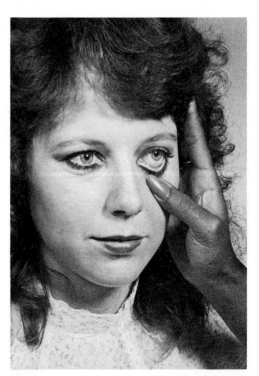

Figure 7-14. *Inspection of the inferior palpebral conjunctiva.*

Table 7-2.   Selected Abnormalities of the Accessory Structures

Finding	Condition	Description
"Black eye"	Palpebral hematoma	Ecchymotic, tender area secondary to lid trauma.
Palpebral redness	Palpebral inflammation or hyperemia	Localized tender inflammation suggestive of involvement of other areas near eye: lacrimal sac—redness of lower lid medially; frontal sinus-nasal part of upper lid.
Palpebral redness	Marginal blepharitis	Generalized redness of the lid margins, which also may occur with flaking or greasy material clinging to the cilia in seborrhea of the lids.
Palpebral swelling	Palpebral edema	May accompany local inflammatory process, e.g., hordeolum (sty) or exist concommitantly with acute diseases, e.g., nephritis, thyrotoxic exophthalmos.
Palpebral pustule	External hordeolum (sty)	Tender, red edematous area produced by inflammation of a sebaceous gland (glands of Zeis or Moll).
Palpebral mass	Internal hordeolum (sty)	Tender swelling caused by inflammation of a sebaceous gland (Meibomian gland) in palpabral conjunctiva, often accompanied by conjunctival hyperemia (bulbar).
Palpebral mass	Chalazion (Meibomian cyst)	Swelling resulting from granuloma of a sebaceous gland in palpebral conjunctiva (Meibomian gland), often accompanied by conjunctival redness (bulbar).
Sclera visible between upper lid and superior limbus	Lid spasm (Dalrymple's sign)	Widening of the palpebral fissure may result from proptosis or lid retraction. Occurs in thyrotoxicosis.
Sclera visible between upper lid and superior limbus	Lid lag (Von Graefe's sign)	Type of lid spasm not apparent by widened palpebral fissure. During extraocular muscle testing as the penlight is moved downward from the primary position, the eyelid lowers more slowly than the eye itself. Occurs in hyperthyroidism.
Failure of lids to close	Lid retraction	The lids remain open, exposing the corneal surface to drying and causing the spillage of tears onto the cheeks. May be partial or complete.
Failure of the upper lid to retract	Ptosis	Eyelid droops due to weakness of orbicularis oculi, impairment of cranial nerve III (oculomotor nerve), or impairment of sympathetic nerves that supply the upper lid.
Out-turning of the lid	Ectropion	Results in exposure of conjunctival membrane.
Inward turning of the lid	Entropion	May result in conjunctivitis secondary to mechanical irritation by the cilia rubbing across the bulbar conjunctiva.
Constant lacrimation and mucoid discharge	Obstructed nasolacrimal duct	Common among newborns, may be accompanied by a purulent discharge and redness, tenderness, edema, and warmth in the nasolacrimal duct region. Gentle pressure against the lacrimal sac toward the orbit (away from the nose) causes expression of material from the punctum.

Table 7-2.   Selected Abnormalities of the Accessory Structures (*continued*)

Finding	Condition	Description
Enlargement and redness of lacrimal gland apparent during lid eversion	Inflammation of lacrimal gland	Accompanied by tenderness upon palpation. May also produce redness of adjacent eyelid area.
Redness or swelling below inner canthus	Inflammation of lacrimal duct	Tender upon palpation and may be accompanied by a purulent discharge from the punctum.

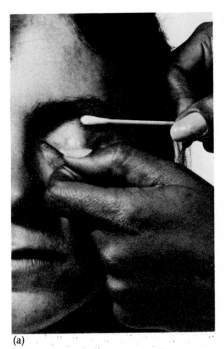 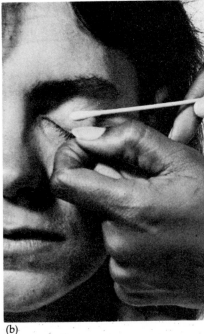 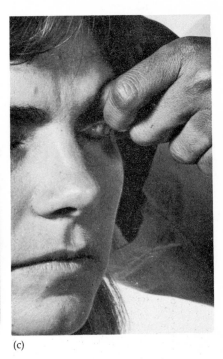

(a)   (b)   (c)

Figure 7-15. *Eversion of the eyelid: (a) the examiner holds some medial eyelashes with the thumb and forefinger and gently pulls downward; (b) presses against the lid with an applicator; and (c) flips the lid upward.*

The cornea is normally transparent, moist, and smooth. A penlight shown on the cornea obliquely from several directions in a darkened room illuminates its normal clarity.

The iris is pigmented a variety of shades dependent on genetic factors. It commonly contains specks of darker-pigmented material called Brushfield spots. A penlight shown on the cornea from the lateral aspect projects a uniform cone of light medially. This technique also provides a rough gauge of the depth of the anterior chamber (Figure 7-16, Table 7-3).

Pupillary Responses. The pupils are round and equal; they adjust to light by constricting in the pres-

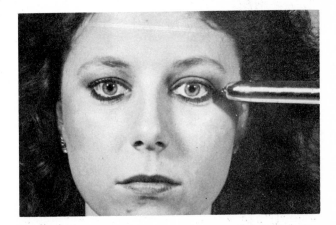

Figure 7-16. *Inspection of the cornea.*

Table 7-3. Selected Abnormalities of the Conjunctiva, Sclera and Cornea

Finding	Condition	Description
"Pink eye"	Global hyperemia (conjunctivitis)	Injected conjunctiva; superficial vessels are readily visible; often accompanied by tearing secondary to bacterial or viral infection, allergy, trauma, chemicals, fungi, invasion by parasites or spirochetes, and a few systemic diseases.
Yellowish, triangularly shaped thickening of the bulbar conjunctiva located on both sides of the cornea (usually larger on the nasal side)	Pinguecula	Increase in elastic fibers of conjunctiva; associated with the trauma of prolonged exposure to airborne contaminants.
Extension of the pinguecula beyond the limbus	Pterygium	Encroachment of the pinguecula on the iris, which interferes with vision.
Ciliary flush	Ciliary injection	Diffuse flush around iris from congestion of the branches of the anterior ciliary artery indicating a disorder of the cornea or inner eye (does not blanch with lid pressure), e.g., glaucoma.
Bleeding under the conjunctiva	Subconjunctival hemorrhage	Red patch from bleeding between the conjunctiva and sclera (does not blanch with lid pressure).
Yellow sclera	Scleral icterus	Homogeneous yellow color of sclerae due to uniform distribution of bilirubin throughout. Occurs in liver disease.
Yellow sclera	Fat deposits	Yellow color more intense at periphery; perilimbal area is white; more apparent among the elderly due to their thinner conjunctival membranes and among people with anemia.
Corneal scratch	Corneal abrasion	Staining of the cornea after instillation of fluorescein indicates corneal abrasion usually due to trauma; stain adheres to areas where surface integrity is disrupted.
Spots on cornea	Corneal opacities	Spots move upward when person elevates eyes. Usually result from trauma or infection.

ence of bright light (myosis) and dilating in dim light (mydriasis). Their reactions to light are normally equal. The pupillary response tests indicate the functioning of cranial nerve III (the oculomotor nerve). The pupils respond to light stimulation in several ways: directly, consensually, and in the accommodation reflex.

In testing the pupils, the room is darkened while a penlight is shown on each pupil. The client is asked to focus straight ahead while the light is directed onto one pupil from the lateral direction. In the direct reaction, pupillary constriction occurs in the eye in which the light is shown. In the consensual reaction, light shown on one pupil also results in constriction of the opposite pupil (Figure 7-17).

Pupillary constriction in the accommodation reaction is one facet of a three-part mechanism. In accommodation, the pupils constrict, the eyes converge, and the lenses thicken as the client glances from a distant object to a near one. In conducting this test, the examiner directs the client to gaze at a penlight held 50 centimeters (20 inches) from the nose. The examiner directs the client to maintain focus on the penlight as it is brought to within 10 centimeters (4 inches) of the nose. The eyes are observed for convergence and pupillary constriction as the penlight nears the nose (Figure 7-18). The examiner records normal findings as follows: PERRLA (pupils equal, round, and react to light and accommodation) (Table 7-4).

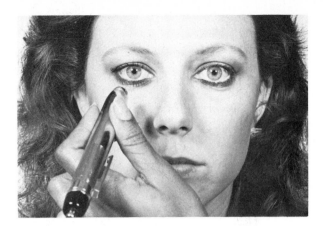

Figure 7-17. *The examiner directs the light into one eye. The pupil of that eye constricts in the direct pupillary reaction, while the pupil of the other eye constricts simultaneously in the consensual reaction.*

Visual Fields. The visual fields are the areas in the range of vision of both eyes. The visual field of each eye is tested separately, and each visual field is divided into a temporal and a nasal portion. Testing provides information regarding the range of peripheral vision. Routine screening is accomplished by the confrontation method, provided the examiner has no visual field defects (scotomata). The nature of visual field cuts, if any, can accurately locate a lesion at various points along the visual pathway.

Confrontation involves comparison of the client's visual fields with those of the examiner. The examiner and client sit facing each other approximately 1 meter (3 feet) apart. To test the temporal field of the left eye, the client occludes the right eye with a card, the examiner covers his or her own left eye with the left hand,

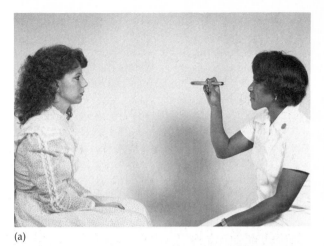

(a)

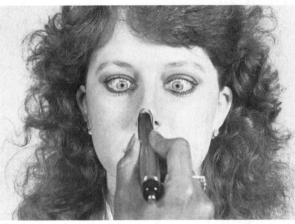

(b)

Figure 7-18. *(a) The examiner directs the client to gaze at the penlight, which is held one meter from the eyes; (b) during the accommodation reaction, the pupils constrict and the eyes converge as the penlight is brought closer to the client.*

Table 7-4. Selected Pupillary Abnormalities

Finding	Condition	Description
Anisocoria (unequal pupils)	Horner's syndrome	Affected pupil is small and regular; associated with ptosis of eyelid and often with loss of sweating on the forehead of the involved side; secondary to interruption of sympathetic innervation, most frequently in the neck.
	Adie's pupil	Large, regular pupil (usually unilateral) which reacts very slowly to light and accommodation; may be accompanied by diminished deep tendon reflexes; benign.
	Argyll-Robertson pupils	Small, irregular, bilateral pupils, which react to accommodation but not to light; often related to tabes dorsalis (central nervous system syphilis).
	Coloboma (post-iridectomy pupils)	Cleft in iris resulting from surgical incision (may be congenital).

and each fixates on the other's open eye. The examiner holds a penlight in the right hand and maintains it at an equal distance between them. The examiner asks the client to identify when the penlight comes into view as it is moved toward the nose from the extreme superior, inferior, and temporal positions. Normally the client first sees the object with each maneuver at the same time as the examiner. To test the nasal field of the left eye, the examiner uses the right hand to cover his or her own left eye and moves the penlight held by the left hand from the extreme nasal, superior, and inferior directions, The other eye is tested similarly (Figure 7-19, Table 7-5).

Extraocular Movements. The eyes normally have the ability to move conjugately through the six cardinal positions of gaze. These directions of gaze are the following: superior medial, superior lateral, lateral, inferior lateral, inferior medial, and medial. The six extraocular muscles of one eye act with their respective pair-mates of the other eye to affect this movement and maintain the axes of the eyes in a parallel relationship (Figure 7-6).

Extraocular muscle testing is performed with the examiner facing the client. The client is directed to maintain the head in a fixed position while gazing at the examiner's penlight as it is moved through the six cardinal positions. Normally the eyes maintain their parallel relationship throughout the entire testing sequence (Figure 7-20).

Abnormal movements such as lid lag and nystagmus are usually recognized during extraocular muscle testing. Nystagmus is a fine oscillatory movement of the eyes and is a normal variation in the extreme lateral gaze only (Table 7-6).

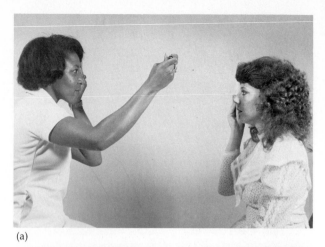
(a)

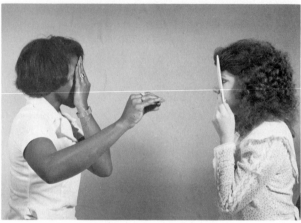
(b)

Figure 7-19. *Testing visual fields by confrontation: (a) temporal field of the left eye; (b) nasal field of the right eye.*

The eyes of some individuals are able to maintain a parallel relationship only when the fusion mechanism is intact. When fusion is disrupted, for example, when one eye is covered, the other eye may deviate.

Table 7-5. Selected Visual Field Abnormalities

Finding	Condition	Explanation
No vision in the right eye	Blindness of the right eye	Right optic nerve lesion or lesion of right eye results in mononuclear blindness.
Visual field loss involving temporal half of each visual field	Bitemporal hemianopsia	Lesion at the optic chiasm involving the fibers that decussate (fibers from nasal half of each retina).
Visual field loss involving the right half of each visual field	Right homonymous hemianopsia	Lesion of the left optic tract involves fibers originating from the same side of both eyes.
Visual field loss involving a portion of the right half of each visual field	Homonymous right upper quadrant defect	Partial lesion of the left optic radiation may interrupt several but not all of the nerve fibers resulting in a corresponding defect.
Visual field loss of the right half of each visual field	Right homonymous hemianopsia	Total involvement of the left optic radiation results in a visual defect like that of a lesion located in the left optic tract.

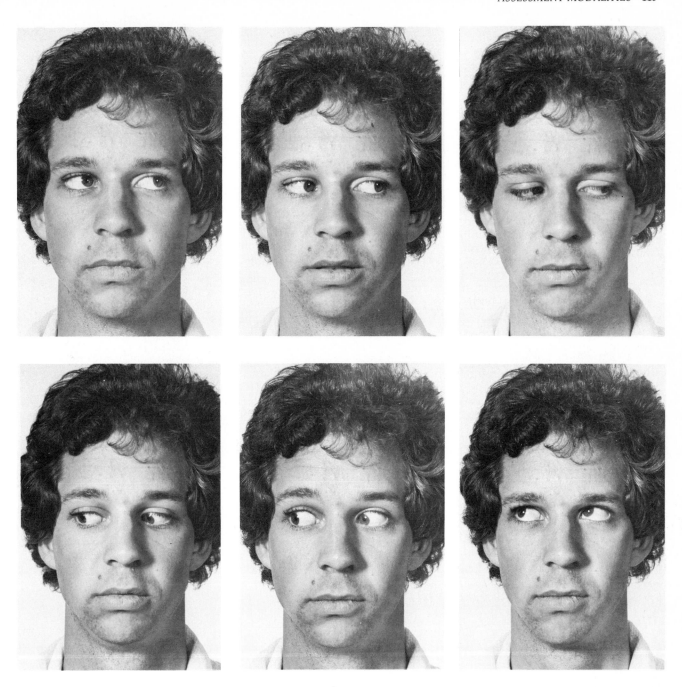

Figure 7-20. Extraocular muscle testing.

This is true in certain types of strabismus, a general term for deviation between the ocular axes. Tests that disrupt the fusion mechanism are known as cover tests and are presented in the life cycle variations section of this chapter.

Palpation

Palpation is used as a rough gauge of ocular tension. Normal ocular tension is a reflection of adequate hy-dration and normal intraocular fluid dynamics. In palpating, the index fingers are placed on the globes with the eyelids closed and the client looking downward. Gentle but firm pressure is then exerted in a back-and-forth horizontal direction (Figure 7-21). Normally the eyeballs have a firm but springy feeling.

It is difficult to appreciate the difference between the hard eyeballs that accompany increased intra-ocular pressure and normal tension until many exam-inations have been performed. Therefore, a more ac-

Table 7-6. Selected Abnormal Extraocular Movements: Nystagmus

Finding	Condition	Description
Oscillatory motion of the eyes End position: Oscillations that occur with fixation in extreme positions of gaze in which the rapid component is necessarily in the direction of fixation. Primary position: Fixation occurs either in the primary position of gaze (eyes in midline) or at a location in the direction of the slow component.	Although horizontal nystagmus occurs among normal persons in extreme lateral gaze positions, nystagmus may suggest one of the following: Multiple sclerosis, encephalitis, brain tumors, eye muscle paresis or paralysis, labyrinthine disorders	Series of repetitive jerky eye movements composed of two components: (1) drifting of eyes away from fixation followed by (2) a rapid return to the original position. Named for direction of rapid component (left) or (right) and pattern of movement (horizontal, vertical, rotatory, or mixed); involvement may be monocular (dissociated) or binocular (associated); described further as fine (amplitude of less than 1 millimeter) or coarse (greater than 3 millimeters) and slow (less than 40 jerks/minute) or fast (greater than 100 jerks/minute).

curate estimate of intraolcular pressure results from tonometry. The two most common conditions recognizable by palpation are glaucoma and fluid volume deficit (Table 7-7).

Tonometry

Intraocular pressure is most accurately measured by tonometry. Normal values range between 12 and 22 millimeters of mercury. For tonometry the client is supine and is asked to keep the eyelids open. An anesthetizing solution is instilled into one eye as the examiner holds the lids apart. The tonometer foot is applied to the cornea, and a reading is taken. The procedure is repeated for the other eye (Figure 7-22).

Auscultation

Auscultation is usually not part of the routine eye assessment. However, in persons in whom occlusive vascular disease is suspected, it is indicated. This includes persons with a family history of cerebrovascular accidents or transient ischemic attacks and patients with a medical history of cerebrovascular accident or unexplained neurologic symptoms. To auscultate, the examiner places the bell of the stethoscope over the ocular orbit, with the eyelid closed, and listens for bruits. A bruit is an abnormal sound produced by the coursing of blood through narrowed blood vessels (Figure 7-23).

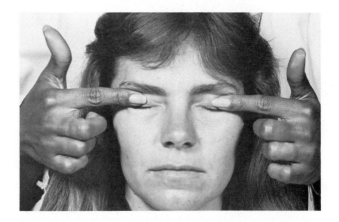

Figure 7-21. Palpation of the eyes.

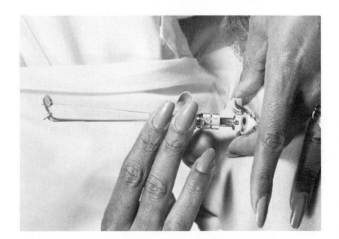

Figure 7-22. Tonometry.

Table 7-7. Selected Conditions Causing Changes in Intraocular Tension

Finding	Condition	Description
Hard eyeballs	Glaucoma—open angle	Chronic painless increase in intraocular pressure due to gradual decrease in drainage of aqueous humor. History of gradual concentric loss of visual fields (tunnel vision) and of seeing colored haloes around lights.
Red eye, pupils fixed in mid-position (5 millimeters), steamy cornea, acute eye pain	Glaucoma—angle closure	Acute increase in intraocular pressure, may be as high as 60-90 ml./Hg. Often accompanied by severe nausea and vomiting. Extreme pressure against optic disc causes reduced vision. May result in blindness if not treated promptly. Necessitates prompt referral to ophthalmologist. If ophthalmoscopy is possible through the steamy cornea, pulsation of the retinal artery is apparent.
Soft, sunken eyeballs	Fluid volume deficit	After 10% loss of body weight due to extracellular fluid depletion, eye pressure changes accompany decreased skin turgor. Among young children the fontanelle is sunken and the sutures are apparent.

Ophthalmoscopy

Ophthalmoscopy involves the examination of the eyes with the use of the ophthalmoscope, an instrument that magnifies, illuminates, and provides a variety of refractive lenses.

While most of the assessment of the anterior structures of the eye is performed during inspection, ophthalmoscopic examination enables more refined observation of the cornea and anterior chamber. Use of the ophthalmoscope is necessary for inspection of the lens, vitreous, and retina. These interior structures are collectively known as the ocular fundus.

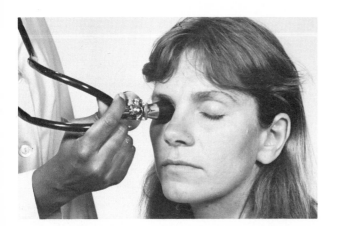

Figure 7-23. *Asucultation over the ocular orbit.*

There are two types of ophthalmoscopes: portable and wall-mounted models. For practice, it is easier to use a portable model, as the cord attached to the wall-mounted instruments poses another obstacle to developing a smooth, coordinated approach. The ophthalmoscope consists of two parts: the head and the body. The body contains the batteries in portable models and serves as a handle in all models. The head projects the light beam and contains a variety of lenses located on two lens wheels. One lens wheel contains a variety of apertures while the other contains lenses of various degrees of refractive power (Figure 7-24).

Among the types of light apertures are two sizes of circular white beams. The light aperture wheel is located on the front portion of the head of the ophthalmoscope; the appropriate setting is selected prior to the examination.

The lens wheel is located on the lateral portions of the ophthalmoscopic head and is rotated by the examiner's right index finger during examination of the right eye and by the left index finger during examination of the left eye. The lens wheel of most models contains 22 lenses. Usually 11 lenses are convex, 10 are concave, and 1 has no correction. This variety of lenses enables examiners with various degrees of visual acuity to examine clients with various degrees of visual acuity. It also enables the examiner to focus on structures at different depths within the eye, that is, anterior, interior, and posterior features.

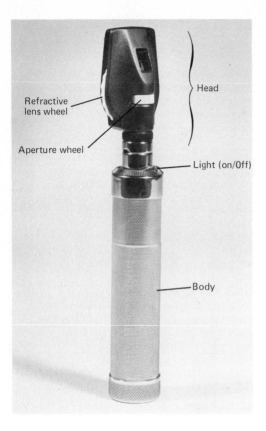

Figure 7-24. *Components of the ophthalmoscope.*

The refractive power of a lens is measured in terms of diopters. The convex lenses are designated by black numerals ranging from +1 through +20 diopters, the zero lens has no correction or refraction, and the concave lenses have red numerals ranging from −1 through −20 diopters. The higher the numeral of the black numbered lenses, the stronger the lens and the more light rays converge. This causes focus closer to the ophthalmoscope. The lower the numeral of the red numbered lenses, the weaker the lens and the more light rays diverge. This results in focus farther from the ophthalmoscope. Thus, the ophthalmoscope can correct various degrees of refractive error in examiner and client. The exceptions are persons with severe refractive errors and those with astigmatism. Astigmatism is the condition in which the lens is not homogeneous and contains various refractive indices (Table 7-8).

For the ophthalmoscopic examination, the room is darkened, and the client is directed to stare straight ahead at a point, for example, the light switch or a mark on the wall. This causes pupillary dilation and keeps the eyes fixed. In most cases a mydriatic is not necessary. However, if the pupils fail to dilate adequately, one of the following agents can be instilled:

10 percent Phenylephrine HCL, 0.5 percent Mydriacil, or 1 percent Cyclogel. The examiner follows agency protocol in using eye drops. Prior to instilling eye drops, the examiner must be certain that the client does not have increased intraocular pressure. Some of the signs and symptoms of increased intraocular pressure are a scarred iris (previous surgery for glaucoma), palpation of hard eyeballs, previous diagnosis or family history of glaucoma, and a history of acute attacks of eye pain or seeing colored haloes around lights.

The client is assured that the examination is not uncomfortable, and that cooperation is essential for a thorough evaluation. The client may blink occasionally. However, if blinking occurs so frequently that the examiner is unable to visualize the fundus, the upper lid is grasped with the thumb and held against the upper orbital rim. The ophthalmoscope is held in the right hand close to the right eye for examining the client's right eye and in the right hand close to the left eye for examining the left eye.

The top of the ophthalmoscope is held against the examiner's forehead approximately 30 centimeters (12 inches) from the eye to be examined; light is directed onto the pupil (Figure 7-25). This results in a circular reddish glow, the red reflex. This represents the reflection of light from the vascular retinal surface through the clear vitreous, posterior chamber, lens, anterior chamber, and cornea. The red reflex is kept in focus as the examiner approaches the client approximately 15 degrees lateral to the line of vision. The examiner's index finger is on the lens disc, which is initially set at +15 or +20 for focusing on the anterior structures. The cornea, lens, and anterior chamber are normally clear and have no opacities or clouding.

The vitreous is best inspected with a +10 or +4 lens, and normally this area is clear. When the examination of the anterior and interior structures of the

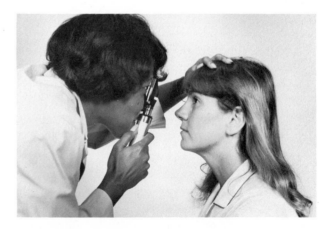

Figure 7-25. *Ophthalmoscopic examination.*

Table 7-8.   Selected Lens Abnormalities

Finding	Condition	Description
Opaque spot	Cataract	With oblique lighting, spot appears grayish against the black pupil; visible through pupil only; causes a black spot type of break in continuity of red reflex.
		Upon opthalmoscopic examination as the client looks upward, the spot moves upward. The spot moves upward also if the location is on the anterior lens. If the spot stays fixed when the client gazes upward, the cataract is located near the lenticular center. Location is in the posterior lens or vitreous if the spot moves downward. Cataracts are common after age 50; if extensive, ophthalmoscopy may be impossible. Client history may reveal better vision at night (pupils are dilated; therefore he is able to see around opacities).
Focus on retinal structures with concave lens of ophthalmoscope (red numbers, −1 through −15)	Myopia (near-sightedness)	Either client's eyeball is too long or the lens is too strong, which causes convergence of light rays at a point anterior to the retina. Client may successfully read newspaper print but do poorly at reading Snellen eye chart.
Focus on retinal structures with convex lens of ophthalmoscope (black numbers, −1 through +20)	Hyperopia (far-sightedness)	Either client's eyeball is too short or lens system is too weak or absent (e.g., after cataract surgery), which results in convergence of light rays at a point behind the retina. Person may test normally with the Snellen eye chart but have difficulty reading newsprint.
Focus on retinal structures at a variety of settings	Astigmatism	Lens system contains various degrees of refraction.

eye is completed, the examiner adjusts the lens disc toward zero (moves the index finger counterclockwise) for examination of the retina.

The examiner rests one hand on the client's forehead and advances toward the client until the head of the ophthalmoscope contacts that hand. The retina is viewed systematically in order to avoid omissions. Most examiners proceed in the following order: optic disc, blood vessels, retinal background, and macula (Figure 7-26). In viewing the retina, the examiner moves the ophthalmoscope and head as a unit and pivots around the client's eye as the fulcrum.

Usually the first structure in view is a blood vessel which can be followed centrally to the optic disc. The examiner rotates the lens disc until the optic disc is clearly in focus. The setting is at zero if examiner and client have normal vision. In a normal retina the rest of the retinal features are in focus at the same setting. When the examiner has a refractive error, compensation is made by turning the lens disc to a refractive lens. A myopic examiner uses one of the concave lenses (red numbers from −1 through −15). The optic disc is normally a reddish-yellow oval or round structure located in the nasal portion of the retina. The disc margin should be sharp or well-delineated, although it may be slightly blurred along the nasal margin. Other variations of normal are scleral crescents and rings. A scleral crescent is a pigment deposit outside the disc temporally; and a scleral ring is a white circle around the disc margin. The disc is also used as a standard of measurement in describing the size and location of other retinal markings.

The physiologic cup is a whitish area central within the disc. The relationship between cup and disc sizes is expressed as the cup/disc ratio and normally equal to 0.2/1.

The retinal blood vessels are evaluated as they emerge from the disc and course peripherally. In comparison with the veins the retinal arteries are smaller (approximately two-thirds to four-fifths their di-

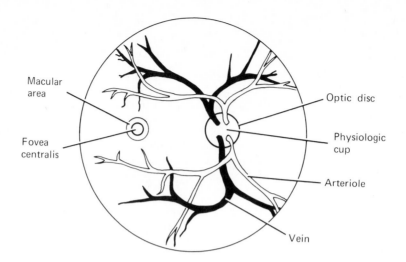

Figure 7-26. Retinal landmarks.

ameter) and lighter red in color; they reflect light in a bright linear fashion as opposed to the veins, which do not refract light or refract light in a patchy manner. As the examiner follows the blood vessels peripherally through all quadrants, their size and contours and the character of the arteriovenous crossings are noted. There is no narrowing or tortuosity of the vessels and no arteriovenous nicking, which is an indentation of a vein or venule at a crossing. Arteriovenous nicking is significant only if it occurs more than one disc diameter outside the disc margin.

The retinal background is observed for its color and the presence of any abnormal markings. Since it is a melanin pigmented tissue that overlies the vascular choroid, retinal color varies with genetic origin and hematologic status. The retina of a person with fair complexion may be pinkish-yellow while that of a dark individual may be almost brown. The pigment is usually evenly distributed but may be patchy. The description of the size and location of abnormal findings can be given using the disc diameter system or the clock method (Figure 7-27, Table 7-9).

Finally the client is asked to look at the light. The macula is identifiable as a more darkly pigmented area two to three disc diameters temporal to the disc and one disc diameter in size. Since light sensitive cones are most numerous in this area, it is the area of maximal visual acuity and central vision. Consequently the client may experience some discomfort during this part of the funduscopic examination; therefore, it is performed last. Within the macula is the fovea centralis, a small depression that is darker than the macula but whose center reflects a speck of bright light. At completion of the ophthalmoscopic examination, a drop of Pilocarpine may be instilled in each eye to constrict the pupils if dilating drops were necessary.

Life Cycle Variations

Childhood

The macula is not fully developed at birth: therefore, newborns are believed to have poor vision. At birth infants have been credited only with light perception,

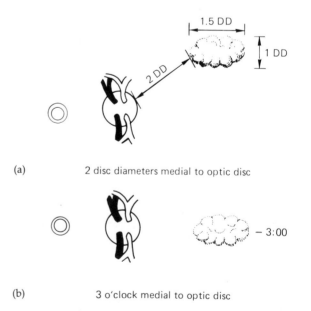

(a)   2 disc diameters medial to optic disc

(b)   3 o'clock medial to optic disc

Figure 7-27. Description of abnormal retinal findings using the disc-diameter and clock methods: (a) lesion is located 2 disc diameters medial to the optic disc; (b) lesion is located at 3 o'clock.

Table 7-9. Selected Retinal Abnormalities

Finding	Condition	Description
Disc margins blurred when rest of fundus is in focus, discs elevated 4 diopters; blood vessels bend as they emerge from disc; punctate hemorrhages and soft exudates present	Papilledema ("choked disc")	Discrepancy is estimated in diopters by subtracting the two settings, e.g., if disc is in focus at +2 and the margin is in focus at −2, +2 −(−2)=4; therefore, the degree of disc elevation is expressed as 4 diopters; occurs with increased intracranial pressure (hemorrhage, brain tumor, hypertension, hydrocephalus, arteriosclerosis); with disc elevation blood vessels can be seen to curve around the disc; hemorrhages and exudates accompany papilledema also.
Fluffy patches and red spots with ill-defined borders	Soft exudates ("cotton-wool patches")	Caused by swelling of terminal nerve fibers of retina; superficial location; occur with papilledema, systemic lupus erythematosis, hypertension.
Small white spots with well-delineated borders	Hard exudates	Caused by deposition of fat or colloid in old hemorrhages; deep location.
Variety of shapes of spots and blotches on retina	Hemorrhages	Appearance determined by source; found in hypertension, subacute bacterial endocarditis, systemic lupus erythematosis, leukemia, sickle cell disease.
Veins stop abruptly on either side of arterioles	A-V nicking (concealment)	Thickened arteriolar walls occlude portions of the veins as they pass under the arterioles; occurs in arteriolar sclerosis
Increased cup/disc ratio	Glaucomatous cupping	Size of cup approaches that of the disc, retinal vessels sink into the disc and under it; occurs with increased eye pressure.
Yellowish-red narrowed column of blood within arteriole	"Copper wire" defect	Narrowed column of blood within thickened arteriolar wall produces yellowish-red color; occurs in moderate arteriolar sclerosis.
Whitish arteriole without visible column of blood	"Silver wire" defect	Arteriolar wall so thick that no blood is visible within it; occurs in advanced arteriolar sclerosis.

although recent studies indicate that they demonstrate a preference for likenesses of the human face as opposed to likenesses of inanimate objects. This finding suggests that the actual visual acuity of newborns is unknown. The assessment of vision in the newborn involves visual reflex testing. Visual reflexes present at birth are the following: direct and consensual pupillary responses to light; a twofold reaction to bright light involving blinking and neck dorsiflexion (optic blink reflex); blinking in response to an object moved quickly toward the eyes; and nystagmus invoked by the rapid movement of vertical black lines across the visual fields.

The vast majority of neonates under 1 week of age demonstrate visual acuity of 20/670. Between 2 and 4 weeks fixation occurs; at 5 to 6 weeks infants demonstrate the ability to track objects; and by 3 months convergence of the eyes occurs, and the baby begins to reach for objects. Further refinement of vision is obvious when eye-hand coordination and the ability to focus develop. Binocularity begins to develop between 4 and 6 months and is firmly established by the end of the first year. By 12 months visual acuity is approximately 20/200. Gradual improvement in vision continues until age six when adult visual acuity is attained.

At birth 75 to 80 percent of newborns are hyperopic due to shorter globes and flatter corneas. This hyperopia may increase until age seven to eight years and then decreases. The lens is more spherical (convex) and exerts a counteractive influence toward the hyperopia.

Since neonates frequently keep their eyelids tightly closed and exhibit the optic blink reflex, the examination is performed in a dimly lit setting. For optimal visualization of the anterior structures and extraocular movements, the examiner holds the baby upright at eye level. The infant's chest is supported with the examiner's thumbs placed under the baby's arms and the hands cupped around the baby's back. The head is supported and fixed by the examiner's index and middle fingers on either side of both ears. The infants eyes turn as a unit with the body during side-to-side rotation. After rotation to one side is complete, the eyes look in the opposite direction after a brief episode of horizontal nystagmus.

The lacrimal gland is poorly developed at birth; therefore, most infants have few or no tears until after three months. Epicanthal folds are found in 20 percent of Caucasian children and disappear spontaneously by age 10 years in 97 percent of cases. These semicircular bands of skin extend vertically from the upper to the lower lid just lateral to the inner canthus. Mongolian folds are horizontal folds of skin and are normal for people of Asiatic origin (Figure 7-28). The presence of prominent inner epicanthal folds accompanied by an outward upper slant of the lids is suggestive of Down's syndrome.

Chemical conjunctivitis frequently occurs after instillation of silver nitrate. This condition is characterized by lid edema and conjunctival inflammation; it sometimes produces a purulent discharge. It is also not uncommon to find small conjunctival and scleral hemorrhages among newborns.

Among newborns the sclera is thin and appears blue since the color of the underlying tissue is more apparent. As the scleral fibers thicken, the eye assumes a whiter appearance. The iris in newborns contains little pigment and accounts for the almost universal blue eyes among Caucasian neonates. By six months, pigment is deposited, and the iris takes on its permanent coloration.

Short periods of nystagmus may be seen in an infant who is not yet focusing. Although searching nystagmus is common immediately after birth, it is sug-

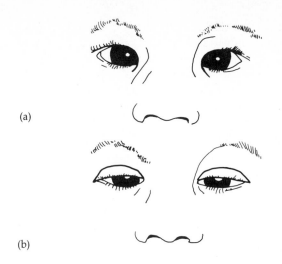

Figure 7-28. *(a) Epicanthal folds; (b) Mongolian folds.*

gestive of blindness if present beyond the first few days. Intermittent convergent horizontal strabismus ("crossed eyes") is a normal phenomenon before three months of age.

When the infant's head is turned through its full range of motion during the first 10 days of life, the eyes remain in their original position. This effect, called the doll's eye test, tests cranial nerve VI (the abducens nerve) and screens for paresis of the lateral rectus muscle in older babies, children, and adults. The setting sun sign or downward deviation of the eyes (hypotropia) may be a finding in normal newborns although it characteristically occurs in hydrocephalus.

Visual fields can be tested by dangling a small toy from various directions, with the head held in the midline. As the toy is brought into the child's field of vision from each direction, the eyes are normally directed toward it when it comes into view.

An ophthalmoscopic examination is done on all infants. This examination is generally performed between two and six months of age. If there are neurologic or ocular abnormalities, the ophthalmoscopic examination is performed earlier. The baby is positioned supine on the examining table, sitting on an adult's lap, or held upright against the adult's shoulder. A mydriatic is essential, such as a 10 percent phenylephrine and 1 percent mydriacyl solution, two drops in each eye every 15 minutes for three times.

Upon initial assessment all newborns are observed for the red reflex. The red reflex is a circular red glow that represents reflection of light by the lens. It is visible when a light is shone on each eye and represents a screening tool for such conditions as cataracts, retrolental fibroplasia, and a persistent posterior lenticular fibrovascular sheath.

In infants ophthalmoscopy is performed in the same manner as for adults although there are some differences in the appearance of the landmarks. These differences include a paler optic disc, poorly developed peripheral vessels, and absent foveal reflex. Small retinal hemorrhages are common; however, extensive bleeding is indicative of severe anoxia or subdural hematoma. Intracranial bleeding also presents a picture of dilated, congested, and tortuous retinal veins. Papilledema is rare under age three since the sutures can separate and compensate for increased intracranial pressure.

Assessment of the eyes among children past infancy is similar to that of adults except for some important aspects. Visual acuity continues to improve. It is approximately 20/40 at three years of age, 20/30 between four and five years, and 20/20 by six or seven. In children under three the Snellen picture chart may be used. Prior to beginning, it is best to ascertain from the parent the child's familiarity with the objects pictured and their names. In children over three the Snellen E chart may be used. The child is asked to indicate verbally or with hand signals the direction the E is pointing.

A crucial aspect of eye assessment in children under six is screening for amblyopia ex-anopsia. This term applies to reduced vision as a result of disuse in an otherwise normal eye. Most commonly it is caused by either strabismus or anisometropia. Strabismus is a general term applied to various degrees and directional components of eye deviation (Table 7-10). Anisometropia refers to a difference of greater than 1.5 diopters in the refractive indices between the eyes. Precise visual acuity measurement is the screening tool for detection of anisometropia.

Both of these conditions prevent binocularity; therefore, two dissimilar images are received by the visual cortex and fusion cannot occur. The cortex then suppresses one of the images, which causes one eye to cease functioning to capacity or to become "lazy." Consequently macular vision never develops in the affected eye.

There are several methods employed to detect muscle weakness. Gross deviations are usually observed during inspection. The corneal light reflex (Hirschberg test) may uncover some more subtle eye devi-

Table 7-10. Selected Abnormalities of the Extraocular Muscles

Finding	*Condition*	*Description*
Malaligned eyes	Strabismus (squint)	General term applied to various types of deviation between the axes of the eyes.
	Tropia Eso-inward deviation Exo-outward deviation	Overt deviation usually apparent during inspection or corneal light reflex (Hirschberg test).
	Hypo-downward deviation Hyper-upward deviation	In the alternate cover test, the affected eye remains in deviated position when occluded. The affected eye makes a corrective movement when the occluder is placed over the normal eye if condition has not progressed to amblyopia exanopsia.
	Phoria (same descriptive prefixes as in tropias)	Latent deviation necessitating maneuver to disrupt the fusion mechanism. During the cover-uncover test the affected eye deviates when the normal eye is occluded. As the cover is removed from the normal eye, the affected eye makes a corrective maneuver to the primary position. Occlusion of the affected eye produces no change in position of the normal eye, but results in deviation of the affected eye.

ations. These deviations are discussed in preceding sections of this chapter. However, some types of deviations are manifest only when the fusion mechanism is interrupted, and they are detectable by the cover-uncover and alternate cover tests.

In performing the cover-uncover test, the examiner asks the child to look at an object about 30 centimeters (12 inches) from the eyes in the midline. The examiner uses an opaque card to occlude one eye while observing for movement of the uncovered eye. Normally there is none. When the card is removed, the examiner observes for movement of the previously covered eye. Normally there is no movement. The procedure is repeated for the other eye for a near object and is repeated for each eye for a distant object (Figure 7-29).

In performing the alternate cover test, the examiner asks the child to look at an object about 30 centimeters (12 inches) from the eyes in the midline. The examiner covers one eye and quickly removes the cover and uses it to occlude the other eye. This card is alternately placed over both eyes several times. Normally there is no deviation (Figure 7-30, Table 7-10).

Pregnancy

During pregnancy, pigmentation of the eyelids and periorbital areas frequently increases. This finding is called chloasma and is consistent with other accumulations of pigmentation in the skin. Vasoconstriction and hemorrhage may occur in the conjunctival vessels as well as in the retinal vessels, particularly during labor. Retinal vascular occlusion and enlargement of the physiologic blind spot have also been reported. In addition, increased thickness of the lens occurs, possibly from the increased fluid content; this thickness may result in transient myopia.

Late Adulthood

With advanced age there is a gradual loss of lid elasticity, which leads to drooping of the eyelids (blepharochalasis). Raised yellow plaques (xanthelasma) occur on the upper and lower lids near the inner canthi, and are frequently associated with hyperlipidemia. They are slow-growing and sometimes disappear spontaneously. The conjunctivae are drier in late adulthood because there is decreased tear production.

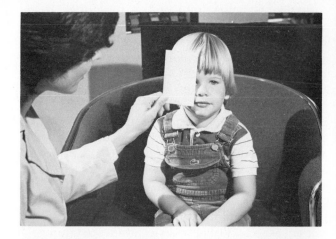

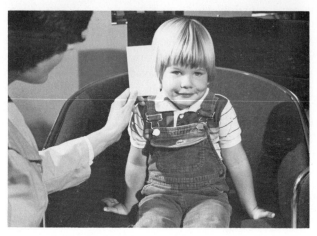

Figure 7-29. The school nurse performs the cover–uncover test on kindergarten student.

The arcus senilis represents an iris change found in most persons over 60 years of age. It begins as a whitish-gray opaque arc separated from the limbus by a narrow clear zone within the cornea. It eventually becomes a full circular band about 1.0 to 1.5 millimeters wide. The presence of an arcus senilis before age 40 frequently is associated with hyperlipidemia. The pupils are slightly smaller in the aged. The lens loses protein over time, is less elastic, and consequently loses the ability to accommodate, a condition known as presbyopia. The lens may show a loss of transparency, which leads to clouding of vision and decreased visual acuity. Ophthalmoscopy may reveal vitreous floaters, choroidal sclerosis, macular degeneration, and retinal exudates. There is also a decrease in the visual fields, speed of dark adaptation, and sensitivity to blue hues.

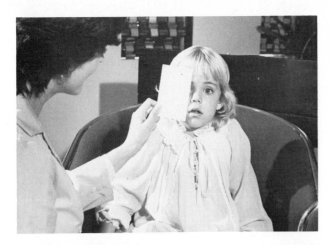
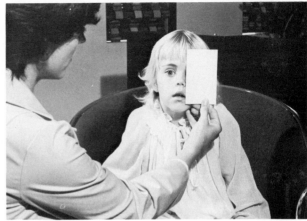
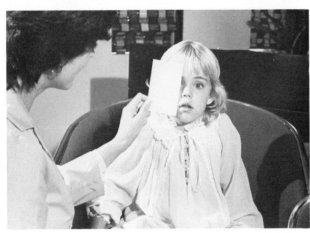

Figure 7-30. *The school nurse performs the alternate cover test on kindergarten student.*

Anatomy and Physiology

Anatomically the ear is divided into three parts: external, middle, and inner ear. The external ear comprises the pinna (auricle) and external auditory canal (ear canal). The pinna is the rigid part of the ear that protrudes from the head; it is composed mainly of cartilage and skin. The landmarks of the pinna are the helix, lobule, antihelix, concha, tragus, and antitragus (Figure 8-1).

The helix is the curved prominent outer rim of the pinna. The lobule is the flabby flap of adipose and areolar tissue at the inferior helix. The antihelix is parallel and anterior to the helix. The concha is surrounded by the curved antihelix. Anterior to the concha is the tragus, a small pointed projection of cartilage that extends posteriorly over the opening of the external auditory meatus. The tragus is continuous with the cartilage found in the external auditory canal.

The external auditory canal is the skin-lined passageway from the pinna to the tympanic membrane. It is an S-shaped canal formed by cartilage and bone. The cartilaginous outer third is thinly lined with skin that contains ceruminous and apocrine glands and hair follicles. The inner two-thirds is narrower and formed by bone.

Functionally the external ear aids in the collection and transmission of sound waves. The pinna is least important and does little to enhance hearing. The external auditory canal provides a passageway through which sound waves travel to the tympanic membrane of the middle ear.

The middle ear is separated from the external ear by the tympanic membrane (eardrum). The tympanic membrane consists of three layers of tissue. The outermost layer is squamous epithelium that originates

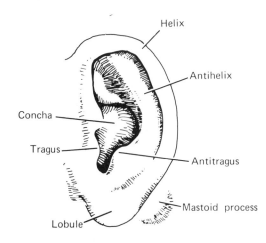

Figure 8-1. Landmarks of the pinna.

Chapter 8

Assessment of the Ear

Objectives

The examiner will be able to do the following:

1. Inspect and palpate the external ear
2. Remove cerumen from the external auditory canal
3. Perform an otoscopic examination
4. Perform screening tests for auditory acuity: whispered and spoken voice tests; watch tick test; Weber, Rinne, and Schwabach tuning fork tests
5. Recognize abnormalities of the ear
6. Record the information obtained

131

from the skin of the ear canal; the middle layer is fibrous tissue; and the inner layer is an extension of the mucosal lining of the middle ear.

The middle ear is the air-filled cavity medial to the tympanic membrane; it contains the ossicles: malleus, incus, and stapes (Figure 8-2). The malleus attaches to the tympanic membrane, and articulates with the incus. The incus articulates with the stapes. The footplate of the stapes covers the oval window, which is the opening into the inner ear. The mucosal lining of the middle ear forms the inner layer of the tympanic membrane. In addition, this lining covers the ossicles and lines the eustachian tube. The eustachian tube opens into the middle ear and connects it with the nasopharynx.

Functionally the middle ear transmits and amplifies sound via the ossicle chain. The ossicle chain transmits sound vibrations from the tympanic membrane to the oval window of the inner ear. The eustachian tube aids in the equalization of air pressure on both sides of the tympanic membrane. By equalizing air pressure, it prevents the eardrum from rupturing.

The inner ear comprises the cochlea and vestibular apparatus. The cochlea is the end organ receptor for hearing. The cochlea resembles a snail shell, is filled with fluid and is lined with a basilar membrane that extends almost its entire length. Rising upon this membrane is the organ of Corti, the neural end organ for hearing. It is from this neuroepithelium that hair cells project. The hair cells are bent or distorted by sound waves entering the cochlea and convert sound waves into electrochemical impulses.

Normal hearing is the end result of the proper functioning and interrelationship of the external, middle, and inner ear. Sound is the stimulus for hearing and travels through the external auditory canal, where it strikes the tympanic membrane. Some sound waves are reflected into the auditory canal while the remaining sound waves cause the tympanic membrane to vibrate. This vibration activates the ossicle chain to transmit sound to the oval window. From the oval window, the sound waves travel through the fluid of the cochlea. Distortion of the hair cells of the organ of Corti creates impulses that stimulate the cochlear portion of cranial nerve VIII (the acoustic nerve). These impulses are interpreted as meaningful sounds by the temporal cortex of the brain.

Two important characteristics of sound are intensity and frequency. The intensity of sound is the amount of energy that flows in a sound wave. It is measured in decibels (dB). The intensity of normal speech ranges from 40 to 65 decibels. Pain is experienced when the intensity of a sound reaches 140 decibels, for example, jet engine noise. The frequency of sound is the number of vibratory cycles per second. Frequency is measured in Hertz (Hz) units. Hearing is most sensitive at frequencies in the range of 500 to 4,000 Hz.

The vestibular apparatus is responsible for balance and equilibrium. The anatomical structures within the vestibular apparatus contain sensory receptors, which respond to positional changes of the body. The nerve fibers of the vestibular apparatus join to form the vestibular portion of cranial nerve VIII (the acoustic nerve).

Assessment Modalities

Preparation

Examination of the ear includes inspection and palpation of the external ear, otoscopic inspection of the tympanic membrane, and an evaluation of hearing

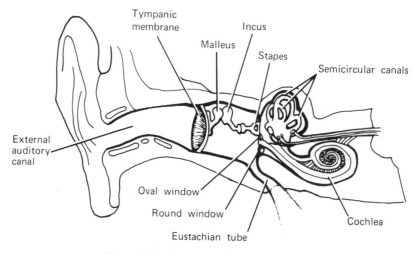

Figure 8-2. Structures of the internal ear.

acuity. Examination of the ear begins with the examiner's initial interactions with the client. The response of the client to directions and questions is often an indication of hearing ability.

Standard equipment for the examination of the ear includes a ticking watch, an otoscope with various sized specula, and a tuning fork. In addition, a head mirror and gooseneck lamp are useful. Use of the head mirror enables the examiner to use both hands for procedures such as cerumen removal (Figure 8-3).

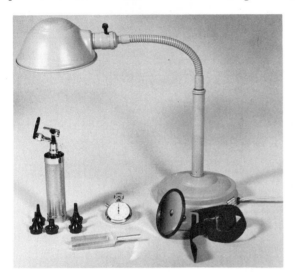

Figure 8-3. *Equipment used during assessment of the ear.*

It is important that the otoscope have freshly charged batteries since an adequate light source is essential. The tuning fork should vibrate at least 256 cycles per second. In addition, a cerumen spoon or ear irrigation set may be needed to remove wax that occludes the canal. The availability of audiometric testing equipment determines whether audiometry is part of the hearing screening. In clinical settings where audiometry is performed, the client is evaluated by a clinician proficient in this type of testing. Testing includes the introduction of pure tones to a client in a soundproofed room. The tones are varied in intensity and frequency by an electronically calibrated instrument. Responses of the client are plotted on a graph, which is used to determine the presence and type of hearing loss.

Inspection and Palpation of the Pinna

Inspection and palpation of the pinna are the easiest parts of the ear examination, yet they are frequently overlooked. Inspection includes assessment for size, position, symmetry, color, and evidence of growths or lesions. The normal pinna varies greatly among individuals and is proportionate to general head and body size. It is positioned so that the tip of the helix

Table 8-1. Selected Abnormalities of the Pinna

Finding	Condition	Description
Nodule on pinna	Sebaceous cyst	Commonly palpated behind the ear as a soft, semifluctuant mass. Usually located within the layers of the skin rather than beneath it. Common finding.
	Gouty tophi	Hard, irregular, painless nodules palpated in helix or antihelix, although they may be seen along the margins of the pinna. Formed by uric acid crystals and observed in clients with long-standing gout.
	Darwin's tubercle	Small, painless elevation in the upper third of the helix. It is harmless but should be distinguished from gouty tophi.
	Neoplasms	Frequently ulcerated, and found on any part of the pinna. Any long-standing lesion should be biopsied. Squamous cell carcinoma more frequently found than basal cell carcinoma.
Small pinna Large pinna	Congenital malformations	Individual variations of the pinna include a pinna that is too small (microtia) or too large (macrotia.)
Prominent pinna	"Lop" ear	Pinna stands out too far from head. Fairly common. Corrected by plastic surgery in which the conchal cartilage is cut and reformed.
Deformed pinna	Cauliflower ear	Due to repeated trauma to pinna. Bleeding occurs between cartilage and perichondrium. If blood is not removed, the cartilage becomes necrotic due to an inadequate blood supply. Aspiration of hematoma soon after injury may help to prevent condition.

lies on the same plane with the lateral corner of the eye and occipital protuberance. It is attached vertically; a deviation up to a 10-degree angle from this vertical plane is normal. While slight variations may exist, normally the pinnae appear symmetrical. The color of the pinna is similar to the color of the surrounding facial skin. The pinna is palpated for consistency. It is normally firm, mobile, non-tender, and free of growths or lesions (Table 8-1).

Otoscopic Examination

Inspection of the external auditory canal and tympanic membrane requires an otoscope (Figure 8-4). There are two types of otoscopes: portable and wall-mounted models. Portable models depend on batteries for power while wall-mounted ones use electrical current. The otoscope consists of two parts: the head and the body. The body contains the batteries in portable models and serves as a handle in all models. The head contains a lamp for illumination, a magnifying lens, and a fitting for the speculum tip. Speculum tips range in size from 2 to 5 millimeters and are usually fitted with disposable liners which reduce the risk of cross-infection.

The examiner inspects the canal prior to inserting the speculum. The forefinger of one hand pulls the tragus anteriorly while the thumb and forefinger of the other hand pull the helix superiorly and posteriorly (Figure 8-5). During this maneuver the examiner estimates canal size for selection of the proper size of speculum and observes for the presence of a foreign body, discharge, or inflammation (Table 8-2).

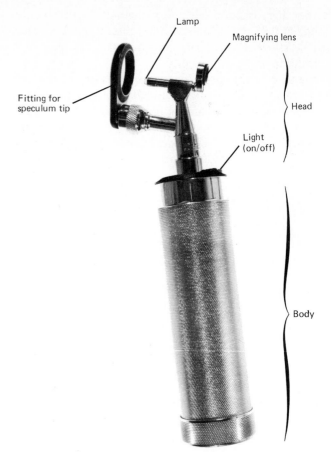

Figure 8-4. *Parts of the otoscope.*

The examiner uses the largest speculum that fits the canal to maximize visualization and prevent excessively deep and painful insertion. The speculum is fitted tightly to the head of the otoscope to prevent it from remaining in the canal when the otoscope is withdrawn.

Table 8-2. Selected Discharge from External Auditory Meatus (Otorrhea)

Finding	Condition	Description
Yellow discharge in outer third of canal	Cerumen	May become impacted. Pain generally not present. Hearing loss if cerumen present in excessive amounts.
Sticky yellow or purulent discharge	Acute external otitis	Pain present when tragus manipulated. Hearing loss may be present. Canal pale and swollen or red. Lymphadenopathy and fever in severe stage.
Malodorous discharge	Chronic external otitis	Itching rather than pain. Hearing usually not affected. Canals red and thickened.
Pustular discharge	Acute suppurative otitis media	Pain present. Hearing is reduced. Prior to rupture of membrane, the membrane bulges and is pink to red in appearance. Fever present.
Serous discharge	Fracture of middle cranial fossa	May be cerebrospinal fluid.
Foul-smelling or nearly odorless discharge	Chronic suppurative otitis media	Painless; hearing impaired. Membrane reveals permanent perforation.
Purulent, white, cheesy, malodorous discharge	Cholesteatoma	Results from marginal perforation of the tympanic membrane.

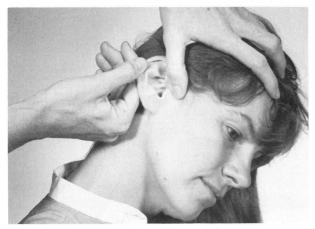

Figure 8-5. Inspection of the auditory canal.

The client is asked to tilt the head away from the examiner; the examiner firmly and gently pulls the helix superiorly and posteriorly with one hand to straighten the canal. The other hand holds the otoscope in a hammer grip. As the otoscope is introduced into the canal, the middle and index fingers are extended against the client's head to provide a brace and prevent overinsertion of the speculum (Figure 8-6).

The speculum is advanced about 8 millimeters into the canal, where cartilage, hair follicles, cerumen, and apocrine glands provide flexibility and protection. Introduction of the speculum beyond this area is painful since the posterior canal is extremely sensitive. Because sensory fibers from cranial nerve X (the vagus nerve) are present in the posterior portion of the canal, some clients cough throughout the otoscopic examination. This can cause client embarrassment unless the examiner explains this phenomenon.

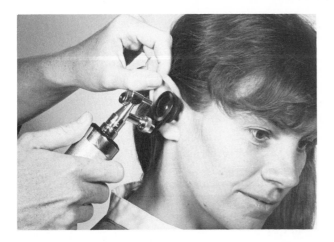

Figure 8-6. Introduction of the otoscope into the external auditory canal.

It is normal during the otoscopic examination to find small amounts of cerumen in the outer portion of the canal. Cerumen may be yellow or brown in appearance depending upon genetic variations and how long it has been in the canal. Fresh cerumen is lighter than older cerumen. In dark-skinned individuals it is darker and usually appears brown or black in color. As cerumen dries, it becomes flaky and is forced out of the canal by the muscular actions of mastication and talking. Excessive cerumen hampers otoscopy. This buildup occurs when an individual has overactive glands that produce too much cerumen or the cerumen produced is so soft that it builds up and remains in the canal rather than drying and flaking out.

Cerumen, if it fills the canal, must be removed by curettement or irrigation. Curettement is the removal of cerumen with a cerumen spoon and is recommended when the wax is soft or history indicates that the client may have a perforated membrane. Curettement requires that the examiner be skilled and that cerumen be removed by direct visualization through the speculum. The spoon is inserted above the impacted cerumen and then carefully withdrawn. Care is taken to avoid perforation of the tympanic membrane and scraping of the canal. Irrigation is the method of choice when the wax is hard and when the examiner is confident that the tympanic membrane is not perforated. Warm tap water is directed toward the posterosuperior wall of the canal with a syringe or water pic. Water that is too cold or too hot may produce dizziness or vomiting. This procedure is more time-consuming than curettement and may cause the client some discomfort.

An unobstructed external auditory meatus enables the examiner to inspect the tympanic membrane. The examiner identifies the anatomical landmarks, color, and position of the tympanic membrane.

The structure of the tympanic membrane and its relationship to the ossicles of the middle ear create important landmarks. The landmarks include the malleus attachments, light reflex, annulus, pars flaccida, and anterior and posterior malleolar folds. The malleus attachments are the short process, long process, and umbo (Figure 8-7).

The examiner begins by identifying the short process. The short process projects into the tympanic membrane at the midline superiorly and creates the appearance of a tiny knob. Continuing inferiorly from this knob is a dense white line, the long process (manubrium or handle) of the malleus. Both processes attach to the tympanic membrane and draw it into the middle, which causes it to appear concave. The long

Table 8-3. Selected External Auditory Canal Growths

Finding	Condition	Description
Nodule near tympanic membrane	Exostosis	Benign, bony projection attached to osseous canal. Appears small with a broader base. Covered with normal epithelium. Often more than one. No discharge.
Reddish, discrete papule or several pustules	Furuncle	Extremely sensitive projection found in outer third of canal. May be localized edema. Pustular discharge if opened.
Bulbous, reddened, pedunculated mass	Polyp	Nonpainful mass in canal wall or middle ear. Bleeds easily. Foul, purulent discharge present. Hearing impairment if polyp originates in middle ear.
Granular, easily bleeding tumor	Carcinoma	May arise in epithelium of canal or middle ear. Pustular drainage may be present. Deep, boring pain. Hearing loss. Facial paralysis in later stages.

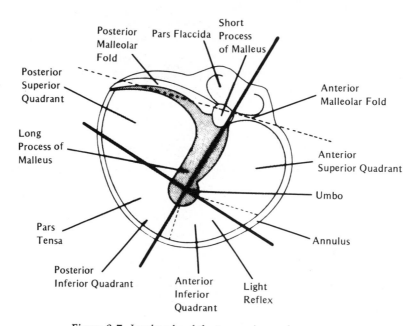

Figure 8-7. Landmarks of the tympanic membrane.

process continues inferiorly and ends at the center of the tympanic membrane, where the umbo attaches. The umbo is the most depressed part of the tympanic membrane. Extending from the umbo in an antero-inferior direction is a triangular-shaped area known as the light reflex or cone of light.

The light reflex is followed to the periphery, where the annulus is observed. The annulus is a fibrous ring which appears denser and whiter than the rest of the membrane except superiorly at the pars flaccida. Special care is taken to follow the annulus systematically around the periphery of the membrane, as perforations often occur in this area. Two bands of tissue extend inferiorly from the pars flaccida to the short process. They are the anterior and posterior malleolar folds.

The normal tympanic membrane, which is free of distinguishing marks other than its anatomical landmarks, is translucent and pearly gray in color. The position of the normal tympanic membrane is oblique with respect to the external auditory meatus, and is slightly conical in shape (Table 8-4).

Assessment of Hearing Acuity

Assessment of the ear is not complete until a hearing screening is performed. A hearing screening utilizes whispered and spoken voice tests and watch tick and tuning fork tests. Audiometric testing provides a precise measuring tool of hearing acuity when one of the screening tests suggests hearing loss. Testing is performed in a quiet environment.

Table 8-4.   Selected Abnormalities of Tympanic Membrane

Finding	Condition	Description
Blue drum	Hemotympanium	Blood in middle ear from basilar skull fracture. Membrane bulges.
Dead white to ashen gray patches	Tympanosclerosis	Deposits of hyaline material in membrane. May vary from small areas to large plaques. No complaint of pain. Hearing unaffected unless there is middle ear involvement or a large area of tympanic membrane involvement.
Pink to red drum with bulging	Acute suppurative otitis media	Presence of inflammatory process causes pus in middle ear. Pressure causes bulging of membrane. Membrane appears pink in mild cases but progresses to a red, thick, dull appearance with severe infection. Both pain and fever present. Hearing is reduced. Landmarks may be obscured. Light reflex may disappear.
Amber drum with depressed membrane	Serous otitis media	Serous fluid in middle ear. Membrane retracted. Collection of fluid in middle ear causes a visible fluid level. Air bubbles may be scattered throughout fluid. Feeling of fullness rather than pain.
Central oval opening with darker center	Acute otitis media with perforation	Tympanic membrane remains intact around perforation. Handle of malleus may project into perforation. Usually heals spontaneously. Central perforation indicates a more benign process than a marginal one.
White cheesy, foul-smelling discharge that originates from marginal opening	Cholesteotoma	Perforation involving annulus or margin of tympanic membrane. Squamous epithelium from the external auditory meatus grows around perforation preventing primary closure. Surgical intervention may be necessary.
Thin, flaccid, more translucent area	Healed perforation	Area of perforation heals but fibrous layer of membrane does not reform.

There is no equipment necessary for whispered and spoken voice tests. The examiner's own voice is used to test the client's hearing. Testing requires that the examiner's lips be approximately 1 meter (3 feet) from the client's ear. The examiner begins by exhaling as strongly as possible and whispering softly. If the client cannot understand what has been said, the examiner uses a medium whisper and finally progresses to a loud whisper. If there is still difficulty in comprehension, a speaking voice is used. Certain precautions are taken to assure that the test is a reliable predictor of hearing. They include the following: the examiner asks questions that require more than yes or no answers; the examiner asks the client to repeat bisyllabic words such as rainbow or boyfriend; and the examiner masks the ear that is not being tested. Masking is achieved by placement and rapid movement of either the examiner's or client's finger in the external auditory canal. The examiner takes care to prevent lipreading by the client (Figure 8-8).

The watch tick test evaluates the ability to hear high-frequency sound by comparing the client's hearing with the examiner's hearing. It presupposes that the examiner has normal hearing. While one of the client's ears is masked, the examiner slowly brings the watch toward the client in a line midway between them from a distance of about 1 meter (3 feet). The examiner observes the client's ability to hear the tick-

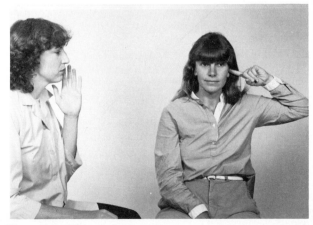

Figure 8-8. Whispered voice test.

ing of the watch. Normally the client begins to hear the ticking at the same point as the examiner.

Tuning fork tests are an important part of the hearing screening since they screen for conductive and sensorineural hearing losses. The examiner selects a tuning fork with a frequency greater than 256 cycles per second. The 128-cycle tuning fork that is used to test vibratory sensation can cause confusion if used for hearing screening since it is sometimes difficult to distinguish between hearing sound and feeling vibration. The examiner strikes the tuning fork quickly and gently against the knuckles. Striking the tuning fork too hard causes the fork to vibrate too long. This may create client fatigue, and cause the client to answer inappropriately in order to bring the test to its completion. There are three types of tuning fork tests used: Weber, Rinne, and Schwabach tests.

The Weber, or lateralization, test is a test of bone conduction. It is performed by placing an activated tuning fork on the midline of the skull at the forehead (Figure 8-9). A client with normal hearing hears only at the midline. Lateralization of sound refers to hearing the sound in one ear only and indicates hearing loss.

The Rinne test is a test of bone and air conduction. It is performed by placing a vibrating tuning fork on the mastoid process until the client can no longer hear it. At that point the tuning fork is held just outside of the opening of the external auditory canal without reactivation of the tuning fork. It is important when performing this part of the test that the broad shaped surface of the tuning fork is held perpendicular to the ear canal (Figure 8-10). The client is asked to indicate when sound can no longer be heard. A client with normal hearing will be able to hear sound twice as long by air conduction as by bone conduction (AC > BC). Clients who respond normally are said to be Rinne positive.

The Schwabach test compares the examiner's hearing by bone conduction with that of the client. The vibrating tuning fork is alternately placed against the examiner's and client's mastoids (Figure 8-11). Normally cessation of sound occurs at the same time for both the examiner and the client (Table 8-5).

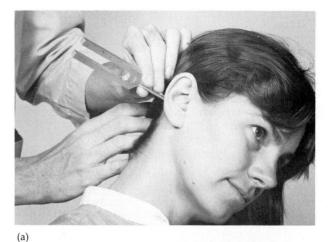

(a)

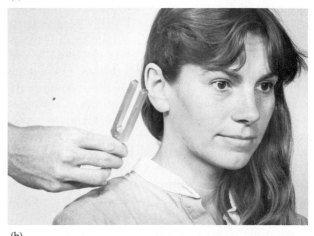

(b)

Figure 8-10. Rinne test: (a) bone conduction; (b) air conduction.

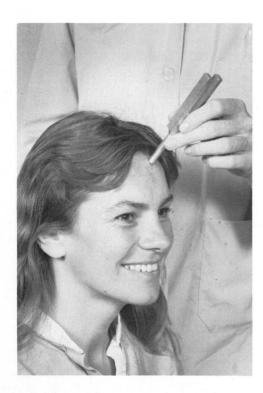

Figure 8-9. Weber test.

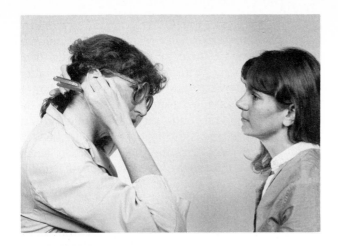

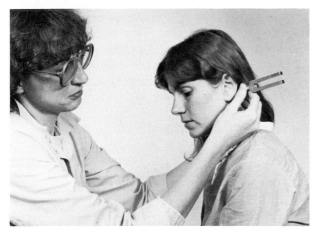

Figure 8-11. *Schwabach test.*

Life Cycle Variations

Childhood

The equipment used in the pediatric ear examination is similar to that used in the adult except that the specula are smaller. In addition, an otoscope that allows for a pneumatic attachment should be available for pneumonoscopy (Figure 8-12). Watch tick and tuning fork tests are not included in the pediatric hearing screening. A small bell is useful for hearing screening, especially when testing infants.

The infant is placed supine on the examining table, and an adult assists by immobilizing the arms and head. The assisting adult grasps the infant's arms at the elbows and holds them against the head (Figure 8-13).

Examination of the toddler or young child is performed while the client sits on an adult's lap. Prior to beginning the examination, the examiner may wish to familiarize the child with the equipment. This is accomplished by showing the equipment and letting the child handle it. For the examination, the child's arms are secured by having an adult hold them against the chest. The adult's other hand is used to hold the head steady.

Foreign bodies are frequently seen in the external auditory canals of toddlers and young children; inspection serves as a precaution to inadvertently forcing a foreign body farther into the canal when introducing the speculum.

In the neonatal period, an otoscopic examination is performed for the purpose of establishing the presence of a patent external auditory canal. Vernix caseosa occludes the canal during the first few days of life, after which the tympanic membrane may be visual-

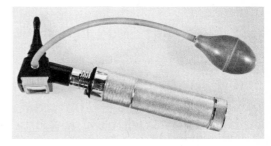

Figure 8-12. *Otoscope with pneumatic attachment.*

Table 8-5.   Selected Hearing Abnormalities

Finding	Condition	Explanation
Weber: lateralization to poor ear. Rinne: negative. Schwabach: sound heard longer by client. Client hears best in noisy room.	Conductive hearing loss	Occurs when sound cannot reach the cochlea due to obstruction of external auditory canal, damage to eardrum or middle ear, or otosclerosis. For this reason bone conduction is greater than air conduction (BC > AC).
Weber: lateralization to good ear. Rinne: positive. Schwabach: sound heard longer by examiner. Client hears poorly in noisy room.	Sensorineural hearing loss	Occurs when cochlear or auditory nerve (cranial VIII) is damaged due to congenital defect, ototoxicity, occupational hazard, Ménière's syndrome, or acoustic neuroma.

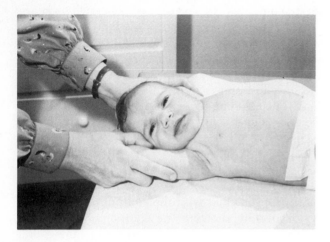

Figure 8-13. *Positioning of the infant during the otoscopic examination.*

ized. In the infant the external auditory canal extends superiorly. To visualize the tympanic membrane, the examiner gently pulls the lobule of the pinna inferiorly. Anatomical landmarks of the membrane are the same as in the adult except that the cone of light appears more diffuse. After the first few months of life, the light reflex becomes cone-shaped.

Examination of the external auditory canal in the toddler may be more difficult. Fear, past experiences with health care providers, and the rapport the toddler has with the present examiner affect the child's acceptance of the otoscopic examination. The anatomical position of the external auditory meatus in the toddler differs from that of the infant. The canal assumes a more inferior and anterior position. To straighten the canal, the examiner gently pulls the pinna in a superior and posterior direction.

Pneumatic otoscopy is a procedure in which air is introduced into the external auditory canal to check the mobility of the tympanic membrane. It is performed when middle ear pathology is suspected and the tympanic membrane is intact. The examiner selects a speculum that is large enough to create an airtight seal in the external auditory canal. The speculum is attached to the pneumatic otoscope and inserted into the canal. The hand bulb of the otoscope is squeezed to introduce a few puffs of air into the canal and the examiner observes the movement of the tympanic membrane. Normally it moves inward with the introduction of air and returns to its original position as air escapes from the canal.

Evaluation of hearing is an important part of the pediatric ear examination. During the first few weeks of life, hearing may be evaluated when the examiner rings a bell or claps hands at a distance of 30 centi-

meters (12 inches) from the infant's ears. A startle (moro) response is normally elicited. The infant may also respond by blinking his eyes (acoustic blink reflex) or momentarily stopping activity. Hearing screening is always performed while the infant is awake and not crying because a sleeping or upset infant may not respond. At approximately four months the infant turns the head and eyes toward the direction from which sound originates. At seven months the infant turns the head in search of a quietly spoken voice. During the toddler years and early childhood the whispered voice test can be used to screen hearing. The examiner stands approximately 8 feet away from the child, gives whispered questions or commands, and evaluates the appropriateness of the child's responses. The examiner may also wish to perform a telephone test. This test compares the child's ability to hear the dial tone of a telephone held at a given distance to that of the examiner's. Audiometric testing should be performed whenever the examiner or parent questions the ability of a child to hear adequately. In addition, audiometric testing should be done on all children at age 3.

Speech development is another indication of the young client's ability to hear. Generally infants begin to make babbling sounds in the fourth month; word usage begins at 9 to 12 months. Speech development may be delayed slightly between 12 to 18 months as the child becomes preoccupied with walking and exploring the environment. Mastery of various sounds develops throughout the first few years; by six most children have intelligible speech. Children should be referred for thorough speech and hearing evaluations any time that speech development appears to lag.

Late Adulthood

A normal consequence of the aging process is a change in the structure and function of the ear. Loss of elasticity of the pinna causes elongation of the lobule and oblique creases traversing the pinna. In some males hair may protrude from the opening of the external auditory canal and grow on the tragus.

Inspection of the external auditory meatus may be more difficult since the canal is often narrower due to an inward collapsing of the canal wall. Cerumen may also occlude the canal. Although cerumen production decreases slightly with age, the cerumen present in the canal has a tendency to be thicker and consequently more difficult to remove, which may affect hearing. Otoscopic inspection of the tympanic membrane reveals a whiter, thicker, duller, and more opaque membrane. There is no evidence, however, that these eardrum changes affect hearing.

Hearing loss is a normal consequence of aging. While subtle changes may occur as early as 40, more noticeable changes do not usually appear until after age 60. Most often the loss is the result of a sensorineural deficit caused by genetic disease, ototoxic drugs, or environmental factors. At first, perception of high frequency sounds is affected; eventually perception of medium frequency sounds is affected. Presbycusis refers to a sensorineural loss in which the person is able to hear normal speech but is unable to understand what is being said. Although presbycusis is the most frequently encountered loss, conductive defects can also interfere with the ability to hear. Hearing screening is performed to determine the type of hearing loss present so that the appropriate rehabilitative measures can be instituted. As in any client with a hearing loss, audiometric testing is employed when a more thorough evaluation is needed.

Anatomy and Physiology

The mouth, pharynx, nose, and sinuses are structures of the head located in proximity to one another with interrelated functions.

The Mouth

The mouth (oral cavity) performs the functions of taste, initiation of carbohydrate digestion, and formation of sounds in speech; it also serves as a passageway for food and air. The structures of the mouth are the lips, the hard and soft palates, the tongue, the floor of the mouth, the openings of the salivary glands, gingivae (gums), teeth, uvula, palatine arches, and palatine tonsils (Figure 9-1).

The lips form the anterior boundary of the mouth. Their varying degrees of closure facilitate speech formation, prevent the loss of fluid and food from the mouth during ingestion, and allow increased air flow during inspiration and expiration.

The roof of the mouth is formed by the hard and soft palates. The hard palate forms the anterior portion and is a fixed structure; the soft palate forms the posterior portion and is mobile.

The tongue, a muscular organ on the floor of the mouth, facilitates speech and mastication and contains the sensory organs for taste. The circumvallate papillae (taste buds) are on the posterior third of the dorsal surface. There are two other types of papillae: the filiform and fungiform. They have no gustatory function and are distinguished from each other by their appearance. The filiform papillae are small, hairlike projections at the tip of the tongue; the fungiform papillae are broad and flat and are located on the central dorsum of the tongue. Taste is mediated by two cranial nerves: cranial nerve VII (the facial nerve) and cranial nerve IX (the glossopharyngeal nerve). The tongue and other muscles of mastication are innervated by three cranial nerves: cranial nerve V (the trigeminal nerve), cranial nerve VII (the facial nerve), and cranial nerve XII (the hypoglossal nerve) (Chapter 18).

The floor of the mouth is formed by mobile connective tissue and muscle attached to the mandible. The ventral surface of the tongue is attached to the floor of the mouth by the frenulum, while the posterior portion, or root, of the tongue is attached to the mandible, hyoid bone, and styloid process of the temporal bone.

The openings of two of the salivary glands (submandibular and sublingual) are located under the tongue. The ducts (Wharton's ducts) of the sub-

Chapter 9

Assessment of the Mouth, Pharynx, Nose, and Sinuses

Objectives

The examiner will be able to do the following:

1. Inspect and palpate the structures of the mouth
2. Inspect the pharynx
3. Obtain a throat culture
4. Inspect the nose
5. Palpate, percuss, and transilluminate the frontal and maxillary sinuses
6. Teach self-examination of the head and neck
7. Recognize abnormalities of the mouth and pharynx
8. Record the information obtained

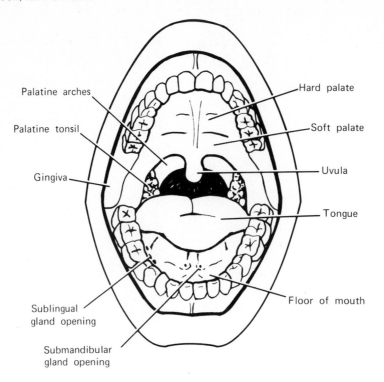

Figure 9-1. Structures of the mouth.

mandibular gland open on either side of the fren-ulum. The sublingual glands are the smallest salivary glands and are located in the floor of the mouth be-tween the sides of the tongue and the mandible. Each has about 20 openings directly superior to the glands themselves. The ducts (Stensen's ducts) of the parotid glands open into the buccal membrane beside the upper second molar teeth.

The gingivae are the tissues that surround the neck of the teeth and cover the bony (alveolar) ridges of the mandible and maxilla. The teeth grow from within the alveolar ridges.

The normal adult has 32 teeth, 16 in the maxilla and 16 in the mandible (Figure 9-2). The teeth are the organs of mastication, give form to the lower face, and aid in speech formation. The root accounts for the largest percentage of tooth size, although it is located under the gingiva in the alveolar ridge. The visible part of the tooth is the clinical crown. Each tooth comprises four tissues: enamel, dentin, cementum, and pulp. The enamel is the hard, calcified outer por-tion of the tooth. The dentin is the calcific tissue that forms the body of the tooth and underlies the ce-mentum and enamel. The cementum is the layer of bonylike tissue that covers the root; and the pulp is the soft vascular center of the tooth.

The uvula is a small, soft projection of connective tissue suspended from the posterior midline of the soft palate. It is the posterior boundary of the mouth,

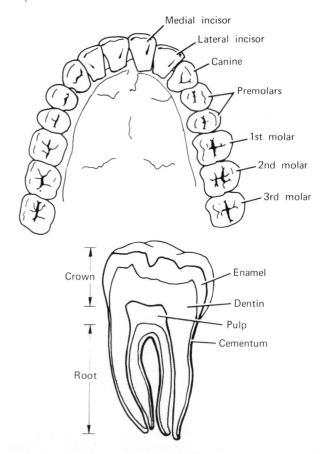

Figure 9-2. (a) Adult dentition; (b) components of the tooth.

moves during phonation, and is innervated by cranial nerve X (the vagus nerve). Lateral and inferior to the uvula on each side are the palatine arches. They are folds of mucous membrane that join the soft palate superiorly and contain the palatine tonsils. The tonsils are anterior oropharyngeal structures, and are small masses of lymphoid tissue that protect against bacterial invaders and form lymphocytes (Chapter 19).

The Pharynx

The pharynx is a muscular membranous tube that extends from the base of the skull to the sixth cervical vertebra, where it joins the esophagus. It is a resonating cavity for speech, a passageway for food and air, and in direct communication with the posterior nares of the nose, the eustachian tube, the mouth, and the larynx. It consists of three sections: the nasopharynx, oropharynx, and laryngeal pharynx (Figure 9-3). The nasopharynx extends from the posterior nares to the soft palate, and drains the secretions of the eustachian tubes. The oropharynx extends from the soft palate to the epiglottis; the laryngeal pharynx, from the epiglottis to the lower border of the cricoid cartilage. The pharynx is innervated by cranial nerve IX (the glossopharyngeal nerve) and cranial nerve X (the vagus nerve), (Chapter 18).

The Nose

The nose is an anterior facial structure that is the major entry and exit for air. It also warms, humidifies, and filters inhaled air. The anterior two-thirds of the

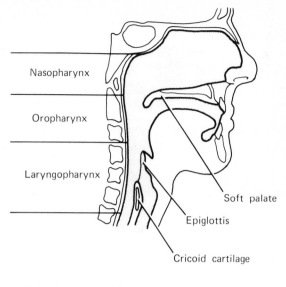

Figure 9-3. *Structures of the pharynx.*

nose is composed of skin and mucous membrane covered cartilage; the posterior third is supported by bone. The nose consists of two nares, a vestibule and septum, three turbinates and their corresponding meatuses, and the openings for the nasolacrimal ducts and paranasal sinuses (Figure 9-4).

Air enters each side of the nose by one of the anterior nares and then moves into the vestibule, a dilated area within the anterior nose. The nasal septum divides the interior of the nose into two lateral compartments; therefore, air entering one side of the nose does not communicate with air entering the other side until reaching the nasopharynx. The septum is carti-

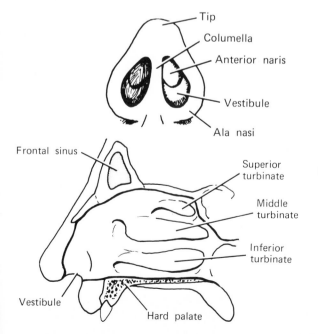

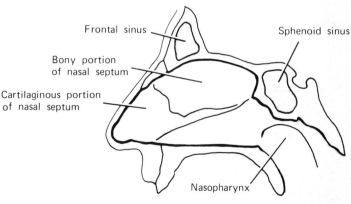

Figure 9-4. *Structures of the nose.*

laginous in the anterior two-thirds and bony in the posterior one-third.

Each side of the nose has three turbinates. The turbinates are bony structures that project medially from the lateral nasal walls. They are covered by a vascular ciliated mucous membrane, which increases the surface area of the nose and greatly enhances the warming, humidification, and filtration of inspired air. The turbinates are named for their location: superior, middle, and inferior. They overlie spaces known as meatuses, with corresponding names. The nasolacrimal duct drains into the inferior meatus. The orifices of the frontal, anterior ethmoid, and maxillary sinuses are located in the middle meatus. The orifices of the posterior ethmoid and sphenoid sinuses are located in the superior meatus. The nose also contains the olfactory receptors for the sense of smell mediated by cranial nerve I (the olfactory nerve).

The Paranasal Sinuses

The sinuses are cavities within the cranial and facial bones containing vascular ciliated mucous membrane. Like the nose, they warm, humidify, and filter air. There are anterior and posterior sinuses. The anterior sinuses are the frontal, maxillary, and anterior ethmoidal sinuses. The posterior are the posterior ethmoidal and sphenoidal. All open into the nose as mentioned (Figure 9-5).

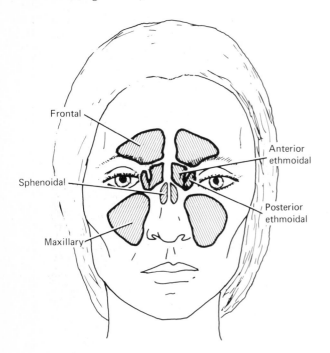

Figure 9-5. The sinuses.

Assessment Modalities

Preparation

For assessment of the mouth, pharynx, nose, and sinuses the client can be fully clothed in a standing, sitting, or supine position. The equipment necessary is the following (Figure 9-6):

Glove

Tongue depressor

Light source (otoscope, flashlight or penlight)

Nasal specula (two types)

Gauze pad

Mirror

Dental floss

Dental mirror*

Head mirror with gooseneck lamp*

The Mouth and Pharynx. The modalities used in assessment of the mouth and pharynx are inspection and palpation. The examiner wears a glove on the hand used to palpate the mouth.

The examiner views the client with the mouth closed. The lips are normally symmetrical, smooth, and pink; they are more darkly pigmented in dark-skinned persons. The examiner asks the client to open the mouth and uses the otoscope for illumination. The mouth is inspected in two open positions: a relaxed open position in which the tongue remains in-

*The dental mirror is not necessary for most oral assessment performed outside dental offices; however, it facilitates visualization of the posterior tooth surfaces and gingivae and the palate.

The head mirror is useful but often unavailable.

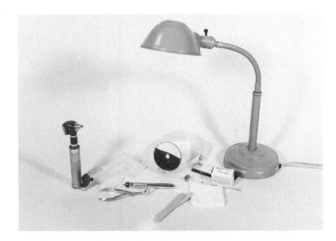

Figure 9-6. Equipment necessary for assessment of the mouth, pharynx, nose, and sinuses.

Table 9-1. Selected Breath Abnormalities

Finding	Condition	Description
Sweet breath	Diabetic acidosis	Acetone-like breath.
Foul breath	Tooth decay, bronchiectasis, tonsillitis, and other upper respiratory infections, necrotizing ulcerative gingivitis (trench mouth)	Breath is offensive, and the client relates that food does not taste the same.
	Diphtheria	Mouselike odor.
	Typhoid	Smell of decaying tissue.
Unusual breath	Alcohol ingestion	Alcohol-type breath.
	Uremia	Ammonia-like odor.

side the mouth and an exaggerated open position in which the tongue protrudes (Figures 9-7 and 9-8).

When assessing the client with the mouth in the relaxed open position, the examiner observes the dorsal and ventral tongue surfaces, the floor of the mouth, the teeth, the gingivae, the roof of the mouth, the buccal mucosa, the uvula, the tonsils, and the oropharynx. (The nasopharynx and the laryngopharynx are not visible without special equipment.) While assessing the mouth, the examiner notes the breath; it is normally nonoffensive (Table 9-1).

The dorsal tongue surface is pink, moist, and roughened by the presence of the papillae. For inspection of the ventral tongue surface and several structures on the floor of the mouth, the examiner asks the client to lift the tongue (Figure 9-9). If the client is unable to do so, the examiner displaces the tongue with a tongue depressor. When examining an unconscious person, there is some danger that the examiner can be bitten; therefore, the examiner places another tongue depressor between the teeth to keep them apart (Figure 9-10). The ventral tongue surface

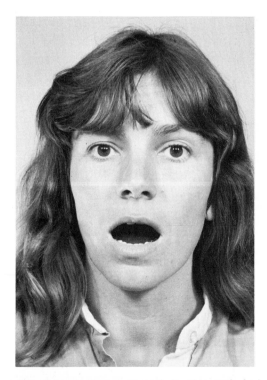

Figure 9-7. Relaxed open position of client's mouth during inspection.

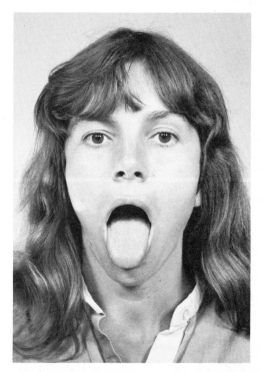

Figure 9-8. Exaggerated open position of client's mouth during inspection.

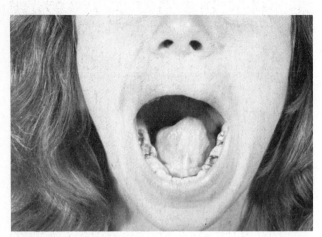

Figure 9-9. Inspection of the ventral tongue surface, frenulum, and openings of the submaxillary glands.

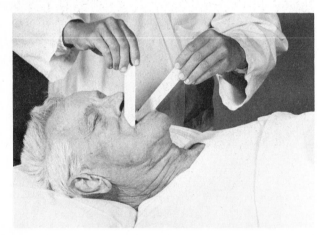

Figure 9-10. In providing oral hygiene, the primary care nurse inspects the mouth of the unconscious person.

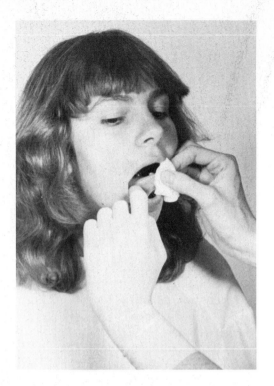

Figure 9-11. Palpation of the floor of the mouth.

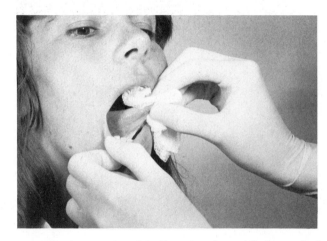

Figure 9-12. Inspection of the lingual surfaces of the lower gingivae and teeth.

is smooth. The frenulum is pink and smooth. On either side of the frenulum on the floor of the mouth are the openings of the submaxillary glands and their ducts. The remaining floor of the mouth is pink, moist, and smooth. When the inspection is completed, the examiner gently holds the tip of the tongue with a gauze pad to displace it and palpates the tongue surface and floor of the mouth. Both normally feel smooth (Figure 9-11).

While maintaining a gentle hold of the tongue, the lower gingivae and teeth are inspected, beginning with their lingual (side next to the tongue) surfaces (Figure 9-12). The teeth are identified by several numbering systems (Figure 9-13).

The examiner releases the tongue and inspects the buccal (cheek) or labial (lip) sides of the lower gingivae and teeth (Figure 9-14). For inspection of the up-

per gingivae and teeth, the examiner tilts the head back and hyperextends the neck (Figure 9-15).

The gingival tissue is inspected for color, contour, and consistency. The gingival tissue is generally coral-colored and stippled, although it is normally more darkly pigmented in dark-skinned persons. It is usually smooth in contour and ends in a knifelike edge, where it covers the individual teeth. Between the teeth (interdental papillae) the gingiva extends no more than 1 to 2 millimeters in a sharp, pointed-looking projection. The consistency of the gingiva is firm and resilient, and tightly bound to the teeth

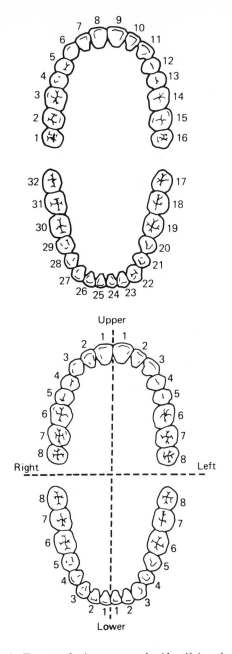

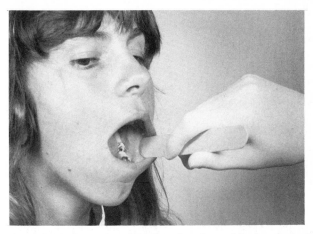

Figure 9-14. *Inspection of the buccal surfaces of the lower gingivae and teeth.*

Figure 9-13. Two numbering systems for identifying the teeth.

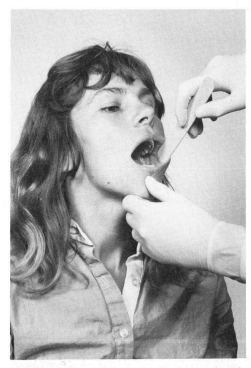

Figure 9-15. *Inspection of the upper gingivae and teeth.*

except at its knifelike edges, known as the free gingival margin (Figure 9-16). (This is the area where the bristles of a soft toothbrush can gently be slipped or vibrated between the gingival tissue and individual teeth.)

The teeth are observed for color, size, form, contour, number, general state of hygiene, and contact relationships. The teeth are normally white, 5 to 12 millimeters in height, straight with respect to one another, and smooth in contour. The incisors and canines have straight biting surfaces, while the molars have smoothly contoured cusps. They are close enough to one another that a piece of unwaxed dental

floss can be passed between any two teeth with steady and firm pressure. Teeth that receive adequate hygiene have no food impacted between them and exhibit the other mentioned qualities.

The techniques mentioned in this chapter are general screening methods. Comprehensive dental examination can only be performed by a dentist using probes, mirrors, and X-ray.

In order to ascertain their fit, the examiner palpates the dentures while an edentulous client wears them.

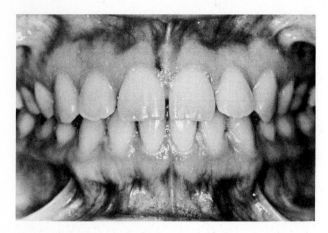

Figure 9-16. Normal gingivae.

They should fit snugly and feel comfortable to the client. The dentures are then removed, and the examiner inspects and palpates the arches (the place along the gums where the dentures fit). The arches are coral-colored, smooth, and nontender.

With the client's neck hyperextended, the examiner inspects and palpates the roof of the mouth. It is pink in color and feels smooth. The hard palate feels bony hard, while the soft palate feels tense and elastic.

After the client returns the head to the normal position, the examiner inspects the buccal mucosa. The buccal mucosa is also pink in color and smooth in contour. The openings of the parotid ducts are visible near the right and left upper second molars. In palpating the buccal mucosa, the examiner uses two fingers; the forefinger palpates internally, while the thumb opposes it from the outside of the mouth (Figure 9-17).

The examiner asks the client to open the mouth completely and stick out the tongue. The tongue protrudes in the midline, a test of the function of cranial nerve XII (the hypoglossal nerve) (Figure 9-18). The examiner uses a tongue depressor to lower the tongue for a clear view of the uvula and oropharynx. As the client says "ahh," the uvula moves upward symmetrically, a test of the function of cranial nerve X (the vagus nerve) (Figure 9-19).

The examiner continues to depress the tongue and inspects each tonsil and the oropharynx (Figure 9-19). Since lymphoid tissue atrophies with aging, fre-

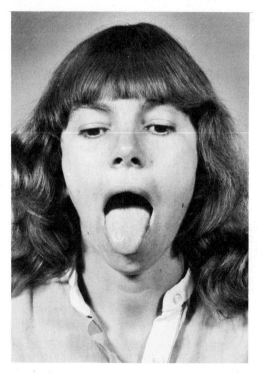

Figure 9-18. The examiner tests Cranial Nerve XII.

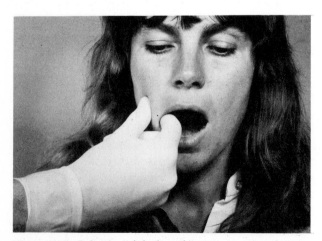

Figure 9-17. Palpation of the buccal mucosa.

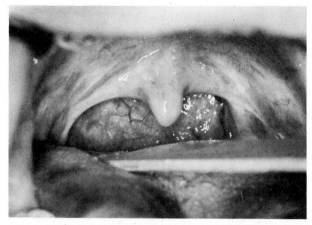

Figure 9-19. After inspection of the tonsils and oropharynx, the examiner tests Cranial Nerve X.

quently the tonsils are small or invisible. When visible, they are pink, rounded masses of tissue in the lateral oropharynx tucked between the anterior and posterior pillars (palatine arches). The posterior wall of the oropharynx is pink. Cranial nerves IX and X (the glossopharyngeal and vagus nerves) are tested during the examination of the pharynx. The examiner touches the pharynx with a tongue blade, which induces the gag reflex.

Throat culture. Many viral and bacterial agents cause acute inflammation of the pharynx (pharyngitis), but infection with beta hemolytic streptococcus can be particularly threatening, as it can cause serious sequelae if untreated. Some possible complications are acute rheumatic fever, glomerulonephritis, cervical adenitis, paratonsillar abscess, otitis media, cellulitis, and septicemia. For this reason a throat culture is usually indicated when a client presents with a sore throat, fever, and pharyngitis (Figure 9-20). The examiner swabs the pharynx with an applicator from a throat culture kit. The applicator is immediately returned to the sterile transport medium. The specimen is then submitted to the lab. Results are usually conclusive within 24 to 48 hours.

The Nose and Paranasal Sinuses. For assessment of the nose, the examiner uses inspection with one of two kinds of nasal specula. The sinuses are assessed by palpation, percussion, and transillumination.

The examiner notes the color, shape, and position of the external nose. It is normally the same color as the remainder of the body skin. The shape varies among individuals and is largely determined by hereditary characteristics. It is normally midline and symmetrical.

To inspect the internal nose, the examiner attaches the short, widened nasal speculum (similar to an ear

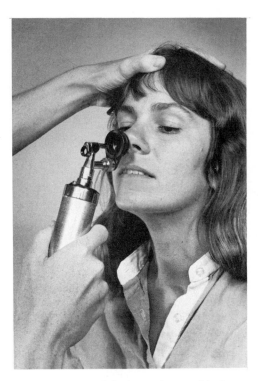

Figure 9-21. Inspection of the internal nose with the otoscope.

speculum) to the otoscope and gently inserts it into one naris, while avoiding the sensitive septum. The other hand is used to stabilize the head in the erect position. The internal nose is inspected for hydration, contours, and color. The inferior and middle turbinates and middle meatus are normally visible, and are moist, smooth and redder than the oral mucosa. The nasal septum is midline. The examiner tilts the head backward to view a more anterior aspect of the same turbinates, and the normal findings are the same (Figure 9-21).

An alternate method of internal inspection uses a nasal speculum and light source (flashlight or penlight). The examiner inserts the blades of the speculum into the vestibule about 1 centimeter and opens them in an anteroposterior direction to avoid the sensitive septum (Figure 9-22). The other hand is used to direct the light source into the nose. The rest of the examination is the same as if using the otoscopic nasal speculum.

An additional method of inspection involves use of a head mirror. When using the head mirror, it is strapped to the head of the examiner and positioned over one eye. A gooseneck lamp is positioned to shine on the mirror, and the mirror reflects light into the nose. The examiner views the nose from a distance of about 14 inches with both eyes open (Figure 9-23).

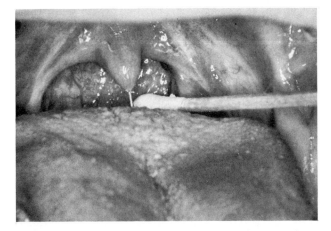

Figure 9-20. The examiner obtains a throat culture specimen, taking care to avoid touching the tongue with the swab.

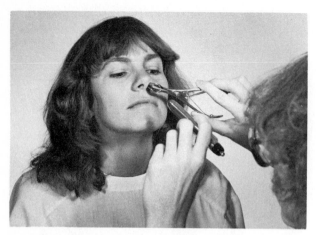

Figure 9-22. *Inspection of the internal nose with the nasal speculum and penlight.*

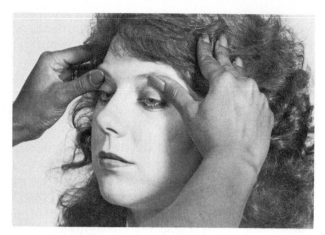

Figure 9-24. *Palpation of the frontal sinuses.*

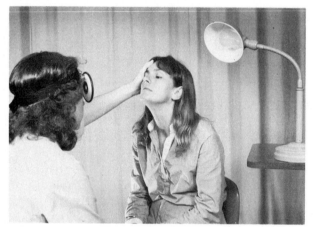

Figure 9-23. *Inspection of the internal nose with the head mirror and gooseneck lamp.*

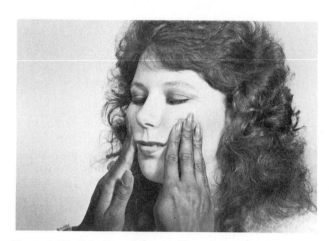

Figure 9-25. *Palpation of the maxillary sinuses.*

The frontal and maxillary sinuses are the only ones accessible to physical examination. For assessment of the frontal sinuses the examiner places one thumb under each eyebrow and exerts pressure in a superior and inward direction. Normally they are nontender. For assessment of the maxillary sinuses the examiner places the thumbs under the maxillae and exerts similar pressure. These are also nontender in the healthy client (Figures 9-24 and 9-25). The examiner percusses over the same areas and in the normal client finds that they are nontender (Figure 9-26).

An additional technique useful in assessing the sinuses is transillumination. Light passes through the sinuses evenly and symmetrically because they are air-filled cavities. Transillumination of the frontal sinuses involves shining a penlight against the frontal area of the head with the room darkened (Figure 9-27).

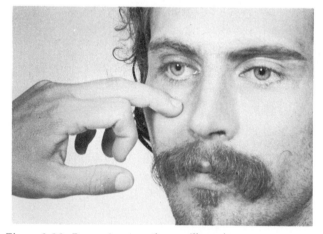

Figure 9-26. *Percussion over the maxillary sinuses.*

Transillumination of the maxillary sinuses involves shining a penlight against the zygomatic bones superiorly with the room darkened (Figure 9-28). Normally, crescents of light are visible below the pupillary red reflexes (Tables 9-2 and 9-3).

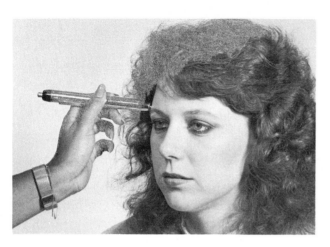

Figure 9-27. Transillumination of the frontal sinuses.

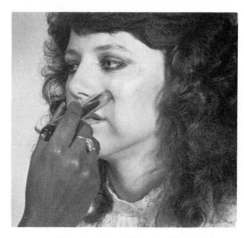

Figure 9-28. Transillumination of the maxillary sinuses.

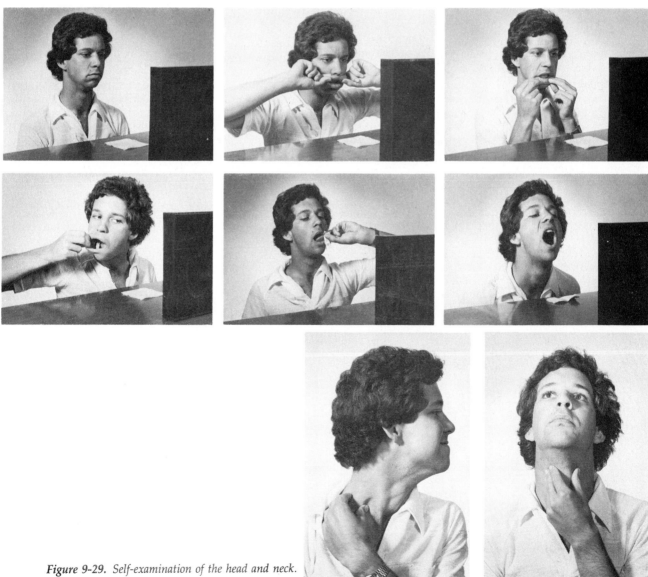

Figure 9-29. Self-examination of the head and neck.

Table 9-2. Selected Abnormalities of the Mouth and Pharynx

Finding	Condition	Explanation
Red, cracked, bleeding dry lips (chapped lips).	Cheilitis	Lip irritation caused by wind, sun, or cosmetic irritants; by febrile stage of any illness; by habitual lip licking and biting.
Diffuse, nonpitting edema of the lips.	Angioneurotic edema	Allergic reaction.
Cluster of small vesicles that ruptures, ulcerates, and then becomes crusted.	Herpes simplex (cold sore, fever blister)	Response to invasion by viral pathogen, Herpes simplex type 1 or type 2.
Tongue has bright red design on dorsal surface that resembles a map; design changes within days.	Migratory glossitis (geographic tongue)	Harmless condition in which the tongue has irregular areas of denuded epithelium.
Distal dorsal surface of tongue appears to have short, black hairs.	Hairy tongue (furry tongue, black tongue)	Hyperplastic filiform papillae and overgrowth of fungal filaments impart a black, hairy appearance.
Dorsum of the tongue is divided by transverse furrows.	Scrotal tongue (congenital furrowing of the tongue)	Congenital, harmless condition.
Dry tongue.	Mouth breather	Moisture lost during respiration, side effect of many medications.
	Sjögren's syndrome	Lack of saliva production (xerostomia).
Dry tongue with longitudinal furrows.	Marked dehydration (loss of 3 liters of extracellular fluid)	Loss of tongue volume is responsible for furrowing.
Chalky, white deposit adherent to teeth	Calculus	Collection of calcified food deposits.
Brownish-black staining of tooth enamel	Tobacco stains	Tobacco discolors the tooth enamel.
Mottled and pitted teeth.	Tetracycline treatment	Tetracycline causes intrinsic discoloration of teeth as it interferes with tooth development.
	Excess fluoride ingestion	Client takes fluoride tablets and drinks fluoridated water.
Loss of stippling of gingivae; inflamed margins of gingivae around teeth; loss of knifelike edges of gingivae over tooth surfaces; and bulbous interdental papillae.	Gingivitis	Changes associated with inflammatory response. Gingivae are edematous, reddened, and tender.
Clusters of tiny vesicles on tongue tip or sides, buccal or labial mucosa.	Aphthous ulcer (canker sore)	Etiology unknown. Thought to be associated with herpes simplex infection, food allergy, and emotional stress.
Bright, red, swollen, and edematous pharyngeal mucosa, very painful condition; tonsillar tissue has more crypts than normal with yellow or white exudate.	Streptococcal or staphylococcal pharyngitis	Local inflammatory response to bacterial pathogen.
Swollen tonsillar tissue with dull red pharyngeal mucosa.	Viral pharyngitis	Mild inflammatory response to viral pathogen.
(Evaluation scale for tonsil size: 1+—tonsil edges seen only; 2+—tonsil edges midway between pillars and uvula; 3+—tonsil edges touching uvula; 4+—tonsil edges meet in midline).	Infectious mononucleosis	Pharynx appears similar to infection with any other virus but associated with marked cervical lymphadenopathy, axillary and inguinal lymphadenopathy, and splenomegaly.
Translucent mass beside the frenulum.	Ranula	Represents a cyst of the sublingual or submaxillary gland. Size estimated by bimanual palpation using one finger under the tongue and the fingers of the other hand in the submandibular region.
Sublingual mass.	Carcinoma	Indurated ulcer or warty growth causes painful movement of frenulum.
Gray to grayish-orange or brownish-blackish areas of varying sizes and depths on tooth surfaces.	Dental caries	Areas of tooth decay associated with inadequate hygiene; also some people have a familial predisposition to caries.
Presence of food particles lodged between teeth.	Food impaction	Associated with inadequate hygiene and too closely spaced teeth.

Table 9-2. Selected Abnormalities of the Mouth and Pharynx (*continued*)

Finding	Condition	Explanation
Improper occlusion or meeting of the biting and chewing surfaces of the upper and lower teeth.	Malocclusion	May be skeletal, functional, or dental in origin.
Shrinkage of gingivae away from crowns of the teeth.	Gingival recession	Atrophy of the gingivae may be caused by poor tooth brushing, hyperfunction, bruxism, hypofunction.
White, pasty substance on teeth.	Dental plaque	Accumulation of bacteria and their by-products on teeth.
Fetid breath, loss of gingivae between the teeth, punched out craters on gingivae covered with a grayish pseudomembrane.	Necrotizing ulcerative gingivitis (trench mouth)	Caused by bacteria and spirochete overgrowth; may involve pharynx and tonsils.

Table 9-3. Selected Abnormalities of the Nose and Sinuses

Finding	Condition	Explanation
Swollen, pale, boggy, grayish-colored nasal mucosa.	Allergic rhinitis	Local response to allergens.
Red, swollen nasal mucosa with nasal discharge; discharge is clear and watery initially and then becomes viscous and mucopurulent.	Acute rhinitis (the common cold)	Local inflammatory response to bacterial or viral pathogens.
Displacement of septal cartilage laterally.	Septal deviation	Usually congenital but may be traumatic.
Small, soft, clear, pedunculated lesion hanging from middle turbinate.	Nasal polyp	Associated with allergic rhinitis.
Pain and tenderness over one or more sinuses.	Acute sinusitis	Inflammation of sinus mucosa; examination of nose reveals red, boggy turbinates and mucosa and frequently a purulent nasal discharge. May be accompanied by swelling of the head, eye pain, proptosis, diplopia, epiphoria, swelling of the eyelids.

Self-Examination of the Head and Neck

The American Dental Association recommends a monthly self-examination of the head and neck. The examiner provides a mirror and instructs the client in performing the eight steps of examination (Figure 9-29).

1. Facial symmetry: The client looks into the mirror with a blank facial expression and checks that both sides of the face look similar. Any lumps, tenderness, or skin changes are palpated, and the client makes a mental or written note of their description.

2. Lips: The client pulls the upper lip out, using the thumb and forefinger of each hand, and inspects the color and texture of inside and outside lip surfaces. The lower lip is pulled out and the same observations are made. The lips are pink, smooth, and dry (but not cracked).

3. Gums (gingivae): The client grasps the upper lip as already described and turns it inside out to expose the upper gingiva. The client turns the lower lip inside out and inspects the lower gingiva. The gingivae are coral-colored and stippled; they normally contain melanin in dark-skinned persons.

4. Cheeks (buccal mucosa): The client uses the right forefinger and middle finger to expose the right inside cheek. The same two fingers of the left are used to inspect the left cheek. The cheeks are pink, smooth, and moist. Next to the second molar teeth are the openings to the parotid salivary glands.

5. Tongue and floor of the mouth: The client checks the tongue's mobility by moving it from side to side, and by extending it. The tip of the tongue is grasped with a gauze pad or clean washcloth and is moved as far to the left as possible. This enables the client to view the right side and the right ventral surface of the tongue, and the right floor of the mouth. The tongue is displaced to the right side, and the client makes a

similar assessment of the left side. After inspection, the client palpates the tongue and floor of the mouth. The tongue is usually pink, moist, bumpy-looking because of the taste buds, mobile to both sides of the mouth, nontender, and smooth on its tip and sides. The floor of the mouth is pink and smooth and has the openings of the two submandibular glands visible in it.

6. The roof of the mouth: The client opens the mouth and hyperextends the neck. The roof of the mouth is inspected and palpated. It normally is pink, smooth, and hard.

7. Lateral neck: The client turns the head to the left, tenses the sternocleidomastoid muscle (the muscle that becomes prominent while clenching the jaws), and palpates up and down the neck on both sides of the muscles feeling for lumps. Normally there are none. The procedure is repeated for the right side.

8. Trachea: The client places the fingers around the Adam's apple (thyroid cartilage) and moves it to each side with and without swallowing. The trachea is in the midline, is movable the same distance from side to side, and moves upward during swallowing.

Life Cycle Variations

Childhood

The normal newborn is edentulous, although some infants appear to have teeth because they have small (less than 3.0 millimeters in diameter) white glistening bumps on their gums or midpalates. These are called Epstein pearls or Bohns nodules; they represent masses of epithelial cells that usually disappear by two to three months. Rarely, newborns are born with one or more deciduous (primary or baby) teeth, which usually present no difficulties.

Babies who have passed through a birth canal infected with Candida albicans (monoliasis, a common form of vaginitis among pregnant women) frequently have thrush, oral candidiasis. This is a condition characterized by a white, cheesy coating on the tongue and buccal mucosa.

A sucking tubercle or sucking blister is frequently apparent on the middle of the upper lip. These occur in breast fed and bottle fed infants and subside spontaneously when the baby begins to eat other foods and to rely less on sucking.

Salivation begins at about three months of age. Infants begin drooling at this time and continue to drool until they learn to swallow the saliva. Drooling is unrelated to teething.

Although the deciduous teeth begin forming during the sixth week of fetal life, they do not begin to erupt until 5 to 9 months of age. There is a wide range of normal for the eruption of the deciduous teeth. Usually the lower incisors appear first. Most babies have 6 teeth at 12 months, 12 teeth at 18 months, 16 teeth at two years, and 20 teeth (the complete deciduous dentition) by two and one-half years (Table 9-4).

Table 9-4. Eruption of Deciduous Teeth

Name	Time of Eruption (Months)
Lower central incisors	6-9
Upper central incisors	8-12
Upper lateral incisors	10-12
Lower lateral incisors	12-15
Anterior (first) molars	12-15
Canines (cuspids)	18-24
Posterior (second) molars	24-30

Teething is a term applied to the period when new teeth are erupting. While teething, babies often have an area of blanching, erythema, or ecchymosis overlying the tooth that is erupting. The deciduous teeth are usually bluish-white in color because the enamel is less translucent and thicker than that of the permanent teeth.

The gingival tissues of primary and mixed dentition are uniformly colored rather than stippled and are less pigmented. In addition the color is pale pink rather than coral-colored. Mixed dentition refers to the period when the deciduous teeth are lost and the permanent teeth appear. This occurs over a period of years from about age 5 to 7 to age 17 to 25 (Table 9-5).

Table 9-5. Eruption of Permanent Teeth

Name	Time of Eruption (Years)
First molars	6-7
Central incisors	7-8
Lateral incisors	7-8
First premolars	9-10
Second premolars	9-10
Canines	12-14
Second molars	12-15
Third molars	17-25

Newborns are evaluated for the patency of both nares and for flaring of the ala nasi. The examiner occludes one naris and feels for the exhalation of air from the other naris. The procedure is repeated for the other side. Since infants are obligate nasal breathers, that is, they cannot compensate for an occluded naris or vestibule by mouth breathing, the examiner must be certain that both nasal passageways are un-obstructed. Flaring of the ala nasi normally accompanies vigorous crying but signifies respiratory distress in noncrying babies.

During childhood the tonsils, like other lymphoid tissue, respond readily to contact with pathogens. Consequently, tonsillar tissue is frequently enlarged, although clients are asymptomatic. As long as tonsillar hypertrophy is asymptomatic and does not impede the passage of air in the pharynx, it is considered a variation of normal. The tonsils decrease in size after puberty (Table 9-6).

Adolescence

As mentioned previously, part of the stage of mixed dentition occurs in adolescence. This is usually less traumatic than the eruption of the deciduous teeth; however, occasionally the eruption of the third molars (wisdom teeth) is problematic. A common problem is impaction of the third molars. When an orderly sequence of primary tooth loss and permanent tooth replacement occurs, the mouth usually accommo-

Table 9-6.   Selected Abnormalities of the Mouth, Pharynx, Nose, and Sinuses

Finding	Condition	Explanation
Large tongue (macroglossia)	Cretinism, Down's syndrome, Hurler's syndrome	Tongue is hypertrophic or protrudes due to genetic disorder.
Fissured, raw angle of lip	Perleche	Children who drool or lick their lips cause maceration of the mucous membrane, resulting in infection, usually with Candida albicans.
Erythematous, edematous fungiform papillae mixed with smaller white filiform papillae (strawberry tongue)	Scarlet fever	Classic enanthem of scarlet fever, which occurs on day 2 or 3 of the illness. Sometimes occurs in measles (rubeola) and other febrile illnesses.
Desquamated, beefy, red filiform papillae with edematous fungiform papillae (raspberry tongue)	Scarlet fever	Classic enanthem of scarlet fever on day 6 or 7. Sometimes occurs in other febrile illnesses.
Small red spots around bluish-white centers on the oral mucosa, especially near the molars (Koplik spots)	Measles (rubeola)	Enanthem of rubeola, which occurs within 9 to 14 days. Occurs prior to exanthem (rash).
Ulcers on tongue and oral mucosa	Hand, foot, and mouth disease	Coxsackie A 5, 10, and 16 viruses cause this enanthem, which occurs simultaneously with characteristic exanthem.
Cleft lip or palate	Congenital anomaly	Failure of closure of lip or palate during fetal development.
Edematous, inflamed Stenson's duct	Mumps or other parotid gland infection	Inflammation of parotid gland results in inflammation of its duct.
Teeth with flattened edges	Teeth grinding (Bruxism)	Children suffering from nervousness, stress, and tension frequently grind their teeth during sleep.
Mottled, stained teeth	Excessive fluoride ingestion Administration of tetracycline under age 10, including to mother while fetus was in utero	Chemical interference with enamel formation.
Decay of teeth	Dental caries	Children prone to caries are those who take a bottle with milk or juice to bed, children with genetic predispositioin to caries, those who practice poor oral hygiene, and those with diets high in sugar and low in calcium.
Foul-smelling breath or nasal discharge	Foreign body lodged in nose	Presence of foreign body causes local inflammatory reaction resulting in transudation of pus into the nasal cavity.
Excoriated, ulcerated ala nasi	Persistent rhinitis	Constant "runny nose" causes maceration and excoriation of ala nasi.

dates adequately. However, when this sequence is disrupted by tooth loss or genetic factors, improper permanent dentition results. This most frequently is manifest as malocclusion, which is often discovered during adolescence and corrected with braces (orthodontics). The complete oral examination with emphasis on the assessment of the teeth and gingivae is essential since many clients do not practice adequate oral hygiene while wearing braces.

A normal condition characterized by gingival enlargement is termed pubertal gingivitis. The gums have an intensified reddened color, bleed easily, and are hypertrophic between the teeth and where their free margins cover the teeth. It is thought to be associated with hormonal changes during puberty.

Pregnancy

The examination of the pregnant woman is similar to that of other adults with the exception of one additional normal variation. A condition called pregnancy gingivitis exists and appears like pubertal gingivitis. It also is due to hormonal changes.

Late Adulthood

As the teeth age, the enamel is abraded and the underlying dentin thickens; therefore, the teeth appear yellowish or grayish-yellow. With advancing age, the gingival tissues tend to recede, which causes the free gingival margin to move toward the root and away from the crown. Whereas the gingivae of the primary and mixed dentition appear less pigmented than the early permanent dentition, the gingivae of the normal elderly client are more uniformly and more darkly pigmented.

Since there is only one set of permanent teeth, aging is associated with increased loss of teeth from caries and periodontal disease. Failing eyesight and failing dexterity are often responsible for deterioration in oral hygiene among many of the aging. Two other factors that contribute to changes in the oral tissues are decreased mobility and financial strain imposed by fixed income, which results in infrequent dental prophylaxis and delayed treatment of correctable conditions.

Similar to the overall trend toward osteoporosis, the resorption of alveolar bone predominates over bone formation, and there is a gradual decrease in the height and width of the alveolar ridge. This is particularly apparent among edentulous persons who wear dentures. As the alveolar ridge decreases in size, the fit of the dentures becomes poorer, and the dentures slide and cause discomfort. This predisposes toward mechanical irritation of the gingivae and resultant inflammation. Poor fitting dentures are also less efficient for mastication.

In addition, decreased mucus secretion and atrophy of the epithelium of the oral mucosa reduce the fit of dentures and resilience of the tissues (Table 9-7).

Table 9-7.   Selected Abnormalities Associated with Dentures

Finding	Condition	Explanation
Flap or roll of tissue on alveolar ridges where dentures rest	Denture hyperplasia	Inflammatory response to denture trauma.
Inflamed, edematous, ecchymotic mucosa under denture	Denture stomatitis	Can result from rough denture fitting surface or poor adaptation of the mucosal tissues to the dentures. Frequently infection with Candida albicans occurs in affected area.

Anatomy and Physiology

The thorax is a cone-shaped, semirigid cage that surrounds the heart and lungs. The cage is constructed of bone, cartilage, and muscle. The bony portions include the thoracic vertebrae, ribs, and sternum, all of which function to protect the heart and lungs and serve as the structural framework for the thorax.

The 12 thoracic vertebrae are irregularly shaped bones in the posterior wall of the thorax. The 12 pairs of ribs are flat, arched bones connected directly to the thoracic vertebrae at a 45-degree angle. The costal cartilages are bars of hyaline cartilage that prolong the ribs anteriorly and add to the elasticity of the chest wall. Only the first 7 ribs are considered true ribs since they are vertebrosternal; they originate from the vertebrae posteriorly and arch anteriorly, and their costal cartilages articulate with the sternum. Ribs 8, 9, and 10 are vertebrochondral; they originate from the vertebrae posteriorly and arch anteriorly, but their costal cartilages join the cartilage of the rib above it. Ribs 11 and 12 are vertebral or floating ribs since their costal cartilages do not connect to anything at the anterior ends (Figure 10-1).

The sternum is a flat bone in the anterior midline of the chest. It has three parts: the manubrium, body, and xiphoid cartilage (Figure 10-1). The junction of the manubrium and body form a bony ridge, sometimes called the sternal angle or angle of Louis, and the second rib articulates with the sternum at this point.

In between the ribs are the intercostal spaces. These spaces take the number of the ribs above them and contain two layers of muscle fibers: the external intercostals and the internal intercostals. The external intercostal muscles are muscles of inspiration. Their contraction elevates the anterior end of each rib, which increases the anterior-posterior diameter of the thorax. The internal intercostal muscles contract mainly during forced expiration and pull the ribs down and in. Although they are not major muscles during quiet breathing, they do play a role in a smooth transition from inspiration to expiration.

The accessory muscles of respiration are the scalene, sternocleidomastoid, trapezius, and pectoralis. These muscles are not normally active during quiet breathing but help to elevate the chest wall to its greatest diameter during forced breathing.

The diaphragm, the principal muscle of respiration, is a dome-shaped muscle that separates the thoracic and abdominal cavities. The center portion of the dome points upward toward the lungs, since intra-

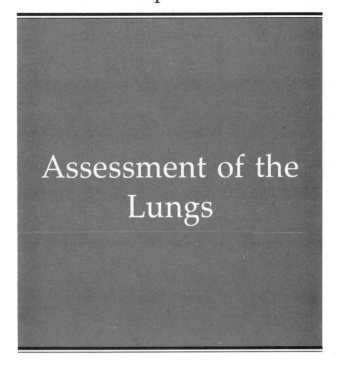

Chapter 10

Assessment of the Lungs

Objectives

The examiner will be able to do the following:

1. Inspect the thorax and respiratory pattern
2. Palpate the posterior thorax to determine respiratory excursion and fremitus
3. Percuss the thorax
4. Auscultate the lungs
5. Measure lung volumes and capacities
6. Recognize abnormalities of the thorax and lungs
7. Record the information obtained

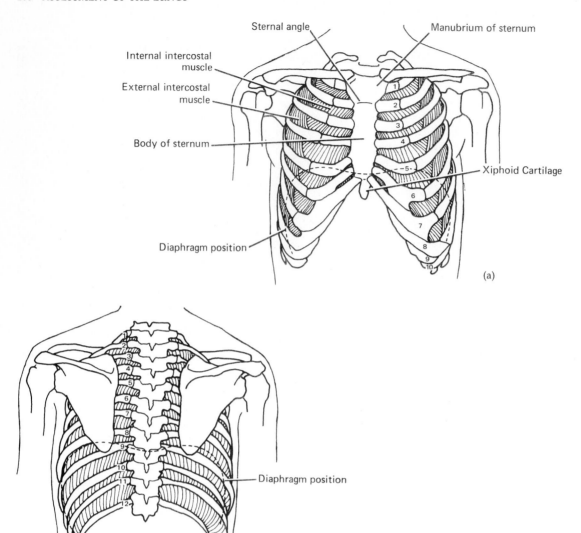

Sternal angle

Manubrium of sternum

Internal intercostal muscle

External intercostal muscle

Body of sternum

Xiphoid Cartilage

Diaphragm position

(a)

Diaphragm position

(b)

Figure 10-1. *Thoracic cage: (a) anterior; (b) posterior.*

abdominal pressure is greater than intrathoracic pressure. Contraction of the diaphragm pulls the dome downward and the superior inferior diameter of the thoracic cavity enlarges. In the posterior chest, the top of the diaphragm is at the 10th thoracic vertebra (T-10) on expiration and the 12th thoracic vertebra (T-12) on a deep inspiration. In the lateral chest it is at the 8th rib at the midaxillary line; in the anterior chest the diaphragm is at the 5th rib at the right midclavicular line and the 6th rib at the left midclavicular line (Figure 10-1).

Within the thorax are the lungs, which are responsible for the exchange of gases between the environment and the blood. The lungs are conical in shape, porous, and highly elastic. They lie freely within the pleural sac except where they are attached by their roots to the bronchi, blood vessels, and pulmonary ligaments. The pleural sac is a serous membrane cov-

ering the lung. It has two layers (the visceral and parietal membranes), with a potential space between them, the pleural cavity. The visceral layer adheres to the lung and actually forms its surface; the parietal layer adheres to the chest wall (Figure 10-2).

Air reaches and leaves the lungs by the tracheobronchial tree. The tracheobronchial tree comprises the trachea (Chapter 6), left and right main bronchi, bronchioles, and alveoli. The trachea extends from the larynx to the manubrosternal junction (angle of Louis) anteriorly and T-5 posteriorly, where it bifurcates into the left and right main bronchi. The left bronchus is approximately 5 centimeters long from its origin to its first branch. It appears to be a branch of the trachea and joins it at a 45-degree angle. The right bronchus (2.5 cm. long) is wider and shorter than the left and appears to be an extension of the trachea. It joins the trachea at a 25-degree angle. Both

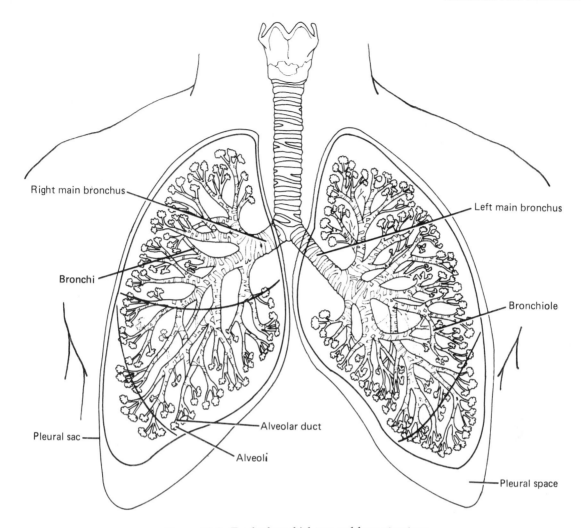

Figure 10-2. *Tracheobronchial tree and lung structure.*

bronchi branch into smaller bronchi, then bronchioles, alveolar ducts, and finally alveoli, where the gaseous exchange between the external environment and the blood occurs. There are over 300 million alveoli in the adult lung.

In the anterior chest the lungs extend from 2.5 centimeters above the middle third of the clavicle to the sixth rib at the midclavicular line. In the lateral chest the lung extends from the apex of the axilla to the eighth rib at the midaxillary line. In the posterior chest the lungs extend from T-1 to T-10 on expiration, and to T-12 on a deep inspiration (Figure 10-3).

The left lung has two lobes, and the right lung, three lobes. The upper and lower lobes of the left lung are separated by the left oblique or diagonal fissure. It begins at T-3 posteriorly and proceeds downward and laterally to the midaxillary line at the 5th rib. The fissure continues anteriorly and terminates at the 6th rib at the midclavicular line (Figure 10-3).

The right lung has three lobes—the upper, middle, and lower lobes—but the middle lobe is present only in the anterior portion of the chest. The right oblique or diagonal fissure separates the upper and lower lobes in the posterior and lateral chest, and the middle and lower lobes in the anterior chest. It begins at T-3 posteriorly and proceeds downward and laterally to the midaxillary line at the 5th rib. The fissure continues anteriorly and terminates at the 6th rib at the midclavicular line. In the anterior chest the upper and middle lobes are separated by the horizontal fissure. It begins at the 5th rib slightly posterior to the midaxillary line and proceeds anteriorly along the third intercostal space to the right sternal border (Figure 10-3).

The lobes of each lung are divided further into bronchopulmonary segments, which consist of a group of alveoli that are supplied by a branch of the bronchi and are not separated by fissures (Table 10-1).

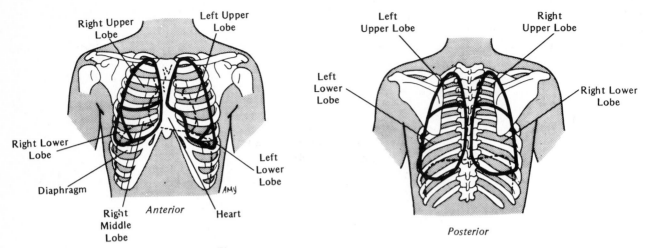

Figure 10-3. *Placement of lungs within the thorax.*

Respiration

Respiration is divided into two processes, internal and external. Internal respiration is the exchange of oxygen and carbon dioxide between the external environment and the blood. External respiration is the process of breathing, which occurs in two phases: inspiration and expiration.

Inspiration is an active muscular process. The chest cage enlarges primarily from the contraction of the diaphragm and secondarily from the external intercostal muscles. With this muscular contraction, the lungs expand to fill the enlarged chest cage. Approximately 500 milliliters of air is sucked into the lungs since air pressure in the lungs is slightly less than atmospheric air pressure. During inspiration, oxygen diffuses into the blood in the alveolar capillaries. Expiration is a passive process from the relaxation of the muscles of respiration. This decreases the size of the chest cage, the lungs recoil, and approximately 500 milliliters of air are pushed out, since the air pressure in the lungs is slightly more than atmospheric air pressure. During expiration, carbon dioxide diffuses into the alveoli and is expired into the external environment.

Forced expiration employs the abdominal and internal intercostal muscles. The abdominal muscles compress the abdominal contents and force the diaphragm up, thereby greatly reducing the superoinferior diameter of the thorax. The lateral and anteroposterior diameters are reduced by the action of the internal intercostal muscles.

The rhythmicity of the respiratory cycle is maintained by nerve reflex control centers in the brain stem. In normal breathing, inspiration takes approximately 2 seconds and expiration takes approximately 3 seconds. Both are shortened in rapid breathing and lengthened in very slow breathing.

The respiratory center is a group of dispersed cells in the brain stem; these affect the nerves that stimulate the muscles of inspiration. The respiratory center is stimulated by a rise in carbonic acid (the circulating form of carbon dioxide) in the cerebral spinal fluid, which causes an increased depth and rate of respirations.

There are also peripheral chemoreceptors located on the aortic arch; these specialized neural bundles are sensitive to changes in the oxygen supply and carbonic acid. If the oxygen supply decreases or carbonic acid increases, the respiratory center is stimulated and is followed by an increased depth and rate of respiration.

There are elastic fibers throughout the lungs that are stretched by inflation. When the lungs exert a pull

Table 10-1.   The Bronchopulmonary Segments

Right Upper Lobe	Right Middle Lobe	Right Lower Lobe	Left Upper Lobe	Left Lower Lobe
Apical	Lateral	Superior	Apical-posterior	Superior
Posterior	Medial	Medial basal	Anterior	Anterior-medial-basal
Anterior		Anterior basal	Superior lingular	Lateral basal
		Lateral basal	Inferior lingular	Posterior basal
		Posterior basal		

on the stretch receptors, an impulse is sent to the respiratory center to end the inspiratory impulse. Expiration begins and the lungs recoil.

The lungs are freed of foreign matter by the action of the cilia and cough reflex. The respiratory passages of the nose, trachea, and lungs are lined with cilia that help in keeping the air passages clean. These cilia aid in moving mucus and foreign matter toward the pharynx. If the foreign matter is large or if the cilia are unable to remove it, the cough reflex is stimulated.

The cough reflex is necessary for life since it keeps foreign matter out of the lungs. The trachea and bronchi are easily irritated, which stimulates the cough reflex. This reflex causes a series of actions. Approximately 2.5 liters of air are inspired, the vocal cords shut, and the epiglottis closes to entrap the air in the lungs. The abdominal and expiratory muscles contract forcefully to increase greatly the pressure within the lungs. Then the vocal cords and epiglottis open wide and the 2.5 liters of air explode from the lungs, up the trachea, and out of the nose and mouth. It is possible for the air to move as fast as 75 to 100 miles per hour. Generally any foreign matter in the bronchi or trachea moves out with the exploding air.

Topographical Anatomy of the Chest

On the anterior chest there are three imaginary lines: the midsternal line and the right and left midclavicular lines. The midsternal line extends from the suprasternal notch to the xiphoid process, through the middle of the sternum. The midclavicular lines extend from the center of each clavicle to the end of the rib cage (Figure 10-4). The most accurate method for communicating findings on the anterior chest is the distance from the midsternal line on a particular rib or intercostal space. Although the midclavicular lines are helpful, they are not precise.

Other surface landmarks on the anterior chest include the right and left supraclavicular fossas, suprasternal notch, angle of Louis, and costal angle. The supraclavicular fossas are the depressed areas immediately above the clavicle. The apices of the lungs are beneath this area. The suprasternal notch is the soft, depressed area immediately above the manubrium. The angle of Louis or manubriosternal junction, is the raised ridge where the manubrium and sternum meet. Generally, in finding the angle of Louis, the suprasternal notch is palpated first, and the fingers continue downward over the manubrium until the ridge is felt, a few centimeters below the suprasternal notch. The flat bone lateral to the ridge is the second rib and its costal cartilage. The costal angle is formed by the costal cartilages of ribs 8, 9 and 10 joining with the xiphoid process. This angle is normally less than 90 degrees (Figure 10-4).

On the lateral chest there are three lines; the anterior axillary line, the midaxillary line, and the posterior axillary line. The anterior and posterior axillary lines are formed by the anterior and posterior axillary folds with the arm adjacent to the body. The midaxillary line is formed through the center of the apex of the axilla with the arm extended overhead (Figure 10-4).

On the posterior chest there are three imaginary lines: the midspinal, or midvertebral line, and the right and left midscapular lines. The midspinal line runs through the center of the spinous processes of the vertebra. The midscapular lines are vertical lines through the middle of the interior angle of the scapula (Figure 10-4). The most accurate method for communicating findings on the posterior chest is the distance from the midspinal line on a particular rib or intercostal space. Although the midscapular lines are helpful, they are not precise.

The only other landmark frequently used on the posterior chest is the vertebra prominens. The vertebra prominens is the prominent spinous process at the base of the neck with the head flexed. This is the location of C-7. If there are two prominent vertebrae, the superior one is C-7, and the inferior one, T-1. Since each rib originates from the thoracic vertebra, the posterior portion of the ribs is identified by first numbering the thoracic vertebra. This is easy to do for T-1, T-2, and T-3, since their spinous processes overlie their vertebral bodies. But beginning with T-4 the spinous processes are oblique and overlie the vertebral body below it. Therefore, the spinous process of T-4 overlies the vertebra of T-5 and the 5th rib, the spinous process of T-5 overlies the vertebra of T-6 and the 6th rib, etc. (Figure 10-4).

Assessment Modalities

Preparation

To begin the examination, the client sits upright. A person too ill to sit unaided is assisted into the upright position. If this is not possible, then the lateral and posterior chest is examined while the person lies in a lateral position. Male clients are disrobed to the waist, and female clients wear a short gown, which is removed for the actual examination.

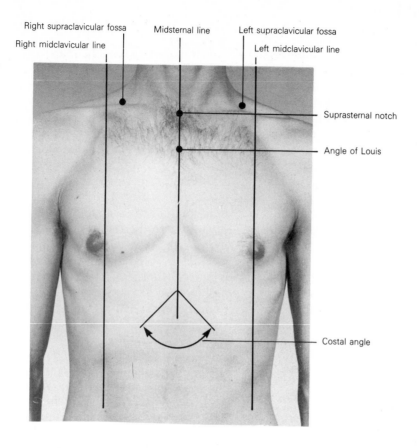

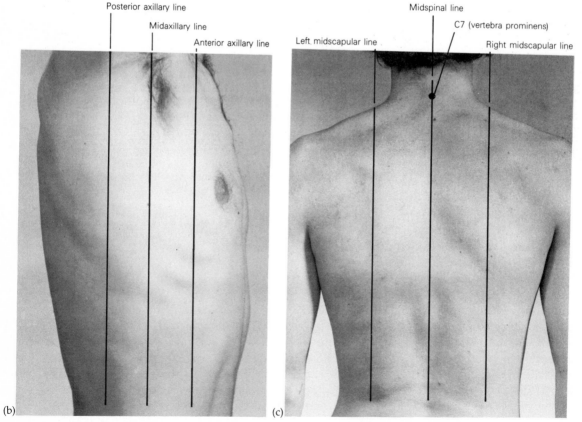

Figure 10-4. *Topographical anatomy of the chest: (a) anterior; (b) lateral; (c) posterior.*

The equipment necessary to assess the respiratory system includes a stethoscope with a diaphragm and a watch with a second hand.

After the client's history is obtained, the examiner proceeds with inspection, palpation, percussion, and auscultation. In any portion of the examination, the client serves as the control. That is, one side is compared with the other, from a superior to inferior direction over the anterior, lateral, and posterior thorax.

Inspection

The examiner begins with a subjective evaluation of the client's comfort or distress and color of the skin and proceeds to inspect the general shape of the thorax and respiratory pattern (Figure 10-5).

Although there is a wide variation in size and shape of chest contour, it is normally symmetrical and slightly convex with the anteroposterior (A-P) diameter less than the transverse diameter. The thoracic index, or ratio of the anterior-posterior diameter to the transverse diameter, ranges from 1:2 to 5:7, depending on the client's body build. The sternum is slightly depressed or level with the ribs, and the intercostal spaces are flat or slightly depressed with no bulging or retractions (Table 10-2). There is generally a slightly greater muscular development on the side of the dominant hand. For instance a right-handed person will have slightly greater muscular development on the right side and slightly less on the left side.

The rate, type and quality of respirations are observed during quiet and forced breathing. The respiratory rate in normal, quiet breathing is 12 to 20 respirations per minute (Table 10-3). The respiratory cycles are rhythmic, with inspiration slightly shorter than expiration. This regular rhythm is interrupted several times per hour with a sigh; a deep, quiet, inspiration. The ratio of the respiratory rate to the heart rate is 1:4. The chest moves in a symmetrical and synchronous manner.

After the respiratory pattern during quiet breathing is observed, the client is instructed to take several deep breaths. The chest movement should be more exaggerated than in quiet breathing. The chest moves symmetrically with no bulging of the intercostal spaces, retractions, or use of the accessory muscles of breathing, although the accessory muscles are normally used for prolonged heavy breathing during exercise.

Palpation

Palpation is performed for respiratory excursion and fremitus. Respiratory excursion is the expansion of the chest wall during a forced inspiration and expiration, generally 5 to 8 centimeters. Fremitus is a vibration produced by the passage of air through the tracheobronchial tree. When the vibrations are heard,

Table 10-2. Selected Abnormalities of Chest Contour

Finding	Description	Possible Conditions
Bulging on intercostal spaces	On expiration the intercostal spaces protrude farther forward than the ribs. Results from difficulty in expiring air from the lungs.	Chronic pulmonary disease, pleural effusion, tension pneumothorax
Retractions	A drawing back of the abdominal, intercostal, or supraclavicular muscles during inspiration. Can include any of the groups of muscles mentioned.	Airway obstruction (tumor, foreign body, secretions, chronic lung disease)
Barrel chest	Increased A-P diameter of the chest, which approaches the size of the transverse chest.	Chronic pulmonary disease
Pigeon breast (chicken breast, pectus carinatum)	Sternum protrudes farther forward than ribs. Increased A-P diameter and decreased transverse diameter of the thorax. Anterior thorax looks like a chicken breast.	Idiopathic rickets
Funnel breast (pectus excavatum)	Sternum depressed below ribs, or ribs extend farther forward than sternum.	Idiopathic rickets
Kyphosis	Excessive curvature of the spine with abnormal thoracic convexity.	Poliomyelitis, Pagets disease, osteoarthritis of the spine, tuberculosis of the spine, osteoporosis
Scoliosis	Lateral curvature of the spine.	Rheumatoid spondylitis, tuberculosis of the spine, idiopathic scoliosis

Table 10-3. Types of Respirations

Type	Definition	Spirogram
Normal	Quiet, rhythmic respirations with a rate of 12-20 per minute.	
Apnea	Temporary cessation of respiration.	
Ataxic	Gross irregularity of rate, rhythm, and depth.	
Bradypnea	Abnormal slowing of respiration.	
Cheyne Stokes	Gradual increase in depth and sometimes rate of respirations, followed by a gradual decrease that results in apnea. Cycles vary in length from 30 seconds to 1 minute.	
Dyspnea	Subjective difficulty in breathing.	
Kussmaul	Exaggerated depth of respirations.	
Sigh	A deep inspiration that interrupts the normal respiratory rhythm.	
Tachypnea	Increased respiratory rate.	

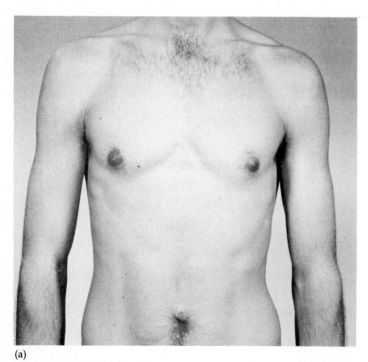
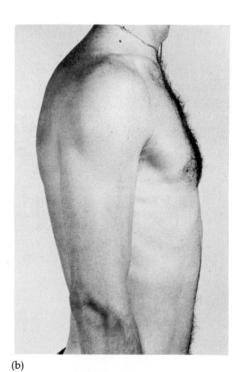

(a)　　　　　　　　　　　　　　　　(b)

Figure 10-5. Normal chest configuration: (a) anterior; (b) lateral.

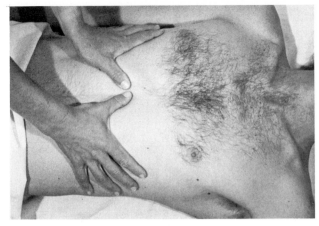

(a)

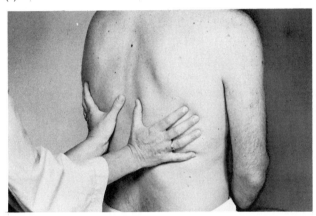

(b)

Figure 10-6. Palpation of respiratory excursion: (a) anterior; (b) posterior.

they are called vocal fremitus. When palpated, they are called tactile fremitus.

Assessment of respiratory movement is done on either the anterolateral or posterolateral chest. The greatest range of motion is felt on the anterior chest.

In palpating respiratory movement on the anterior chest, the client is supine with the examiner's hands palms down and placed lightly on the client's lower anterolateral chest. The examiner's thumbs are along the costal margin pointing toward the client's head with the fingers extended across the anterolateral chest (Figure 10-6). The client is then instructed to take several deep breaths; the amount of movement and symmetry of expansion is observed with each respiration. The thumbs move apart during inspiration and together during expiration. The symmetry of expansion is evident by the rise and fall of the examiner's hands.

In palpating respiratory movement on the posterior chest, the client assumes a sitting position. The examiner places his hands on the lower chest at approximately the 10th rib. The thumbs are parallel to the spine and point toward the head; the fingers extend to the lateral rib cage (Figure 10-6). As with the anterior chest, the client is instructed to take several deep breaths; the symmetry of expansion and distance of movement between the thumbs are observed with each respiration. The thumbs move only if the hands are lightly placed on the chest wall. If the pressure from the hands is too great, the symmetry of expansion may be palpated, but the thumbs will not glide apart on inspiration. (Table 10-4).

Tactile fremitus is palpable on all healthy clients. The normal varies greatly due to several factors: chest wall thickness, voice pitch, and the position of the bronchi in relationship to the chest wall. Generally, thin clients have more fremitus, and obese and muscular clients have less fremitus. Also, lower-pitched voices produce more fremitus, while higher-pitched voices produce less fremitus. In addition, the closer the bronchi are to the chest wall, the greater the fremitus is.

Table 10-4.   Selected Abnormalities of Respiratory Movement on Palpation

Finding	Description	Conditions
Decreased respiratory movement	Barely perceptible chest wall movement (expands less than 3.5 cm. during inspiration). Due to the inability to take a deep inspiration.	Acute pleurisy Chest pain Chest trauma
	Since the lung does not expand, the chest wall does not expand. If only one lung is affected, the respiratory excursion is asymmetrical.	Consolidation Fibrosis Atelectasis Pneumothorax
	Associated with a rigid, maximally expanded chest wall.	Chronic obstructive pulmonary disease
Asymmetrical respiratory movement	Asymmetrical movement of the examiner's hands during inspiration and expiration since the two lungs do not expand symmetrically.	Pneumonectomy Constrictive disease of only one lung or unequal disease involvement of both lungs

Before palpating fremitus, the examiner instructs the client to say "1-2-3, 99," or "blue moon." It is important for each syllable to be said with the same pitch and intensity. If the examiner has difficulty palpating fremitus, the client is instructed to speak in a louder and deeper voice.

As the client recites the syllables, the examiner palpates corresponding parts of the chest wall with the palmar or ulnar aspects of both hands, the ulnar aspect of both fists, or the palmar aspects of the fingertips. The examiner proceeds in a superior to inferior direction (Figure 10-7). The greatest intensity of fremitus is felt on the anterior and posterior chest at the base of the neck, along the trachea, and overlying the major bronchi since they are in close proximity to the chest wall. The least intensity of fremitus is felt at the lung bases and over the scapulae. Over the lung bases there are only very small airways relatively far from the chest wall. Since the scapulae increase the thickness of the chest wall at their location, fremitus is not easily palpable there (Tables 10-5, 10-6).

The other forms of fremitus are palpated in the same manner as vocal fremitus (Table 10-6).

Percussion

Percussion is performed to assess the density of normal and abnormal chest structures and to determine diaphragmatic excursion. Mediate percussion is used to assess the lungs (Chapter 2). The examiner places the pleximeter firmly against the chest wall in the intercostal spaces and parallel to the ribs. Only the distal phalanx touches the chest wall. The palm of the hand and the remaining fingers are kept off the chest wall to avoid damping of the percussion sound (Figure 10-8).

The examiner percusses the anterior chest first, beginning in the supraclavicular fossa and continuing with each intercostal space of the rib cage. Also, the two sides of the chest are compared at each level, so that the client functions as a control. In female clients the breasts are displaced as necessary.

Resonance is the sound normally heard over most of the lung; however, hyperresonance may be a normal finding in very thin individuals. On the left side, percussion over the heart produces a dull sound. It is generally at the second or third intercostal space at the left sternal line and extends to the fifth intercostal space at the midclavicular line. The examiner continues percussing until stomach tympany is elicited.

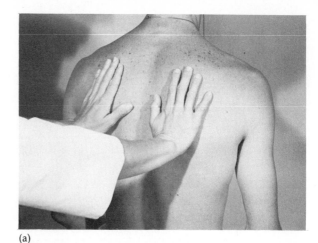

(a)

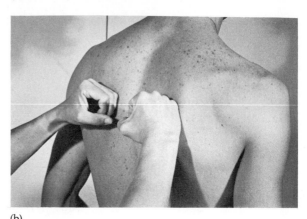

(b)

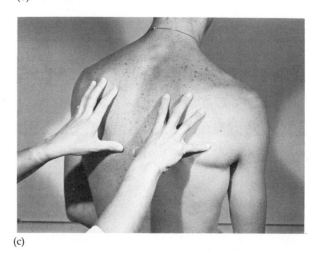

(c)

Figure 10-7. *Palpation of fremitus: (a) palmar aspects of both hands; (b) ulnar aspects of both fists; (c) palmar aspects of fingertips.*

On the right chest, the liver produces a dull sound. This dullness extends from about the fourth intercostal space to about the sixth intercostal space in the midclavicular line. Below the sixth intercostal space, the sound is hyperresonant because of the gas-filled intestines and no liver (Figure 10-9).

Table 10-5. Selected Abnormal Variations in Vocal Fremitus

Finding	Description	Possible Conditions
Increased vocal fremitus	Chest wall vibrates more than usual upon phonation since a solid tissue with elasticity conducts vibrations better than a porous tissue.	Consolidated lungs as in pneumonia, lung tumor, or pulmonary fibrosis
Decreased to absent vocal fremitus	Chest wall vibrates less than usual upon phonation. A nonelastic solid medium decreases sound conduction.	Pleural fibrosis
	Adds another medium through which the vibration must pass before it reaches the chest wall. This decreases the intensity of the vibration. Also a liquid or air medium does not conduct sound vibrations as well as a porous medium.	Fluid or air in pleural space
	Causes decreased sound production and therefore less air vibrates throughout the respiratory tree.	Obstruction of major bronchi

Table 10-6. Other Forms of Fremitus

Finding	Description	Possible Conditions
Tussive	Palpable vibrations on the chest wall that are produced by coughing.	Upper respiratory tract infection
Rhonchal fremitus	Palpable coarse vibrations on the chest wall that are produced by a narrowing of the major airways from either stenosis or thick secretions. Vibrations produced from secretions may decrease after a productive cough.	Secretions in the large airways (bronchitis, pneumonia)
Pleural friction rub	Palpable vibrations on the chest wall that are produced by the rubbing together of the inflamed and roughened surfaces of the pleura. Sometimes it is best felt in the inferior anterolateral portion of the chest since this is the area of greatest thoracic excursion. The examiner feels a grating sensation that is synchronous with both inspiration and expiration. Sometimes it is felt only on inspiration.	Pleuritis
Crepitations (subcutaneous emphysema)	Palpable coarse, crackling vibrations on the chest wall that are produced from pressure on the subcutaneous tissue. This causes a movement of fine beads of air in the subcutaneous tissue. It is sometimes possible for the crackling to be heard.	Injury or surgery of the thorax that allows air to escape from the respiratory tract into the subcutaneous tissue (tracheotomy, chest tubes, any surgery on the lung)

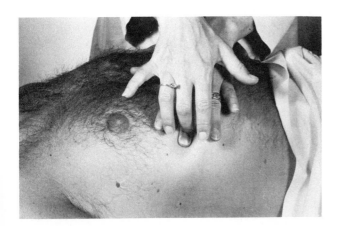

Figure 10-8. *Chest percussion.*

After the anterior chest is percussed, the client's hands are placed upon the head, which facilitates percussion of the right and left lateral chest walls. Normal lung resonance is heard from the apex of the axillae to the costal margins at the seventh intercostal spaces in the midaxillary lines (Figure 10-9).

For percussing the posterior chest, the client leans forward with the head flexed and forearms crossed at the waist. This separates the scapulae and maximizes percussion of the posterior lungs. The apex of the lung is percussed first by identifying the 5 centimeter band of resonance across the shoulders (Figure 10-9). The examiner begins at the neck along the superior border of the trapezius and percusses from the side of the neck to the shoulder until the flat sound changes to a resonant sound. Then the shoulder is percussed

Table 10-7.   Selected Abnormalities in Percussion

Finding	Possible Conditions	Explanation
Hyperresonant sound over lung fields	Emphysema	Air trapping and loss of elasticity in the lung produce a hyperresonant sound.
	Pneumothorax	Presence of air in the pleural cavity produces a hyperresonant sound.
Dull percussion sound over lung fields	Pneumonia with consolidation Atelectasis Large tumor Pulmonary edema	Diseased area of lung is more solid, which produces a dull percussion sound. A mass needs to be over 3 cm. in diameter to produce percussion changes.
Dull percussion sound over lung fields that changes with a change of position, shifting dullness.	Pleural effusion	A fluid-filled pleural space of greater than 250 ml, which responds to the striking blow with a dull sound. With a change in position, the fluid moves to the lowermost area; therefore, the dullness shifts. Fremitus is decreased in this area.
Decreased diaphragmatic excursion	Bronchitis Emphysema Respiratory depression	Diaphragmatic excursion of less than 3 cm. since the diaphragm is not moving more than this on inspiration and expiration.

in the direction of the neck until the flat sound changes to a resonant sound.

Each intercostal space is then percussed. The posterior chest is less resonant than the anterior chest due to increased muscular development. One side is compared with the other until the normal resonance becomes dull from percussing beyond the lower lung borders. At this point the diaphragmatic excursion is percussed (Table 10-7).

Diaphragmatic excursion is the movement of the diaphragm during a forced inspiration and expiration. In measuring it, the client is instructed to take a deep breath and hold it. At this time the examiner percusses the lower margin of resonance on the posterior chest. The diaphragm is located where the sound changes from resonance to dullness. A mark is made on the client's chest; the client is instructed to exhale as deeply as possible and hold it. The lower margin of resonance is again percussed and a mark is made on the posterior chest. This procedure is then repeated on the other side of the posterior chest. The distance between the two lines is the diaphragmatic excursion. Normal diaphragmatic excursion is 3 to 6 centimeters and is often slightly higher on the right due to the liver (Table 10-7, Figure 10-10).

Auscultation

In auscultation, the examiner listens to air movement throughout the chest with the diaphragm of the stethoscope.

The client is instructed to take deep, slow breaths through the mouth. Breathing through the nose pro-

duces unwanted noise; breathing too fast may produce hyperventilation with dizziness and lightheadedness. The examiner auscultates in a superior to inferior direction over the anterior, lateral, and posterior chest, listening to a minimum of one respiratory cycle at each location. The examiner then compares the location where lung sounds cease with where vocal fremitus ceases and the percussion note changes from resonance to dullness. All of these sounds should be at the same level and correspond with the lung borders.

The normal breath sounds heard over the chest wall are vesicular, bronchial (tubular), and bronchovesicular (Figure 10-11). These sounds differ according to the relative duration of inspiration and expiration, pitch and intensity.

Vesicular breath sounds are produced by air moving in and out of the alveoli. They are soft, low-pitched whishing sounds heard over most of the lung. The inspiratory phase is slightly longer than the expiratory phase. Sometimes these breath sounds are simply referred to as normal breath sounds.

Bronchial, or tubular, breath sounds are sounds produced by air moving through the trachea and are loud, high-pitched sounds heard over the upper portion of the anterior chest in the midline. The expiratory phase is slightly longer and louder than the inspiratory phase.

Bronchovesicular breath sounds are a combination of bronchial and vesicular breath sounds. These sounds are produced by air moving through the large bronchi and are moderately loud, medium-pitched sounds. They are heard over the manubrium and large bronchi in the anterior chest, and in the interscapular area in the posterior chest. The inspiratory

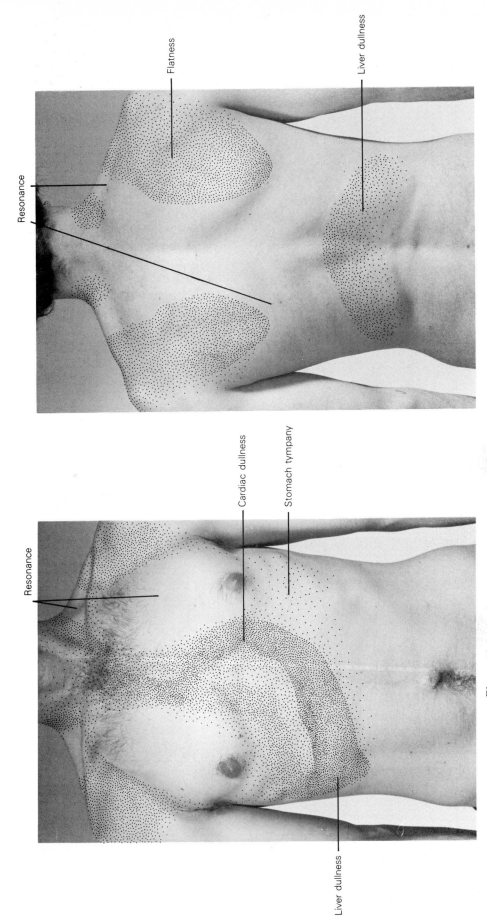

Figure 10-9. *Surface projection of normal percussion sounds.*

Resonance

Flatness

Liver dullness

Cardiac dullness

Stomach tympany

Liver dullness

Resonance

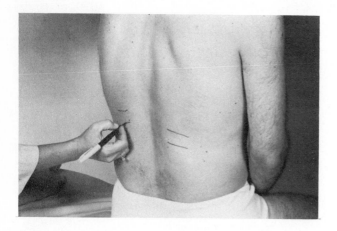

Figure 10-10. *Percussion of diaphragmatic excursion.*

Voice sounds are transmitted to the chest wall and can be auscultated with a stethoscope. Normally, voice sounds are muffled nondistinct syllables, but they are altered in a variety of chest diseases (Table 10-10). These sounds are elicited by having the client say "99, 1–2–3," or "e–e–e."

Lung Volumes and Lung Capacities

Lung volumes and lung capacities are important screening devices in the early detection of pulmonary disease. They are measured whenever there are abnormal findings in the physical examination, such as decreased respiratory excursion, diaphragmatic excursion, or breath sounds. By measuring lung volumes and capacities, the quantity of air flowing through the respiratory system can be documented. These measurements also are used to evaluate the effect of respiratory therapy and progression of a diseased state.

Lung volumes are primary compartments. When two or more volumes are combined, they are referred to as lung capacities (Figure 10-12, Table 10-11). The standard lung volumes are tidal volume (TV), inspiratory reserve volume (IRV), expiratory reserve volume (ERV), and residual volume (RV).

Tidal volume is the amount of air inhaled *or* exhaled during *quiet* breathing, and is approximately 500 milliliters of air. The client is instructed to take normal breaths; the examiner measures three to five inspirations or expirations with the spirometer. The average volume is used.

Inspiratory reserve volume is the additional volume of air that can be inspired above the normal tidal volume. It is approximately 3,000 milliliters of air. The client is instructed to inhale normally, then not to

and expiratory phases are equal in duration and loudness.

Bronchovesicular and bronchial breath sounds are normally heard only in the areas mentioned. If they are heard over other areas of the lung, they are abnormal sounds. (Table 10-8).

Adventitious breath sounds are abnormal sounds superimposed upon the normal breath sounds. Great confusion exists in the terms used to identify these sounds. Often the same term is used to describe different sounds. In recent years attempts have been made to make the terms more descriptive and accurate. In general, adventitious sounds arising from within the lungs are divided into two broad categories: continuous and discontinuous sounds. A third category arises from the roughened visceral and parietal pleura and are called pleural friction rubs (Table 10-9).

Table 10-8. Selected Abnormal Breath Sounds

Finding	*Description*	*Possible Conditions*
Decreased breath sounds	Breath sounds are normal but faint, even when the client takes very deep breaths through an open mouth.	Decreased air flow though the respiratory tree (bronchial obstruction, muscular weakness), increased thickness of the chest wall (obesity), or fluid separating the lungs from the chest wall (pleural effusion)
Absent breath sounds	No breath sounds are heard since the impediment to air flow through the respiratory tree is so great that no air is flowing.	Airway obstruction
Increased breath sounds, bronchovesicular or bronchial breath sounds in an abnormal location	Abnormally loud breath sounds heard over diseased areas.	Consolidation of lung tissue as in pneumonia. Chronic Obstructive Pulmonary Disease

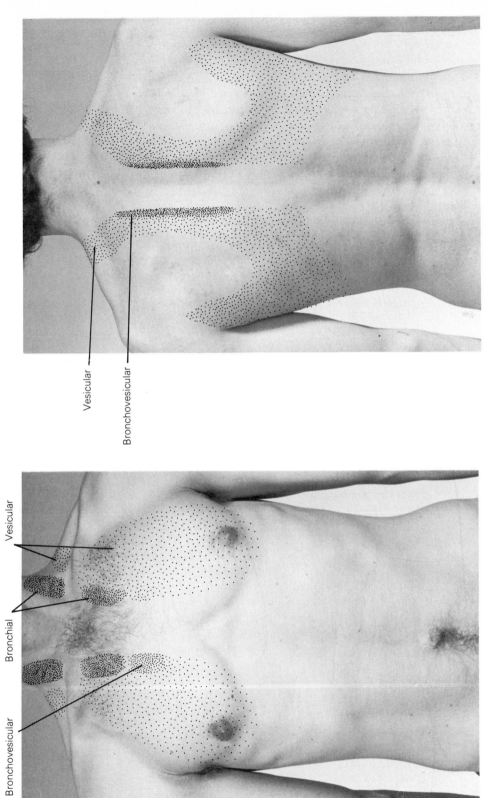

Vesicular

Bronchovesicular

Vesicular

Bronchial

Bronchovesicular

Figure 10-11. Surface projection of normal breath sounds.

173

Table 10-9.   Adventitious Breath Sounds

Finding	Description	Possible Conditions
Discontinuous sounds (rales, crackles)	These sounds are produced by air movement through fluid-filled alveoli. These crackling or bubbling sounds often are exaggerated with deep breathing and are not cleared by coughing. Rales occur during inspiration and expiration, although they are often heard only on inspiration. These sounds can be further defined as fine, medium, or coarse, but this classification is very subjective and often inadequate. Fine rales are soft, crackling noises heard generally at the end of inspiration, while medium rales are louder and often occur in early or midinspiration. Coarse rales are the loudest, have a more bubbling quality, and occur most often in expiration, although they can occur during inspiration.	Pulmonary edema, emphysema, pneumonia, atelectasis
Continuous sounds Rhonchi	These sounds are the result of a partial bronchial obstruction from secretions. These coarse, low-pitched sounds are heard during inspiration and expiration but may be heard on inspiration only. The sounds may decrease or disappear after coughing.	Bronchitis, emphysema, pneumonia
Wheezes	These sounds are the result of a partial bronchial obstruction from a narrowed airway. They are high-pitched, musical sounds occurring during inspiration and expiration, but they may be heard on inspiration only.	Asthma attack, tumor, foreign body
Pleural friction rubs	These sounds result from the inflamed pleural surfaces rubbing together to produce a grating sound. These sounds are unaffected by coughing and are heard during inspiration and expiration, although they are usually loudest at the end of inspiration. Pleural friction rubs can be heard over the entire chest, but are heard most frequently over the lower lateral and anterior chest wall where chest motion is greatest.	Pleuritis

exhale but to inhale as much additional air as possible through the spirometer.

The expiratory reserve volume is the additional volume of air that can be expired after the end of a normal tidal volume. It is approximately 1,100 milliliters of air. The client is instructed to exhale normally, then to blow out as much additional air as possible through the spirometer.

The residual volume is the amount of air remaining in the lungs after a forceful expiration and is approximately 1,200 milliliters of air. Residual volume cannot be measured by direct spirometry but requires indirect methods performed by pulmonary specialists.

The standard lung capacities are the inspiratory capacity (IC), inspiratory vital capacity (IVC), vital ca-

Table 10-10.   Altered Voice Sounds

Finding	Description	Possible Conditions
Bronchophony	Increased loudness and clarity of the spoken voice. Associated with increased vocal fremitus, dullness to percussion and bronchial breath sounds.	Consolidation
Whispered pectoriloquy	Increased loudness and clarity of the whispered voice. Is a form of exaggerated bronchophony. Normally whispered words cannot be heard on auscultation of the lungs.	Consolidation
Egophony (e to a changes)	Spoken e sounds like an a on auscultation of the lungs. A modified form of bronchophony. Normally, the spoken e–e–e is heard as a muffled e–e–e, but with consolidation it is heard as a rather nasal a–a–a.	Consolidation

pacity (VC), functional residual capacity (FRC), and total lung capacity (TLC).

Inspiratory capacity is the sum of the tidal volume and inspiratory reserve volume (approximately 3,500 milliliters). It is the amount of air that a person can forcibly inhale, beginning at the *normal* expiratory level and then inflating the lungs fully. The client is instructed to take a normal breath and at the end of expiration to take as deep a breath as possible through the spirometer.

Inspiratory vital capacity is the *maximum* sum of the inspiratory reserve volume, tidal volume, and expiratory reserve volume (approximately 4,600 milliliters). It is the amount of air that a person can forcibly inhale from the point of *maximum* expiration. The client is instructed to exhale completely and then to take as deep a breath as possible through the spirometer.

Vital capacity is the same volume as inspiratory vital capacity, except that the client is instructed to take as deep a breath as possible and then to expire this maximum volume of air through the spirometer.

Functional residual capacity is the sum of the expiratory reserve volume and the residual volume (approximately 2,300 milliliters). It is the volume of air remaining in the lungs at the end of a normal expiration and is not measurable by direct spirometry.

Another relevant air volume is dead space air (approximately 150 milliliters). This air is within the respiratory passages and has no alveoli (nasal passageways, pharynx, trachea, and bronchi). Although this air is inspired and expired, it never reaches the alveoli for gaseous exhange with the blood. Dead space air is equal to approximately 1 milliliter for each pound of body weight. The amount of air that actually reaches the alveoli is the tidal volume minus the dead space volume (500 milliliters − 150 milliliters = 350 milliliters).

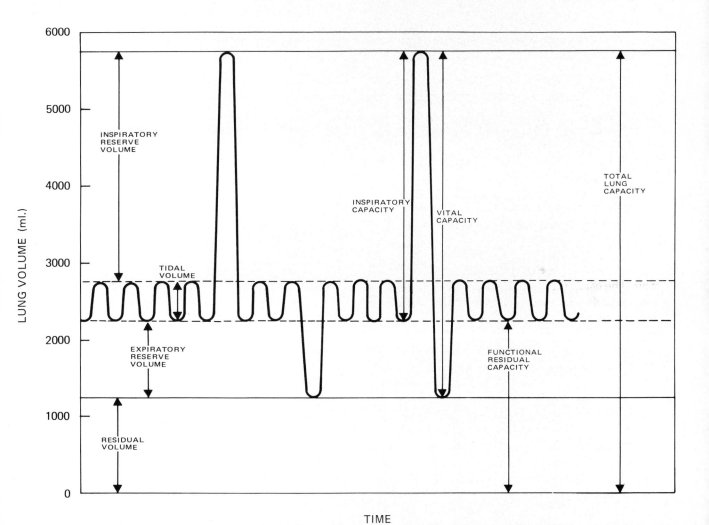

Figure 10-12. *Lung volumes and lung capacities.*

Table 10-11. Selected Abnormal Lung Volumes and Capacities

Lung Volume or Capacity	Possible Conditions	Explanation
Decreased total lung capacity; decreased functional residual capacity; decreased residual volume	Restrictive lung diseases (pulmonary fibrosis, pneumonectomy, pulmonary edema, diaphragmatic paralysis, neuromuscular dysfunction)	Functioning lung tissue is displaced or compressed by fibrosis or fluid.
Decreased expiratory reserve volume	Obesity	The decreased size of the interior chest diameter on inspiration interferes with the ability of the lungs to expand fully and fill with air.
Increased functional reserve capacity; increased or normal residual volume, increased or normal total lung capacity	Obstructive lung disease (emphysema, asthma)	Functioning lung tissue is replaced by fibrosis, and the lungs are hyperinflated even during quiet breathing.
Increased dead space	Obstructive lung disease Ventilatory assistance	There are more respiratory air passages without functioning alveoli. Although the tidal volume may be normal, less air is perfused by the pulmonary capillary blood supply.
Decreased dead space	Pneumonectomy Tracheotomy	Removal of a portion of the conducting airway increases that portion of the tidal volume that reaches the alveoli.
Decreased vital capacity	Obstructive lung disease Restrictive lung disease Poor effort	Functioning lung tissue is replaced by fibrosis, compression, or fluid. The lungs are not fully expanded.
Increased vital capacity	Aerobically conditioned athletes	The strength of respiratory muscles is increased in athletes. This increased strength allows increased expansion of the chest cage and therefore increased lung expansion and vital capacity.

Life Cycle Variations

Childhood

From birth through early childhood, inspection provides as much information about the respiratory system as the other assessment modalities combined. The examiner begins by inspecting the general shape of the thorax and proceeds to the respiratory pattern.

The newborn chest is cylindrical in shape, with an anteroposterior diameter equal to the transverse diameter. At approximately age one the transverse diameter is greater and continues to enlarge faster than the anteroposterior diameter until about age six (Table 10-12). Also, the chest circumference is equal to, or slightly smaller than, the head circumference in the first two years of life. After that, the chest circumference is larger than the head circumference. Chest circumference is measured during midinspiration at the xiphoid cartilage. In children under age five, the measurement is done while the child is lying down; after age five the child stands for chest circumference measurement (Figure 10-13).

Table 10-12. Thoracic Index (Ratio of Anteroposterior and Transverse Diameter of Thorax)

Age	Thoracic Index
Newborn	1
1 year	1: 1.25
6 years	1: 1.35

Respirations in the newborn vary greatly in rate and depth. They are counted for a full minute to obtain an accurate rate (Appendix 3). It is best to obtain the respiratory rate when the infant is sleeping, since the respiratory rate increases greatly with excitement. Until the infant is about one-month old, Cheyne Stokes breathing is normal.

Often an infant has paradoxical breathing, that is, diaphragmatic breathing with abdominal protrusion

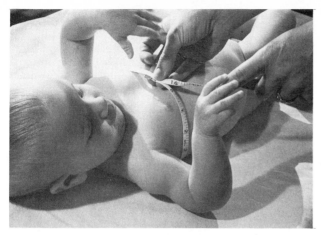

Figure 10-13. Measurement of infant chest circumference.

while simultaneously drawing in the lower thorax on inspiration, while the opposite occurs on expiration. The abdominal breathing continues until about age six or seven when it changes to thoracic breathing. Sometimes in the child under six, there is no intercostal motion at all with inspiration and expiration and the respiratory rate is checked with a hand on the abdomen or with a stethoscope.

Palpation is performed over the entire anterior, lateral, and posterior chest with the palm of the hand lightly but firmly on the chest. The rib cage is soft and pliant. Tactile fremitus is best palpated while the infant cries; the older child is asked to say his name, "1-2-3," or "99."

For both percussion and auscultation, the infant's or child's head is in the midline to avoid any misleading sounds. The percussion technique for assessing children is the same as that for adults; however the normal percussion note over the lung fields is hyperresonance from the thin chest wall.

In auscultation, it is best to use a pediatric bell stethoscope since it fits more easily in the intercostal spaces. Generally the young child is encouraged to play with the stethoscope during the history and is instructed not to handle the tubing during the actual examination to avoid production of misleading sounds. Breath sounds in children are louder and harsher than in adults, and the normal lung sound is bronchovesicular. Breath sounds are rarely absent since the chest is so small and the sounds transmit so well. Rales are often normal in the newborn and are thought to be from alveolar opening. In infants, it is sometimes preferable to auscultate during crying to take advantage of deep inspirations. The older child is instructed to blow hard against the examiner's hand during auscultation. With this maneuver, the child takes a deep breath through his mouth and then exhales against the examiner's hand.

Adolescence

During adolescence, the respiratory rate slows down to the adult rate or even slower due to a decrease in somatic growth. The examination of the chest and respiratory system is virtually the same as that for adults, although some adolescents are sensitive about privacy, and the many changes taking place in their bodies.

Pregnancy

As the uterus enlarges, the diaphragm moves upward and the thoracic cage widens. The mother's tidal volume and respiratory rate increase, as does alveolar ventilation and oxygen consumption. In addition, breathing becomes more costal and many women complain of dyspnea during the third trimester. The dyspnea is actually maternal hyperventilation from the effects of the hormone progesterone. These changes in breathing help to maintain oxygenation of maternal and fetal blood.

Late Adulthood

Growth and development of the lungs cease when somatic growth stops. Degeneration of the lungs does not generally begin until the fifth decade of life; although there are structural changes in the lungs, they are still capable of maintaining adequate gaseous exchange throughout the life span. This of course occurs only in the absence of pulmonary disease.

With aging, there are structural changes of both the lungs and the rib cage. There are fewer alveoli; those remaining are larger with thicker elastic fibers. There is a senile kyphosis, decreased transverse diameter, decalcification of the ribs, increased calcification of the costal cartilages, and a partial contraction of the muscles of inspiration. All these factors cause a less elastic lung and a stiffer rib cage, which decreases the mobility, or compliance, of the lungs, chest wall, and force of expiration. It is normal for the aged to have minimal dyspnea with activity. This dyspnea is recorded according to a numerical grade that is a description of when the dyspnea begins (Table 10-13).

With the normal process of aging, there is a decreased ability to cough effectively because of the more rigid thoracic wall and weaker muscles of expiration. Although this does not greatly affect the healthy client, it does affect the debilitated client. An

Table 10-13.   Grades of Dyspnea

Grade	Onset of Shortness of Breath
1	Walking rapidly on level ground, walking up small hill, walking up stairs
2	Walking on level ground at normal pace for age
3	Walking on level ground at slow pace
4	Doing activities of daily living, e.g., washing, dressing
5	Sitting quietly with no physical activity

aged client is more susceptible to respiratory complications from bed rest and surgery. Therefore, the examiner needs to look for beginning changes in physical signs.

It is very difficult to determine normal changes in lung volumes since the research on healthy non-smokers living in areas without significant air pollution is not readily available. It is felt that some lung volumes and capacities do change in the elderly because of the anatomical changes in their lungs and chest wall. Although the tidal volume remains the same, the anatomical dead space increases so that less air is exchanged in the alveoli. This correlates with the decreased oxygen needs of the body tissues. With the decreased lung compliance, the vital capacity decreases (up to 50 percent), the residual volume increases (up to 50 percent), but the total lung capacity remains relatively unaltered.

On palpation, the respiratory excursion is decreased and the trachea may be deviated from upper dorsal scoliosis. It may be difficult to auscultate the lung fields adequately, since the elderly client may be unable to take very deep breaths. Therefore, the normal breath sounds are softer, especially in the lung bases where the distal alveoli and airways may have closed.

Anatomy and Physiology

The cardiovascular system is a network that provides an uninterrupted supply of nutrients to the cells. This system has two main components: the heart and the vasculature (arteries, veins, and capillaries).

The primary function of the heart is to pump blood throughout the vessels of the circulatory system. The heart is a double-barreled muscular pump located in the mediastinum between the lungs and above the diaphragm. Generally it lies in an oblique line beneath and slightly to the left of the sternum.

The heart is contained in the pericardium, a strong fibrous sac. Between the pericardium and heart is a small amount of serous fluid, which reduces the friction of the constantly moving heart. The pericardium is secured to the diaphragm, sternum, pleura, esophagus, and aorta. The heart is composed of three layers: the epicardium, myocardium, and endocardium. The epicardium is a thin, smooth lining that covers the outside of the myocardium and interfaces with the pericardium. The myocardium is a specialized muscular layer of the heart. The endocardium is a thin, delicate lining that lines the heart chambers and the surfaces of the heart valves (Figure 11-1).

The heart contains four blood-filled chambers: right atrium, right ventricle, left atrium, and left ventricle. The two atria are adjacent, thin-walled entry chambers in the superior portion of the heart and share a medial wall, the atrial septum. The atria comprise the base of the heart. The two ventricles are adjacent, thicker-walled muscular chambers below the atria and share a medial wall, the ventricular septum. The two ventricles comprise the apex of the heart.

Blood flow through the heart is regulated by four valves: two atrioventricular valves (AV) and two semilunar valves. The AV valves are outlet valves for the atria, and the semilunar valves are outlet valves for the ventricle. These valves maintain forward flow of blood at all times. This function is entirely dependent on pressure gradients; the valves open and close passively (Figure 11-2). When the pressure above the valves is higher than the pressure below, the valves open. When the pressure below the valves is higher than the pressure above, the valves close.

The atrioventricular valves are the tricuspid and mitral valves. The tricuspid valve is composed of three leaflets that are thin and translucent; it separates the right atrium from the right ventricle. The mitral valve (bicuspid valve) is composed of two leaflets that are thicker and less translucent; it separates the left atrium from the left ventricle. The semilunar valves are the pulmonic and the aortic valves. They are com-

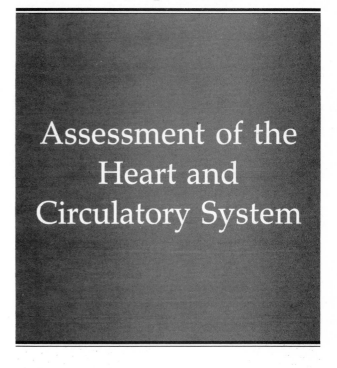

Chapter 11

Assessment of the Heart and Circulatory System

_____ Objectives _____

The examiner will be able to do the following:

1. Inspect the precordium
2. Palpate the apical impulse
3. Percuss the cardiac outline
4. Auscultate the four cardiac auscultatory areas
5. Palpate and auscultate the carotid pulses
6. Inspect the jugular veins and estimate venous pressure
7. Recognize a normal electrocardiogram
8. Recognize abnormalities of the cardiovascular system
9. Record the information obtained

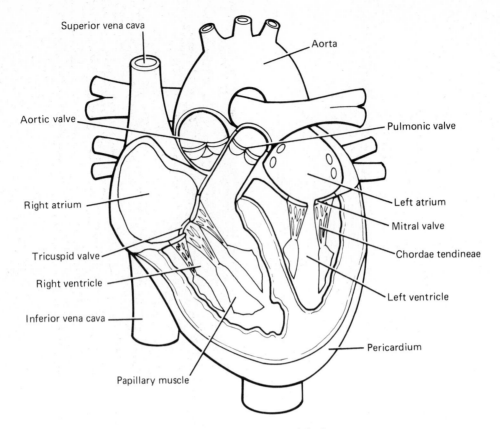

Figure 11-1. Anatomy of the heart.

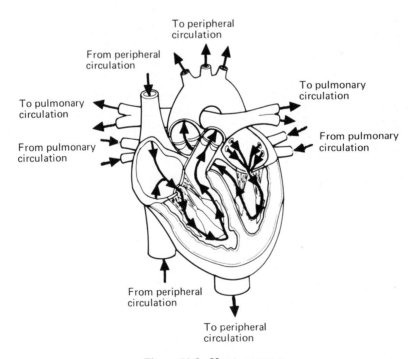

Figure 11-2. Heart pressures.

posed of fibrous cusps shaped like half-moons. The pulmonic valve contains two cusps and separates the right ventricle from the pulmonary artery. The aortic valve contains three somewhat thicker cusps, and separates the left ventricle from the aorta.

During ventricular systole, the ventricles contract which increases intraventricular pressure. This closes the atrioventricular valves and opens the semilunar valves. During ventricular diastole, the ventricles relax, which decreases intraventricular pressure. This decreased pressure opens the atrioventricular valves, and closes the semilunar valves (Figure 11-2).

Attached to the valve leaflets are the papillary muscles and chordae tendinae. The papillary muscles are fingerlike projections on the ventricular wall. They hold the AV valve leaflets together and down at the onset of ventricular systole, which prevents regurgitation of blood into the atria. The chordae tendinae are strong cords of fibrous tissue that extend from the tip of each papillary muscle and attach to the valve leaflets above. They permit the leaflet to spring upward and together during ventricular systole, which evenly distributes the forces of systole and prevents regurgitation of blood.

Blood flows through the heart and lungs in a consistent and rhythmic manner. Blood enters the right side of the heart from the systemic circulation via the superior and inferior vena cava. It passively flows into the right atrium, through the tricuspid valve, and into the right ventricle. From the right ventricle, blood is pumped through the pulmonic valve to the lungs for oxygenation via the pulmonary artery. Oxygenated blood leaves the lungs via the pulmonary vein. The blood passes into the left atrium and then through the mitral valve into the left ventricle. The left ventricle pumps blood to the periphery through the aortic valve and aorta.

The blood supply to the heart becomes clinically significant when it is impeded or blocked. The heart muscle and neuromuscular tissues are supplied by the right and left coronary arteries and their subsequent branches (Figure 11-3). The left coronary artery arises from the posterior aortic sinus. It courses between the root of the pulmonary artery and the left atrium. On entrance to the atrioventricular groove, the left coronary artery has a large branch known as the left anterior descending (LAD), which typically arises as a direct continuation of the main left coronary artery. The LAD branch courses down the anterior interventricular septum sulcus and curves around the apex of the heart. It distributes branches to both ventricles.

The left circumflex branch arises from the main trunk of the left coronary artery at an acute 90-degree angle. It ascends into the left atrioventricular sulcus and courses to the margin of the left ventricle, where it turns down toward the apex of the heart.

The right coronary artery arises from the anterior aortic sinus. It courses between the base of the pulmonary artery and right atrium and travels in the right atrioventricular sulcus to the margin of the right ventricle. It curves inferiorly around the right apex to the posterior heart. The two main branches of the right coronary artery are the marginal and the interventricular. The marginal arises from the main artery as it curves around the apex, and the interventricular arises on the posterior heart shortly before termination of the main right artery.

After distribution throughout the cardiac muscle, blood enters the coronary veins and is collected in the coronary sinus before returning to the right atrium for circulation to the lungs. Coronary artery flow occurs during ventricular diastole when the pressure in the aorta is high. The contraction of ventricular muscle prevents coronary flow during systole.

Cardiac output is the amount of blood pumped by the heart per unit of time and is the product of stroke volume and heart rate. Stroke volume is the amount of blood pumped out of the heart with each heartbeat. Normally it is about 70 milliliters/beat. Therefore,

$$\text{Cardiac Output} = \text{Stroke Volume} \times \text{Heart Rate}$$
$$4{,}900 \quad = \quad 70 \quad \times \quad 70$$

Normally, while at rest, the heart pumps about 4 to 6 liters of blood each minute. However, during vigorous exercise the heart can increase this output five or more times. This is possible from an increased heart rate and increased stroke volume, or a combination of the two.

Provided stroke volume remains constant, any increase in heart rate consequently produces an increase in cardiac output. The heart rate is controlled by a balance between the inhibitory influence of the vagus nerve (cranial nerve x), and the excitatory influence of the sympathetic nervous system. While at rest, the heart rate is mainly controlled by the effect of the vagus with only a slight contribution from the sympathetic system. During stress or exercise, the sympathetic influence increases, which causes an increased heart rate and cardiac output, while the parasympathetic control wanes. Increased heart rate with sympathetic stimulation effectively increases cardiac output up to about 200 beats per minute. Beyond 200 beats per minute, the ventricular filling time becomes so shortened that a drop in cardiac output occurs.

Stroke volume output can be regulated to produce a change in cardiac output. This phenomenon is

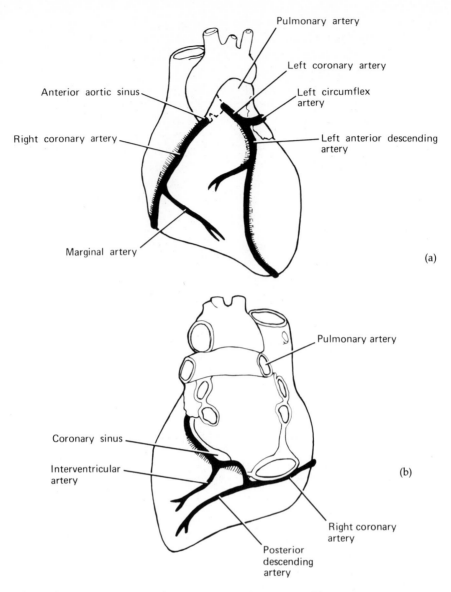

Figure 11-3. Cardiac blood supply: (a) anterior; (b) posterior.

based on the "law of the heart" (Starling's law). Starling's law states that the force of cardiac contraction is determined by the presystolic muscle fiber length. This is based on the physiology of muscle fiber length. Essentially it means that the greater the muscle fiber is stretched, the greater will be the force it produces at contraction. Therefore, if there is an increased venous return to the pulmonary circulation, the left ventricle accommodates this increased blood volume by maximal stretching of fibers. Increased fiber length results in an increased force of contraction, thereby expelling the larger blood volume. This holds true within certain physiological limits of fiber length capacity, after which the force of contraction diminishes and cardiac output falls.

Conduction System

The conduction system of the heart is responsible for the transmission of electrical impulses throughout the myocardium. It includes the sino-atrial node, atrioventricular node, Bundle of His, and Purkinje fibers (Figure 11-4). The sinoatrial (SA) node is an area of specialized muscular tissue located in the wall of the right atrium beneath the junction of the superior vena cava and the right atrium. The SA node is supplied by the right coronary artery in 55 to 60 percent of human hearts. The other 40 to 45 percent are supplied by branches of the left circumflex artery. This tissue is well supplied with nerve fibers and ganglia cells. The

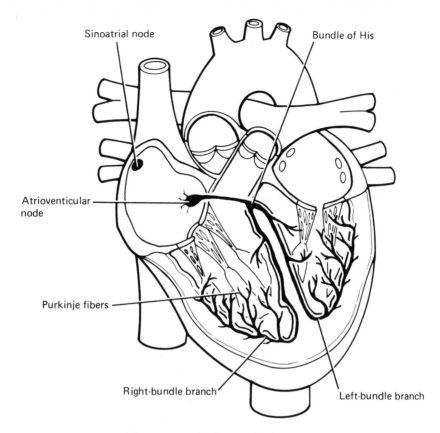

Sinoatrial node

Bundle of His

Atrioventicular node

Purkinje fibers

Right-bundle branch

Left-bundle branch

Figure 11-4. Cardiac conduction system.

electrical impulse that initiates myocardial muscle depolarization originates in the SA node and travels to the AV junction. When the impulse reaches the atrioventricular junction, it excites another area of specialized tissue: the atrioventricular (AV) node. This tissue conducts impulses at a slower rate, so there is a delay of conduction from the atria to the ventricles of about 1/10 of a second. This pause between atrial and ventricular depolarization allows atrial systole to provide additional filling volume to the ventricles before the ventricles contract.

The electrical impulse then travels down the conduction pathway to the Bundle of His, a channel of nervous tissue within the ventricular septum and walls. The conduction pathway then divides into one right and two left bundle branches. The electrical impulse continues down each side of the septum; it curves with the contours of each ventricle and travels up the ventricular walls opposite the septum. Here the conduction pathway branches into very fine Purkinje muscle fibers. These fibers contract very weakly, as they are composed of few contractile fibrils. Rather, they permeate the mass of ventricular muscle and serve as a system of rapid transmission of impulse throughout the heart.

Peripheral Circulation

The peripheral circulation is composed of the arterial and venous systems. The arterial system contributes to the resistive feature of the peripheral circulation. Peripheral resistance is the impediment to blood flow in a vessel; it is largely a product of the tone of the muscular walls of the arterioles.

By selective constriction and dilation, the arteries vary blood flow to the appropriate tissue beds in accordance with tissue needs. This activity is controlled by the autonomic nervous system. During decreased cardiac output, the arteries support arterial blood pressure through constriction.

Normally the veins serve as a storage system for about 65 to 70 percent of the blood volume. Venous tension is controlled by autonomic impulses from the vasomotor center located in the brain in the floor of the fourth ventricle. Sympathetic stimulation produces a more marked effect on the maximum ability of the veins to constrict than on arterial vasoconstriction. This effect on venomotor tone can be observed in the instance of hemorrhage. In the absence of reflex compensatory mechanisms, a fall in blood volume results in a decreased venous return to the heart and a decreased cardiac output. As blood volume falls, venous tone increases due to sympathetic stimulation, the blood return to the right heart improves, and cardiac output is maintained within the realm of venoconstrictor capacity. Consequently, the blood flow is maintained even with a decreased volume.

Assessment Modalities

Preparation

The client is supine, semirecumbent, and sitting upright for various portions of the examination. A person too ill to sit unaided is assisted into the upright position. Male clients are disrobed to the waist; and female clients wear a short gown, which is removed for the actual examination.

The equipment necessary to assess the heart and circulatory system includes a stethoscope with a bell and diaphragm, a sphygmomenometer, and a watch with a second hand. After the history is obtained, the examiner proceeds with inspection, then palpation, percussion and auscultation.

Inspection

Inspection begins with the client in the supine position. The examiner stands at the foot of the examining table or bed and looks at the anterior chest. The symmetry of chest contour is observed (Chapter 10). Then the examiner moves to the client's right side and observes the precordium for pulsations. Observations of motions are facilitated by a tangential view with the aid of a light shadow (Figure 11-5). Usually the apical impulse is observed in the fifth interspace, medial to the left midclavicular line as a slight retraction at the same rate as the heart beat. Chest wall pulsations are often hidden by the developed female breast and in clients with an increased anterior posterior diameter of the chest.

Chest wall pulsations are produced by ventricular contractions. During contraction, the left ventricle moves anteriorly and strikes the chest wall. This is called the apical impulse or point of maximum impulse (PMI) and is visible in over 50 percent of normal adults.

Palpation

The chest wall is palpated to further assess the apical impulse and identify the presence of other impulses. The examiner identifies the apical impulse by standing to the right of the supine client and placing the palm of the hand over the precordium (Figure 11-5). If the apical impulse is not palpable, the client is instructed to lean to the left, and the maneuver is repeated.

The apical impulse is palpated with two fingers, the index and middle finger on one hand. Normally the impulse is felt at the fifth left intercostal space at the

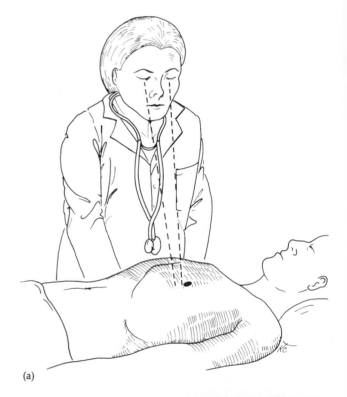
(a)

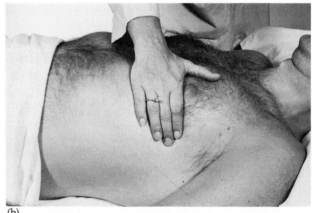
(b)

Figure 11-5. *Apical impulse: (a) inspection, (b) palpation.*

midclavicular line. The size, rate, duration, and force of impulse are estimated.

The normal apical impulse occupies only one intercostal space, is the size of a penny, but may be as large as a quarter. The rate of the impulses are the same as the heart rate, 60 to 100 impulses each minute. The apical impulse generally rises rapidly and falls away from the chest wall in less than a third of the duration of systole. The force is felt as a light tapping pulsation.

After the apical impulse is assessed, the examiner places the palm of the hand over the precordium along the left sternal edge (Figure 11-5). Normally no significant impulses are palpated; occasionally a faint tap is noted (Table 11-1).

Table 11-1. Selected Abnormal Cardiac Pulsations

Finding	Description	Possible Conditions
Lift or heave	Diffuse pulsation felt along the left sternal edge. Due to increased pressure or enlargement of the ventricle.	
	Palpable pulsation on the chest wall near or lateral to the apex.	Left ventricular hypertrophy
	A diffuse impulse or rising of the palpating hand. Is often also palpated in the epigastrium with three fingers being pushed slightly forward and down into the costal angle.	Right ventricular hypertrophy
Thrill	Purring vibratory sensations from an increased or turbulent blood flow; a palpable heart murmur. The examiner palpates with the palmar surface of three fingers in the upper sternal regions along the left heart border and at the apex. The suprasternal notch and infraclavicular areas are also palpated for thrills.	Heart murmur
Displaced apical impulse	Apical impulse displaced below the fifth intercostal space or lateral to 10 cm. left of the midsternal line.	Cardiac enlargement

Percussion

Percussion of the heart serves to locate the left and right heart borders, although this technique is seldom used because it is unreliable. Actual heart size is best detected with a chest X-ray. During percussion of the heart borders, the pleximeter finger is kept parallel to the border being percussed. The pleximeter is moved approximately 2.5 centimeters (1 inch) at a time until the percussion note changes from resonance to relative dullness. At this point the finger moves at smaller intervals to determine the location of the change in the percussion note.

The left heart border is generally percussed in the fifth intercostal space 10 centimeters from the midsternal line, or just medial to or at the left midclavicular line. Normally cardiac dullness is not detected to the right of the sternum.

The first area of relative cardiac dullness occurs in a region where the heart border is partially covered by lung tissue. As the heart nears the chest wall, the percussion note progresses to a flat sound.

Auscultation

When the heart valves close, they produce characteristic sounds, which are heard during cardiac auscultation. It is also thought that blood flow and muscle tension may contribute to the production of heart sounds. Although the valves are situated in a small area on the anterior chest wall, their characteristic sounds are not heard directly over their specific location (Figure 11-6). The sound created by the aortic valve is heard at the base of the heart in the second right intercostal space at the sternal margin (aortic auscultatory area). The sound created by the pulmonic valve is heard at the base of the heart in the second left intercostal space at the left sternal margin (pulmonic auscultatory area). The sound created by closure of the tricuspid valve is heard at the apex of the heart in the fourth or fifth intercostal spaces at the left sternal margin (tricuspid auscultatory area). The sound created by closure of the mitral valve is heard at the apex of the heart in the fifth left intercostal space at the left midclavicular line (mitral auscultatory area).

Successful auscultation requires concentration and listening for one specific item at a time. First the heart rate is determined at the apex and then the normal heart sounds and any pathology are assessed. Auscultation of heart sounds begins at the base of the heart over the aortic and pulmonic auscultatory areas and proceeds to the apex of the heart at the tricuspid auscultatory area.

Auscultation begins with the client in a sitting position while the examiner sits or stands to the right.

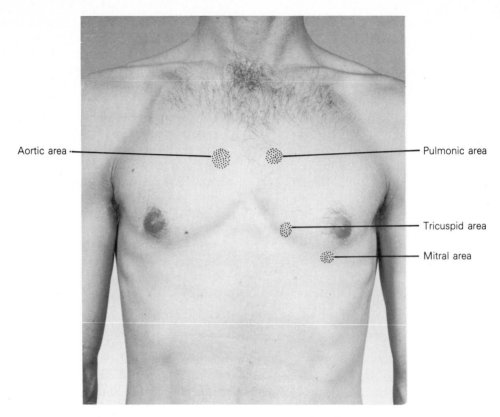

Aortic area

Pulmonic area

Tricuspid area

Mitral area

Figure 11-6. Auscultatory areas of the heart.

The aortic, pulmonic, tricuspid, and mitral auscultatory areas are auscultated in sequence (Figure 11-7).

Since normal heart sounds are relatively low-frequency sounds, the examiner begins with the bell of the stethoscope. The bell is placed directly onto the chest wall with light pressure so that the skin produces a seal. In a supine client the weight of the stethoscope head establishes the seal. If too much pressure is applied, the tightened skin creates a diaphragm over the bell.

First Heart Sound. The first heart sound, S-1, closely precedes the onset of ventricular systole (Figure 11-8). With ventricular contraction, the intraventricular pressure rises above atrial pressure, and the atrioventricular valves close. It is postulated that the two components of S-1 are mitral and tricuspid valve closure.

S-1 is heard over the entire precordium, but it is heard best at the apex of the heart over the tricuspid and mitral auscultatory areas. In these areas S-1 is heard as a "lubb" sound synchronous with the carotid upstroke; it is louder, duller, lower-pitched, and slightly longer than the second heart sound (S-2). At the base of the heart S-1 is softer than S-2, but S-1 is louder on the left side than on the right side.

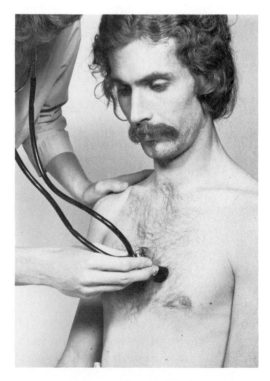

Figure 11-7. Auscultation of the heart.

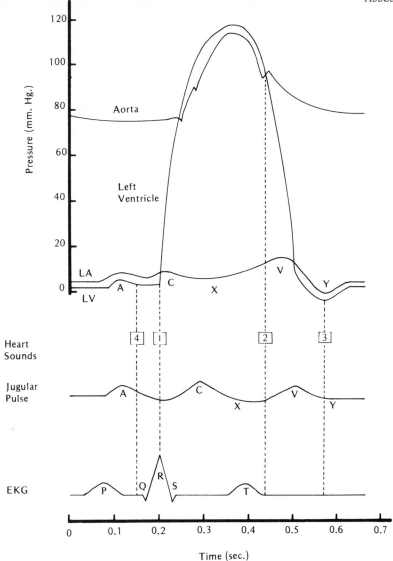

Figure 11-8. *Schematic representation of heart sounds.*

Generally S-1 is heard as one sound. On rare occasions two distinct components of S-1 are heard; this is referred to as physiologic splitting. The split sounds have the same quality as the unsplit sound. Since left heart events precede right heart events, the first component of a split S-1 is mitral valve closure and the second component is tricuspid valve closure. The normal splitting of S-1 is best heard over the tricuspid auscultatory area.

Second Heart Sound. The second heart sound, S-2, occurs after ventricular systole when the pressure in the aorta and pulmonary artery exceeds ventricular pressure. This hemodynamic event causes closure of the semilunar valves. The two components of S-2 are aortic and pulmonic valve closure.

S-2 is heard over the entire precordium as a "dupp" sound that is synchronous with the descent of the carotid pulse wave. S-2 is best heard over the base of the heart in the aortic and pulmonic auscultatory areas, where it is louder, higher in frequency, and shorter in duration than S-1. At the apex of the heart S-2 is softer than S-1.

Normally the aortic valve closes 0.02 to 0.04 seconds before the pulmonic valve during expiration; this time lapse increases to 0.04 to 0.06 seconds during normal inspiration. The time lapse in valve closures produces a splitting of S-2 which is best heard over the pulmonic auscultatory area. Although a split S-2 may be heard in a recumbent client, it is usually more easily auscultated in a sitting client. The normal increased splitting of S-2 on inspiration is termed physiologic splitting. This normal splitting of S-2 is produced during inspiration since the increased venous inflow of blood to the heart at this time causes the pulmonic component of S-2 to be delayed somewhat.

Third Heart Sound. The third heart sound, S-3, is occasionally a normal finding in otherwise healthy clients and occurs during early ventricular filling, approximately 0.12 to 0.16 seconds after S-2. It is produced from the rapid distention of the ventricles from blood when the mitral and tricuspid valves open after S-2. The vibrations produced from the ventricular filling are of a very low frequency and intensity and are often inaudible. S-3 is best heard over the apex of the heart during expiration with the client in the left lateral position.

Fourth Heart Sound. The fourth heart sound, S-4, is heard most commonly in young people with thin chest walls, but is rarely a normal heart sound. S-4 occurs just before S-1 and occurs with the atrial ejection of blood into the ventricle. The distention of the ventricles with blood at this time may cause vibrations of the AV valves, their supporting structures and the ventricular walls, and hence S-4. S-4 is heard before S-1 at the apex of the heart as a low-frequency and low-intensity sound.

Extra Sounds. Extra heart sounds are superimposed on the four basic heart sounds and suggest some underlying pathology. Each auscultatory area is listened to for the presence of abnormal sounds (Table 11-2).

Table 11-2. Extra Heart Sounds

Finding	Description	Condition
Ejection click	A sharp clicking sound heard best over the base of the heart. Occurs during early systole when the aortic or pulmonic valves open at the start of the ejection of blood. It is often difficult to differentiate an ejection click from a split S-1.	Aortic valve disease, pulmonary artery or aortic disease, normal variant.
Midsystolic click	A sharp clicking sound heard in mid to late systole and often moves with respirations; the click is closer to S-1 in inspiration and closer to S-2 in expiration. Heard best over the apex of the heart.	Mitral prolapse.
Gallop sounds	A low-pitched, sequential sound from the intensification of S-3 or S-4. It may also occur with a rapid heart rate. A protodiastolic gallop is from the intensification of S-3 and has the rhythm and accents of the word *Ken-tuck-y*. A presystolic gallop is from the intensification of S-4 and has the rhythm and accents of the word *Ten-nes-see*. A summation gallop or quadruple rhythm is from the intensification of S-3 and S-4 and occurs with a slow heart rate. Gallop sounds are best heard at the apex of the heart and along the left sternal border. These sounds occur as the ventricle distends from the rapid inflow of blood in early diastole when the ventricles have decreased compliance.	Diseased ventricle with heart failure.
Widened, split, S-2	The split of S-2 varies with respirations but is greater than 0.1 second on inspiration and greater than 0.04 seconds on expiration.	Increased pulmonary blood flow (atrial septal defects). Decreased pulmonary pressure (pulmonary stenosis). Early aortic valve closure (mitral insufficiency, ventricular septal defect).
Fixed, split S-2	The split of S-1 or S-2 does not vary with respirations.	Atrial septal defect. Pulmonary stenosis.
Paradoxical split	The split of S-1 or S-2 becomes wider and more pronounced on expiration and decreases on inspiration.	Left bundle branch block. Delay in aortic valve closure (aortic stenosis, hypertension).
Pericardial friction rub	A scratchy, creaking high-pitched sound heard throughout the cardiac cycle or during systole or diastole.	Pericardial disease.

Murmurs. Murmurs are audible vibratory noises that result from turbulent blood flow within the heart. They sometimes have musical qualities and have a definite relationship to the heart cycle. Transient murmurs occur in normal hearts and are thought to be the result of hemodynamic factors. These murmurs are often the result of vibrations in normal valves from a rapid blood flow and are called innocent murmurs. Rapid blood flow past an abnormal valve in diseased states produces pathological murmurs (Table 11-4). Murmurs are described in terms of their primary location, radiation, phase of the cardiac cycle in which they are best heard, intensity, frequency, and quality.

Murmurs are generally auscultated and identified over the four valve-related areas and they radiate in the direction of the blood leak. Variations in sound transmission in different tissues can also determine the direction of the radiation. The phase of the cardiac cycle in which murmurs are heard are identified as systole, diastole, or continuous (throughout systole and diastole). The intensity or loudness of a murmur is evaluated on a scale of 1 to 6 (Table 11-3).

Table 11-3. Grades of Murmurs

Grade of Murmur	Description of Murmur
1/6	Barely audible
2/6	Clearly audible but quiet
3/6	Loud but not palpable
4/6	Loud and palpable with a thrill
5/6	Loud, palpable, and audible with stethoscope just off the chest wall
6/6	Loud, palpable, and audible without a stethoscope

The frequency or pitch of a murmur is described as high-, mid- or low-pitched. A high-pitched murmur sounds like rapid expirations with the mouth open. A midpitched murmur sounds somewhat like rapid expiration through pursed lips, and a low-pitched murmur has a rumbling or drum roll quality to it.

Table 11-4. Murmurs

Finding	Condition	Description
Systolic ejection murmur		Produced by vibrations in various structures from the ejection of blood from the left or right ventricles into the aorta or pulmonary artery. After S-1 there is an interval when pressure in the ventricle rises rapidly while both valves are closed, called the isometric contraction phase of systole. Pressure rises but ventricular volume is constant since both valves are closed and blood is not expelled. When the ventricular pressure rises above the pressure in the aortic or pulmonary artery, the aortic and pulmonary valves open and blood squirts out into the aorta and pulmonary artery. This produces an ejection click.
	Aortic stenosis	Auscultated at the aortic auscultatory area and radiates into the neck down the left sternal border and sometimes to the apex. Has variable intensity. If it is loud, a thrill may be felt in the aortic area and the neck. Has a medium pitch, often harsh quality, and occurs midsystole. Is associated with a diminished S-2 early ejection click, a thrusting, sustained, apical impulse with a slowly rising carotid pulse contour and narrow pulse pressure.
	Pulmonic stenosis	Auscultated at the pulmonic auscultatory area and the third left intercostal space. Radiates toward the left shoulder and upward toward the neck vessels, especially on the left. Has variable intensity. If it is loud, a thrill may be felt in the pulmonic area. Has a medium pitch, often harsh quality, and occurs midsystole. Is associated with a widely split S-2 and diminished to absent pulmonic component of S-2, early ejection click, and a left parasternal lift.
Systolic regurgitant murmur		Pressure in the ventricle exceeds pressure in the atrium. Is associated with blood regurgitation into the atrium from the ventricle because of incompetence of the AV valves. The blood leaks back and various structures vibrate.

Table 11-4.   Murmurs (continued)

Finding	Condition	Explanation and Description
	Mitral insufficiency	Auscultated at the mitral auscultatory area and radiates into the left axilla. Has a variable intensity but is often loud and may be associated with an apical thrill; does not increase with inspiration. Has a high pitch, blowing quality, and occurs pansystolic. Is associated with a decreased S-1, S-3, and the apical impulse thrusts, is sustained, and is displaced downward and to the left.
	Tricuspid insufficiency	Auscultated at the tricuspid auscultatory area and may radiate to the right of the sternum and to the left midclavicular line, but not into the axilla. Has a variable intensity that increases with inspiration. Has a high pitch, blowing quality, and occurs pansystolic. Is associated with a left parasternal lift and systolic pulsations in the jugular venous pulse and sometimes in the liver.
	Ventricular septal defect	Auscultated at the left sternal border in the 4th, 5th, and 6th intercostal spaces. May radiate over the precordium but not into the axilla. Is often very loud and accompanied by a thrill. Has a high pitch that is often harsh and occurs pansystolic. Associated signs vary with the severity of the defect and with associated lesions.
Diastolic insufficiency murmur		Due to leakage of the aortic or pulmonic valves. Results from a stretching of the vessel so that the three leaflets fail to meet, or from leaflet disease that produces shortened leaflets that do not meet in the closed position.
	Aortic insufficiency	Auscultated at the aortic auscultatory area. Radiates down the left sternal border, sometimes the right sternal border, and may radiate as far as the apex. Has a variable, often faint intensity with a high pitch and blowing quality. Occurs during any phase of diastole. Is associated with an aortic systolic murmur, S-3, wide pulse pressure, and a sustained, thrusting, apical impulse displaced inferiorly and laterally.
	Pulmonic insufficiency	Auscultated at the pulmonic auscultatory area. Generally does not radiate. Has a variable, often faint intensity with a medium to high pitch, blowing quality. Occurs during any phase of diastole. Is generally associated with normal heart sounds.
Diastolic filling murmurs		Due to blood filling the ventricle from the atrium. The valve leaflet edges are stuck together by inflammatory material, which interferes with diastolic filling. The leaflets may become rigid and perhaps impregnated with calcium. The A-V valve does not open until the falling pressure in the ventricle reaches the atrial pressure level.
	Mitral stenosis	Auscultated at the mitral auscultatory area and generally does not radiate. Has a variable, soft intensity that can be accentuated in the left lateral decubitus position or exercise. Has a low pitch with a rumbling quality and occurs later in diastole after ventricular pressure has fallen to atrial pressure. Often at this time the murmur decreases or disappears. Is associated with an opening snap of the mitral valve and an accentuated S-1 in the mitral auscultatory area.
	Tricuspid stenosis	Uncommon. Auscultated at the tricuspid auscultatory area and generally does not radiate. Has a soft, low-pitched rumbling quality that occurs in mid- to late diastole. Is associated with an opening snap of the tricuspid valve and an accentuated S-1 in the tricuspid auscultatory area.

Examination of the Blood Vessels

Palpation and Auscultation of the Carotid Pulses.
Since the carotid arteries are central vessels, they provide the best estimate of the character of arterial pulsation. They are palpated one at a time with slight pressure to prevent an undesirable decrease in blood pressure and blood rate. The examiner stands behind or in front of the client and uses the index, middle, and ring fingers of one hand (Figure 11-9). Firm but gentle pressure is used because each carotid artery contains a carotid sinus, an area heavily innervated by parasympathetic nerve fibers. When stimulated by excessive compression, a slowing of the pulse occurs as part of the carotid sinus reflex. The normal pulse is 3+ in quality; that is, it has a strong pulsation (Chapter 2).

During auscultation the examiner lightly places the bell over the area of each carotid and listens for any sounds while the client is breathholding. With normal blood flow, no sounds are heard (Figure 11-10, Table 11-5).

Blood Pressure Determination. Systolic blood pressure is a reflection of stroke volume and the rigidity of the aorta and other major blood vessels. Diastolic blood pressure reflects peripheral resistance, the minimal continuous load against which the heart contracts in pumping blood throughout the vascular system (Chapter 2).

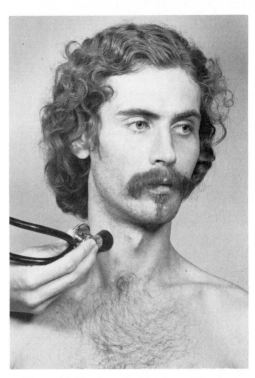

Figure 11-10. Auscultation of carotid pulses.

Inspection of the Jugular Veins. The examiner observes the superficial (external jugular) and deeper (internal jugular) venous pulsations by viewing the neck tangentially with the client supine and the head of the bed or examining table elevated 30 degrees (Figure 11-11).

Venous pulsations are differentiated from arterial pulsations in the neck by the following criteria:

1. A venous pulse is easily compressed by gentle pressure, in contrast to the carotid arterial pulse, which requires firm pressure to obliterate.

2. The normal venous pulse descends on inspiration and rises on expiration, but the carotid arterial pulse remains unaffected by respiration.

3. The venous pulse usually collapses in the sitting position, while the carotid arterial pulse is not affected by changes in position.

4. The venous pulse normally has more components than the arterial. It consists of three positive deflections—the a, c, and v waves—and two negative deflections—the x and y descents (Figure 11-8). Normally this is when the venous pulse waves are most prominent. If venous pressure is high, the pulsations may be better observed if the client is sitting.

The predominant wave in the neck is the a wave, which reflects the pressure transmission caused by atrial contraction. The a wave begins just before the

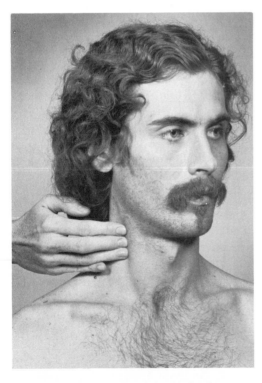

Figure 11-9. Palpation of carotid pulses.

Table 11-5. Selected Abnormalities of the Carotid Pulses

Finding	Condition	Explanation
Slow rise/slow collapse pulse (plateau pulse)	Aortic stenosis	Examiner feels vessel filling prior to the top of the pulse against the fingertips; pulse has a booming quality and seemingly delayed or prolonged recovery phase. Also characterized by decreased amplitude of pulses. Results from slow ejection of blood through a narrowed aortic valve.
Decreased amplitude (Grade I pulse)	Hemorrhagic shock	Pulse is weak due to decreased blood volume.
Alternate beats of the pulse are weak (pulsus alternans)	Myocardial weakness	May not be clinically obvious until blood pressure is taken; as cuff pressure lowers beyond a critical level, the number of sounds doubles.
Rapid rise/rapid collapse (bounding pulse, grade 4 pulse, "water-hammer pulse")	Hypertension, thyrotoxicosis, arteriovenous fistula emotional states	Associated with high pulse pressure; the upstroke and downstroke of the pulse waves are very sharp.
Bruits—high-pitched noises	Carotid artery stenosis	Noises caused by turbulent blood flow pattern in a blood vessel due to partial obstruction.
Thrills—palpable vibrations	Carotid artery stenosis	Vibrations caused by disturbed blood flow pattern in a blood vessel due to partial obstruction.

first heart sound. It can be observed by palpating the jugular pulse, while auscultating at the apex of the heart. Another effective method is for the examiner to

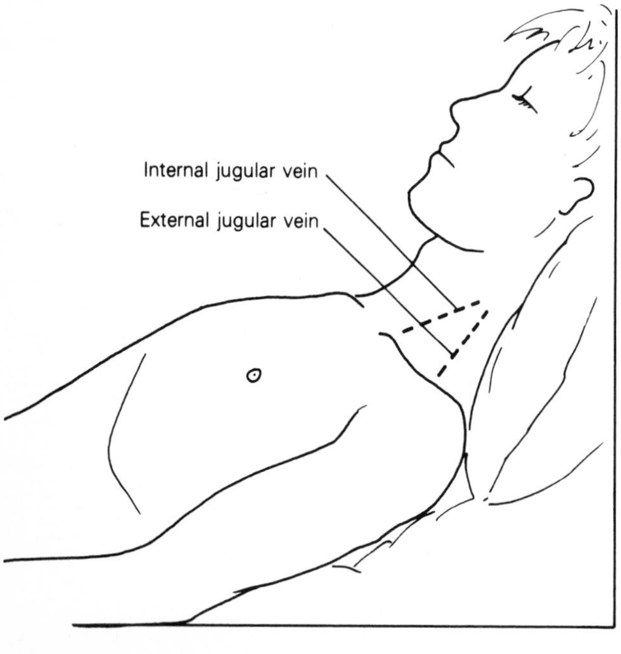

Figure 11-11. Inspection of jugular veins.

palpate the carotid pulse as the a wave occurs just prior to carotid pulsation.

The c wave is a reflection of the onset of right ventricular contraction as the tricuspid valve bulges upward and of adjacent carotid artery pulsation. The c wave begins at the end of the first heart sound. It is usually not visible in the neck veins.

The v wave represents atrial filling with the atrioventricular valve closed. It is usually small and considered a passive filling wave.

The x descent is a negative wave following the c wave, representing atrial diastole.

The v wave is followed by a y descent, a negative wave produced when the tricuspid valve opens, allowing blood to pour into the right ventricle.

Venous Pressure.   In the venous circulation, pressures range from 5 to 12 centimeters of water. The level at which this pressure is measured in relation to the atrium is critical. The venous pressure is accurately measured with a catheter placed into a large vein and attached to a manometer or strain gauge. A fair estimation of venous pressure can also be made by observation of the neck veins. When a person is lying flat, the neck veins are distended. When sitting at a 45-degree elevation from the horizontal position, the neck veins normally collapse or are visible only a centimeter or two above the clavicle. In making a simple bedside estimation of venous pressure, the examiner observes the client sitting comfortably after removing any constrictive clothing. The client is then lowered to a 45-degree angle. Normally the venous pressure rises no more than 2 centimeters above the sternal angle of Louis (Table 11-6).

Assessment of the Conduction System

The conduction system is assessed through an interpretation of the electrocardiogram (ECG). The electrocardiogram gives a schematic representation of the electrical events in the heart, which are recorded on standardized graph paper. This graph paper records time sequences and amplitude of the heart's electrical activity (Figure 11-12). The horizontal lines measure time. Each small square represents 0.04 seconds; five small squares represent 0.20 seconds. The vertical and horizontal lines for every grouping of five squares are darker, which makes it easier to identify the five square groupings. Fifteen of the 0.20 size squares represent three seconds. This amount of time is identified by short lines in the upper horizontal margin of the paper. The vertical lines measure electrical

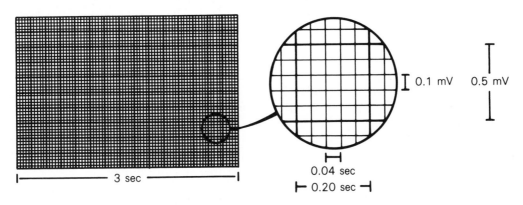

Figure 11-12. *Electrocardiogram graph paper.*

Table 11-6.   Selected Abnormalities of the Jugular Veins

Finding	Condition	Explanation
Absence of a wave	Atrial fibrillation	Since atria are not effectively contracting, the a wave is not visible.
A waves occurring at 300/minute	Atrial flutter	Atria contract at rate of 300/minute.
Unusually large a waves	Tricuspid stenosis, severe pulmonary stenosis, pulmonary hypertension	Presence of obstructing lesions impedes blood flow from the right atrium to the right ventricle.
	Myocardiopathies, nodal rhythm, prolonged AV conduction time	Right atrium contracts against a closed tricuspid valve.
Large, positive c-v waves	Congestive heart failure with tricuspid insufficiency	Hypertrophied right ventricle and stretched tricuspid valve cause leakage of blood back into the atrium during ventricular systole.
Prominent x and y waves	Constrictive pericarditis	Venous pressure is elevated and the neck veins are markedly distended.
Venous distention above 4 cm. while client is reclining at 45 degrees	Right heart failure Constrictive pericarditis Obstruction of the superior vena cava	Impaired return of blood to the right atrium results in distended jugular veins.
Positive hepatojugular reflex	Right heart failure, constrictive pericarditis	With the client sitting at a 45-degree angle and breathing normally, the examiner exerts pressure over the right upper abdominal quadrant, which causes the neck veins to distend and venous pressure to rise more than 1 cm.

amplitude. The height of the vertical lines represents millivolts (mV.); one small square equals 0.1 mV, and five small squares equal 0.5 mV.

The ECG provides information regarding the rate and rhythm of myocardial activity. One ECG complex consists of a series of waves given the arbitrary symbols of P, Q, R, S, T and U wave (Figure 11-13). The P wave is a positive deflection produced by the spread of electrical energy throughout the atria—atrial depolarization. The P-R interval is the amount of time for the electrical impulse to travel through the atrium to the ventricle. The P-R interval ranges from 0.12 seconds to 0.20 seconds. The QRS complex respresents ventricular depolarization, the spread of electrical energy throughout the ventricles. The Q wave is the first negative deflection, the R wave is the first positive deflection, and the S wave is the negative deflection after the R wave. The QRS wave is less than or equal to 0.09 seconds. The T wave is the positive deflection after the QRS and corresponds to ventricular repolarization. The U wave is a positive deflection after the T wave, which is smaller than the P wave, and is not always present.

A rhythm strip is a series of ECG complexes. The baseline is the line produced when no electrical activity in the heart is recorded. In the interpretation of a rhythm strip, various factors are considered. In a normal rhythm strip there are upright P waves with a P-R interval between 0.12 seconds and 0.20 seconds. The P-R interval from one complex to the next is constant. The P wave is always followed by a QRS less than or equal to 0.09 seconds in duration. Each QRS complex is similar in duration and form. The R-R interval is equal to the heart rate and is consistent from complex to complex. The T wave is upright and the S-T segment is at the baseline. Sometimes a small positive deflection, the U wave, occurs after the T wave.

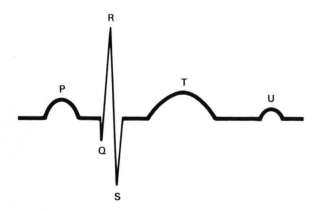

Figure 11-13. The ECG complex.

Although the ECG represents the electrical activity of the heart, it does not assess the efficiency of the heart (Table 11-7).

Life Cycle Variations

Childhood

In infancy the heart is located higher in the chest cavity than in later years. The apical impulse is easily visible in newborns and is palpated in the fourth left intercostal space just lateral to the left midclavicular line. After two years of age, the apical impulse is palpated in the fifth left intercostal space in or medial to the left midclavicular line. Percussion in infants is difficult because of the thick layers of subcutaneous fat on the chest wall and the barrel shaped thorax. S-1 and S-2 are higher in pitch and shorter in duration in children.

An S-3 is a common finding particularly during periods of rapid growth, and it occurs in early diastole. It is best heard at the apical area and is of low intensity and frequency. S-4 may also be a normal finding in children and occurs with atrial systole.

Thirty to fifty percent of children have innocent murmurs with a grade of 1/6 or 2/6. More than half of normal newborn infants have transient soft systolic murmurs during the first 48 hours of life. This is most probably due to turbulent pulmonary and straight artery flow. Other innocent cardiac murmurs include systolic ejection murmur, innocent pulmonic murmurs, venous hum, supraclavicular bruits, and cardiorespiratory murmurs.

A systolic ejection murmur is most commonly heard between the ages of three and seven years. It occurs during systolic ejection and has a musical quality similar to the vibrations of a tuning fork. The murmur lasts for a brief period and is at its loudest in the lower left sternal border with the child supine. The murmur is less audible in the sitting position and is intensified by fever, excitement, or exercise.

Innocent pulmonic murmurs commonly found in children and adolescents are caused by the normal turbulent flow of blood into the pulmonary artery. They are high-pitched, blowing, brief, early, and midsystolic murmurs with an intensity of grade 1/6 to 3/6. With the child in the recumbent position, they are most audible in the second left intercostal space at the sternal margin. These murmurs increase in intensity with full, prolonged expiration; excitement; fever; or exercise.

Table 11-7. Selected Variations in Heart Rates and Rhythms

Type	Definition	ECG representation
Normal sinus rhythm (NSR)	Regular or very slightly irregular cardiac rhythm of 60 to 100 normal ECG complexes per minute.	
Sinus bradycardia	A sinus rhythm with less than 60 normal ECG complexes per minute.	
Sinus tachycardia	A sinus rhythm greater than 100 normal ECG complexes per minute.	
Paroxysmal atrial tachycardia (PAT)	A series of rapidly repeated premature atrial beats with an absent or abnormal P wave. The P wave may precede or follow the QRS complexes. Has a regular rate between 150 and 250 per minute.	
Atrial flutter	Atrial rhythm of 250-350 complexes per minute. Has a distorted P wave that gives the complexes a saw-toothed appearance.	
Atrial fibrillation	No discernible P waves. Irregular, wavy line precedes the QRS complex. QRS complexes are irregular in rhythm and may vary in amplitude.	
Sinus arrhythmia	Sinus node forms impulses irregularly. The rate increases with inspiration and decreases with expiration. Is a variation of normal.	
Premature atrial contraction (PAC)	An otherwise normal complex that occurs early. Is determined by a shortened P-P or R-R interval.	
Junctional rhythm	An abnormal P wave that occurs closely before or after the QRS complex, or no P wave present with a normal QRST sequence at a rate of 40-60 complexes per minute.	
Premature junctional contraction	A normal but premature QRS with an abnormal P wave just before or after the QRS. Sometimes no P wave is present.	
Premature ventricular contraction (PVC)	Bizarre, premature QRS complex with no P wave.	
Ventricular tachycardia	A series of 3 or more unifocal PVCs in a row.	
Ventricular fibrillation	A complete absence of QRS complexes. ECG tracing shows an unevenly waving line with no form.	
Heart block— First degree	P-R interval greater than 0.20 seconds.	
Second degree	QRS complexes are dropped up to a maximum of every third beat.	
Type I, Wenkebach	P-R interval gradually lengthens until there is a P wave with no QRS.	
Type II, Mobitz	P-R interval constant, normal, or prolonged with dropped QRS waves.	
Third degree or complete heart block	Atria and ventricles contract independently of each other because there is no conduction of P waves.	
Bundle branch blocks (BBB)	Abnormally prolonged and sometimes abnormally formed QRS wave.	
Artificial pacemaker rhythm	Artificial "blips" that precede the QRS wave and indicate that the pacemaker is "firing" and stimulating ventricular depolarization.	

A venous hum is caused by increased blood flow in the jugular veins. It can be heard in the neck area of the anterior upper chest as a soft hum during systole and diastole. The murmur can be intensified or obliterated by altering the head position or with light compression over the jugular veins. These characteristics of a venous hum make it easy to distinguish it from similar sounding pathologic murmurs.

Supraclavicular bruits are most likely caused by turbulent blood flow at the junction of the brachiocephalic vessels. They are most audible above the clavicles, particularly the right, and in the suprasternal notch. They sometimes radiate below the clavicles. These murmurs are best heard with the child sitting erect and looking straight ahead. They are brief in duration in early systole and diminish with hyperextension of the shoulders and also with compression of the subclavian or carotid artery.

Cardiorespiratory murmurs are sounds possibly caused by the pressure of the heart against the lung. They are superficial, high-pitched, well-localized, and systolic in timing. These murmurs may be mistaken for those produced by late systolic mitral regurgitation.

The straight back syndrome may also cause innocent cardiac murmurs. This syndrome involves the loss of concavity of the upper thoracic spine with consequent decrease of the anterior posterior chest diameter. This condition results in innocent systolic ejection murmurs. Sometimes the murmur is intensified in late systole.

The heart rate of newborn infants is rapid and subject to wide variation. The average heart rate ranges from 120 to 140 beats per minute. It increases up to 170 or more with crying and activity and decreases to 70 to 90 during sleep. As the child grows older, the heart rate becomes slower (Appendix 2). During childhood, the heart rate is labile; that is, it increases rapidly with physical exertion and emotional stimuli.

Sinus arrhythmias and premature ventricular contractions are relatively common in children and they have no pathological significance.

Adolescence

The assessment of the heart and circulatory system of an adolescent is essentially the same as the adult examination. Heart rate, blood pressure, and location of pulses and heart sounds have reached adult characteristics, although the innocent murmurs of childhood may persist.

Pregnancy

Some of the vascular changes during pregnancy are functions of normal hormonal alterations. Increased estrogen levels contribute to a decreased vascular resistance of the uterus, which aids in the supply of an adequate blood flow to meet the increasing metabolic demands of the embryo. Vascular resistance is also decreased in other tissue beds; consequently, there is a compensatory increase in cardiac output, heart rate, and blood volume. The resting heart rate is elevated and is common in all pregnant women. There is an increased occurrence of paroxysmal atrial tachycardia.

The female sex hormones also cause relaxation of the vein walls, which is evidenced by spider angiomas. Pressure of the expanding uterus causes increased pressure on the inferior vena cava, which causes increased pressure in the legs. This often results in the supine hypotension syndrome, characterized by a sudden, severe drop in venous return, cardiac output, and blood pressure. Supine hypotension can be alleviated by the client lying on her left side.

Cardiac output increases to 30 to 40 percent above normal early in pregnancy and is maintained until the 32rd week of gestation. At 38 to 40 weeks of gestation, the cardiac output declines to nonpregnant levels. This is due to the obstructed venous return from the enlarged uterus.

Blood volume increases 20 to 100 percent above normal during the latter half of pregnancy. Increased hormone levels (estrogen, progesterone, and adrenocorticoid hormones) promote fluid retention and are secreted in large quantities during the latter half of pregnancy. Decreased capillary pressures throughout the mother's body also contribute to increased blood volume. This is felt to result from the blood shunted through the placenta, which lowers total body perfusion pressure.

Late Adulthood

Excluding myocardial and endocardial disease, the heart experiences little anatomical change with increasing age. There is an increase in age pigment but its effect on function is unknown.

The cardiac output decreases 30 to 40 percent between age 25 and 65 years. Stroke volume is reduced, and the resting heart rate remains the same or increases to a small degree. During stress the heart rate increases but does not achieve the same tachycardia as in youth. In addition to a decreased maximum heart rate, more time is required to return to basal rates. The isometric phase of contraction is prolonged, which requires increased energy and oxygen consumption by the heart.

During exercise, the stroke volume increases considerably, which compensates for the inability of the heart to achieve maximum acceleration of heart rate. Cardiac output is therefore increased and is reflected in the resultant rise in arterial blood pressure.

With age, arteries exhibit progressive chemical and anatomic changes correlated directly to changes in function. The elastic fibers gradually straighten, fray, split, and fragment. These changes are partially caused by calcium deposits, which lend a brittle character to the arterial walls. There is a progressive decrease of elastin with aging, which renders the arteries less resilient. An increase in collagen fibers adds to the compromised vascular compliance. This loss of elasticity is reflected in the aorta by a sharp rise in intra-aortic systolic pressure with each contraction.

There is an increase in peripheral resistance with age, despite the reduction in cardiac output. This arteriosclerotic rigidity of vessel walls is reflected in a rise in blood pressure. There is a systolic overshoot due to loss of elasticity, as well as a rise in diastolic pressure with an increased total peripheral resistance.

Anatomy and Physiology

The two breasts or mammary glands are located on the anterior chest wall overlying the pectoralis major, serratus anterior, and external oblique muscles. The superior border of the developed breast is generally at the second or third rib with the inferior border at the sixth or seventh costal cartilage. The lateral borders are at the sternum and anterior axillary line. A "tail" of breast tissue, called the axillary tail of Spence, extends to the anterior axillary fold (Figure 12-1). The size and shape of the breasts vary greatly, although they are basically symmetrical, conical, and protuberant in the postpubescent female and act as accessory organs in the reproductive system. In children and adult males the breasts are small and flat and remain functionless.

Female Breasts

The external breast is composed of skin, areola, and nipple (Figure 12-1). The skin is smooth and soft and extends from the circumference of the breast to the areola. The areola is the pigmented area containing raised sebaceous glands (glands of Montgomery) surrounding the nipple. These glands secrete a liquid substance that protects and lubricates the nipple during lactation. Light rubbing of the areola or nipple produces nipple erection from the contraction of the radial and circular muscle fibers in the subcutaneous tissue. The nipple is a large, conical projection at the summit of the breast, with well developed dermal papillae. Although the exact nipple location in the developed breast varies, it is slightly below the center of the breast at approximately the fourth intercostal

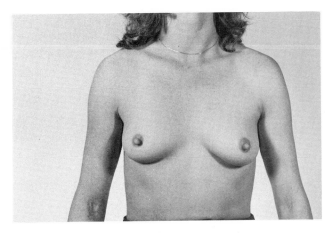

Figure 12-1. *The external developed female breast.*

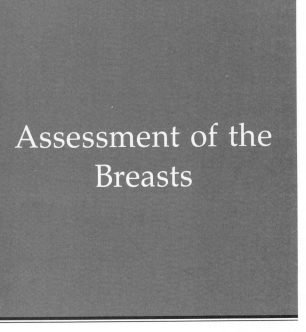

Chapter 12

Assessment of the Breasts

_____ Objectives _____

The examiner will be able to do the following:

1. Inspect and palpate the breasts
2. Health teach self-examination of the breasts
3. Recognize abnormalities of the breasts
4. Record the information obtained

space in the midclavicular line. At the summit of the nipple are 3 to 20 openings from the milk ducts.

The internal breasts are composed of modified sebaceous glands, fibrous tissue, and fat (Figure 12-2). The glandular tissue is made up of 12 to 20 lobes separated and supported by fibrous tissue, including the suspensory ligaments (Cooper's ligaments). These ligaments connect the superficial fascia to the skin. Each of the lobes terminates in its own excretory duct, which opens onto the surface of the nipple. The main collecting ducts enlarge to form milk sinuses at the base of the nipple; during lactation, the sinuses dilate into reservoirs for milk. Each lobe further divides into 20 to 40 lobules with each lobule dividing into 10 to 100 acini or alveoli. The acini are the milk producing glands and are controlled by hormonal factors. Since most of the breast is composed of fat, the individual size of an adult female breast is not an indication of the quantity of glandular tissue.

Hormones play a significant role in breast physiology. Breast growth, which occurs at puberty and pregnancy, and involution, which occurs after menopause, are directly related to estrogen and progesterone levels. Estrogen stimulates the growth of breast epithelium, which causes the development of more and larger glands. The action of progesterone is less understood, but it too causes growth of the mammary glands plus the development of secretory characteristics of the acini. Prolactin from the anterior pituitary gland is secreted at the termination of pregnancy and stimulates milk production. Suckling stimulates oxytocin secretion, which causes the acini to contract and express the milk into the duct system and out through the nipples.

Assessment Modalities

Preparation

Inspection and palpation are the examination modalities used in the assessment of the breasts and axillae. It must also be stressed that both male and female

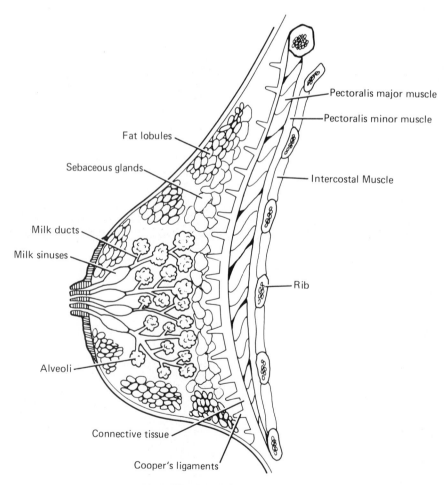

Figure 12-2. The internal developed female breast.

breasts are examined, since males account for approximately 1 percent of all breast cancer.

The client is disrobed to the waist, which insures adequate exposure for inspection. Some female clients have anxiety regarding breast examination and potential breast lesions and may be embarrassed to have the breasts exposed and examined.

Inspection of the Female Breasts

It is important to inspect the breasts in various positions, since some findings may be apparent in one position but not in another. The basic positions for breast inspection are the following (Figure 12-3):

1. Sitting upright with arms resting at sides.
2. Sitting upright with arms extended overhead.
3. Sitting and leaning forward at least 45 degrees.
4. Sitting upright and tensing the pectoral muscles. This is accomplished by pushing the palms of the hands together or placing hands on hips and pushing in.
5. Lying down with arms at sides.
6. Lying down with arms overhead.

The examiner observes the breasts for size, symmetry, contour, color, hair pattern, and venous pattern (Table 12-1). Any variation from normal is more significant if it is of recent onset, since it may suggest acquired disease. Any abnormal observation is documented with the location, size, shape, and date first noticed. If there is drainage, the color, amount, odor, and consistency are documented, as well as if the discharge is unilateral, bilateral, and from one or many ducts.

Normal breast size varies greatly and obesity is the most important factor affecting both breast size and shape. Obese women have large and pendulous breasts, often unequal in size. The breast on the dominant side is slightly larger from the more developed pectoralis major muscle. The inequality has no significance unless it is of recent origin.

The breasts are relatively symmetrical; this includes symmetrical placement of the areola and nipple, venous pattern, and contour. They are conical with no bulging, flattening, indentation, or skin retraction, and the skin is consistent with the client's genetic heritage, remainder of the body, and exposure to the

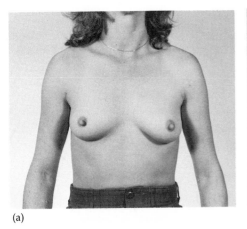
(a)

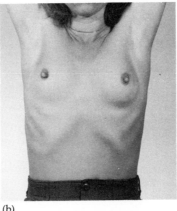
(b)

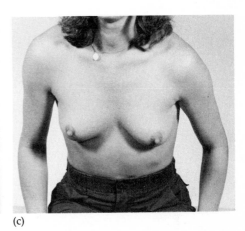
(c)

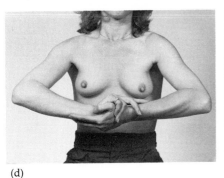
(d)

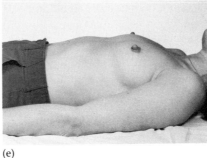
(e)

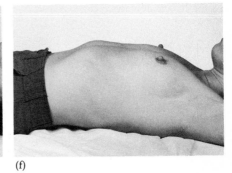
(f)

Figure 12-3. Basic positions for breast inspection: (a) sitting with arms at sides; (b) sitting with arms overhead; (c) sitting and leaning forward; (d) sitting and tensing the pectoral muscles; (e) lying with arms at sides; (f) lying with arms overhead.

Table 12-1. Selected Abnormalities of the Breasts

Finding	Description	Possible Conditions
Mass—any bulging, flattening, and dimpling or irregular contour	Occurs singly or in multiples of mobile, round, well-defined masses that disappear periodically and vary in size. Is often associated with pain and tenderness and is rarely associated with nipple discharge or retraction.	Benign cyst Fibrocystic disease Galactocele
	Generally occurs as a single, fixed, poorly delineated, hard mass that does not disappear or vary in size. Generally not associated with pain or tenderness and sometimes produces nipple discharge and inversion. Often associated with palpable nymph nodes.	Malignant tumor
Retraction	Dimpling of breast tissue and is more apparent with tensing of the pectoral muscles. The mass is fixated to overlying skin and therefore pulls skin inward or the mass exerts abnormal pressure on the breast ligaments and causes the skin to dimple.	Benign tumor Malignant tumor Fat necrosis
Inflammation	Localized area of inflammation associated with induration, tenderness, and possible low-grade fever.	Lactational mastitis
	Localized area of inflammation associated with induration, tenderness, edema, fever, and possible purulent discharge.	Abscess
	Edematous, reddened, indurated breast. May or may not be localized and generally associated with nipple retraction.	Malignant tumor
Peau d'orange	Enlarged, more pronounced, and deep follicular openings of the breast skin from stretching by the underlying tumor. Skin looks like an orange peel.	Malignant tumor Mastitis
Nonsymmetrical breast contour	An abnormal bulging or flattening of the breast. More apparent with tensing the pectoral muscles.	Benign tumor Malignant tumor Fat necrosis Trauma Free silicone injection into breasts
Unilateral dilated superficial veins	Enlarged and easily visible superficial veins. The growth of the tumor places a larger demand for blood, and the vessels dilate to accommodate the need for more blood volume to the area.	Benign tumor Malignant tumor
Breast pain	Cyclic pain occurs several days premenstrually in teenagers and young adults. Also occurs with sensation of breast enlargement.	Premenstrual breast enlargement
	Well-localized, noncyclic pain unrelated to menses.	Benign tumor Breast trauma Abscess
	Sharp, stabbing noncyclic pain with no apparent cause. Generally malignant tumors are painless.	Malignant tumor
Breast hair in female	Moderate to dense hair extending beyond the areola. Hair in the midline is especially significant.	Endocrine disorders
Abnormal lactation	Abnormal stimulation of the normal causes of lactation. Occurs mainly in females but can occur in males.	Breast trauma, pituitary disorder (tumor, surgical removal, inflammation)
Scars	Bilateral (inframammary) or subareolar scars.	Augmentation mammoplasty
	Complete circumareolar scars.	Reduction mammoplasty
Enlarged male breasts	Firm, slightly nodular, enlarged breasts. Often occurs unilaterally.	Gynecomastia

sun. Sparse hair surrounding the areola is common and is of no significance. A venous pattern, if present, is diffuse and symmetrical.

Menstrual Changes. There are various breast changes during the menstrual cycle. The breasts are least engorged and smallest in size during days four through seven from decreased circulating estrogen. Three to four days prior to menstruation the mammary glandular tissue engorges from higher levels of estrogen. This causes the breast to be larger and more dense, sensitive, tender, and nodular. Many women experience bilateral premenstrual breast fullness, although it is common for the breast changes to occur in only one breast or even in a portion of a breast. The cause of breast engorgement is not completely understood but is probably from an increased extracellular fluid tension.

Inspection of the Areolae and Nipples

The examiner observes the nipples and areolae for placement, color, contour, and inversion, and the chest for the presence of supernumerary nipples (Table 12-2). The nipples and areola are slightly below the center of the developed breast in the midclavicular line, at approximately the fourth intercostal space. Any asymmetrical placement or pointing suggests retraction. The degree of pigmentation varies among individuals and is related to complexion and estrogen

levels. Generally the areolae range in color from light pinkish in fair-skinned people to dark brown in dark-skinned people. Any recent change in color is directly related to estrogen levels. Pregnancy and puberty darken the areolae and nipples, menopause lightens them. The areola is relatively rough from the presence of sebaceous glands and the nipple is protruberant with many papillae.

Longstanding, bilateral nipple inversion is often seen as a variation of normal. If disease is not present, the inverted nipples can generally be momentarily everted by squeezing the areola at the base of the nipple between the thumb and index finger (Figure 12-4).

Supernumerary nipples occur from the axilla to the groin on the "milk line" (Figure 12-5). In the embryo an epithelial ridge forms from the axillae to the groin. Later in uterine development, the ridge atrophies except at the pectoral region where a breast, areola, and nipple develop. Absence of breasts is from atrophy of the ridge, and supernumerary nipples are from portions of the ridge that do not atrophy. The most common area for supernumerary nipples is the axillae. The second most common location is just below the normal breast. There may be a nipple, nipple and areola, or glandular breast tissue only. This variance results from a minor error in development; the only significance of a nipple or nipple and areola is in dis-

Table 12-2. Selected Abnormalities of the Nipples and Areolae

Finding	*Description*	*Possible Conditions*
Nipple retraction Inverted nipple Deviation of nipple axis	Recent and unilateral nipple inversion that is fixed; nipple cannot be everted. The fibroses from the tumor shortens the duct system of the breast and causes the nipple to point toward the tumor. If the tumor underlies the nipple, the fibrosis pulls the entire nipple inward. If the tumor is lateral, above, or below the nipple, the nipple points in that direction. A deviated nipple is a subtle sign of retraction. Often the inverted or deviated nipple is also broad and thick.	Benign tumor Malignant tumor Subareolar abscess
Fissures	Cracked, painful nipples. Inflammation may be present.	Local infection Inadequate lubrication during lactation
Discharge	Pus, serous, or bloody fluid drains from the nipple or is expressed on palpation. Discharge from many ducts occurs more frequently with benign conditions while discharge from only one duct is more ominous.	Benign tumor Malignant tumor Fibrocystic disease Paget's disease Abscess Fat necrosis Mastitis
Scaling	Scaling of nipples progressing to reddened and excoriated nipples to complete erosion of the nipple.	Paget's disease
Tender nodule	Montgomery glands inflamed, tender, and palpable. Often associated with fissures or ulceration.	Abscess

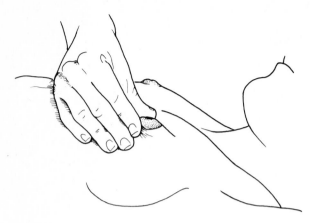

Figure 12-4. Nipple eversion.

tinguishing it from a mole. The only significance of glandular breast tissue is in distinguishing it from a tumor.

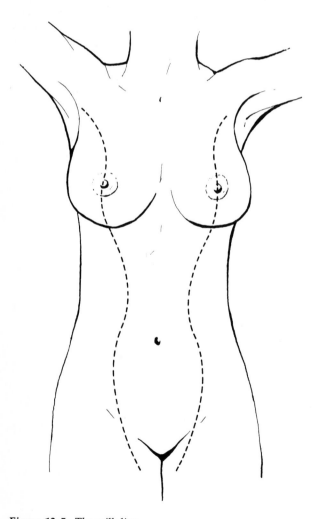

Figure 12-5. The milk line.

Palpation of the Female Breasts

It is ideal to palpate the breasts with the client supine and then sitting, but if this is not possible due to client or time limitation, the sitting position may be omitted. In both positions the examiner palpates the breasts with the client's arms at her sides and extended overhead. All females with a current or past history of breast masses, a family history of breast cancer, or very large pendulous breasts must have their breasts palpated while sitting and supine. This technique ensures complete palpation of the entire breast tissue.

In the supine position, the breast is distributed across the chest wall. This distribution is augmented by placing a small pillow under the shoulder on the side being examined, the ipsilateral side. By abducting the ipsilateral arm and placing the hand under the neck, the pectoral muscles are tensed and the breast is further flattened and more evenly distributed (Figure 12-6).

The breast is palpated against the rib cage with the palmar aspects of the fingertips of one or both hands. Gentle but firm pressure is applied while moving the fingers in a pulsating or rotary movement. The palpation must be gentle enough so that it is not unpleasant for the client but firm enough to discover any underlying pathology.

There are several methods used for palpating the breast. The most important consideration is that the entire breast be palpated. The examiner selects one method and uses this same system on all clients. This system includes definite beginning and ending points; therefore, no part of the breast is overlooked.

One method for breast palpation is to start at the circumference of the breast and palpate to the nipple in three or four concentric circles, covering the entire breast (Figure 12-7). Particular attention is paid to the

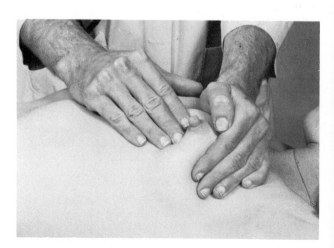

Figure 12-6. Breast palpation.

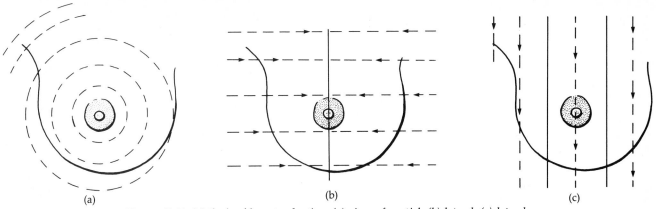

Figure 12-7. *Methods of breast palpation: (a) circumferential; (b) lateral; (c) lateral.*

tail of Spence and the upper outer quadrant since the majority of breast masses occur here. This is the method that the American Cancer Society uses in teaching breast self-examination. Another method is to divide the breasts laterally in half and palpate in a series of six to eight parallel transverse lines across the breast beginning superiorly and proceeding inferiorly (Figure 12-7). First the medial breast tissue is palpated, then the lateral tissue. A third method is to divide the breast laterally in thirds and palpate in three lateral lines down the breasts, beginning at the clavicle (Figure 12-7). If the client is concerned that her method of breast palpation differs from the examiner's, she is taught the principle of using one method each time and palpating the entirety of both breasts.

In the case of very large, pendulous breasts, it may be necessary to palpate the breasts bimanually. In this situation the examiner uses one hand to support the breast and the other hand to palpate the breast against the supporting hand. Bimanual palpation is performed with the client sitting upright or supine.

If a client complains of a lump in one breast, the examination begins with the other breast to maintain the examiner's objectivity regarding the mass. In this way the examiner establishes a baseline for the client's breast. Also, the examiner does not want to overlook any pathology in the "normal" breast. Often, if a client complains of a lump in one breast and a mass is palpated, the other breast is not palpated as carefully. It is never assumed that the client discovered all of the pathology in her breasts. By doing a careful examination in the unaffected breast first, any pathology present will be noticed more easily.

The breasts are palpated for consistency and masses. Normal breast tissue feels firm and elastic with no masses, areas of tenderness, or hyperthermia. The lobes are sometimes more distinct premenstrually.

Masses are palpated for size, depth, shape, de-

marcation, consistency, and degree of fixation to the underlying muscle and location. The size is approximated by the distance in millimeters between the palpating fingers for all three planes: length, width, and thickness. Also included is an estimation of how deep into the breast tissue the mass extends. The shape is described as round, discoid, elongated, or irregular. In terms of demarcation some masses have very distinct borders while others seem to fade into the surrounding tissue. The consistency is described as elastic, soft and compressible, rubbery, firm or hard in quality. It may be difficult to determine the consistency of small masses accurately. The degree of fixation to underlying muscle is assessed while the client is sitting with arms at her sides. Then the pectoral muscles are tensed by pushing the palms of the hands together or by placing hands on hips and pushing in. The three degrees of fixation are as follows:

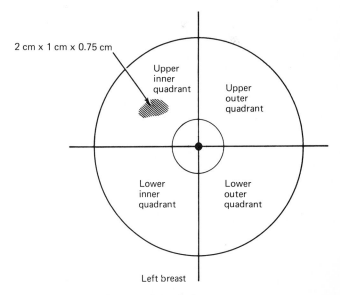

Figure 12-8. *Sample recording of a breast mass.*

first-degree fixation—an elevated, movable mass becomes fixed when the pectoral muscles are tensed.

second-degree fixation—pectoral contraction causes sharp fixation and immobility of the mass.

third-degree fixation—a mass that is clearly fixed to the pectoralis, even during relaxation.

The location is recorded by drawing a sketch of a breast with a horizontal and vertical line intersecting at the nipple. This topographically divides the breast into four quadrants; upper lateral, lower lateral, upper medial, and lower medial. An alternative method of division is to compare the breast to a clock, with the nipple at the center. In this way the vertical line represents 12 and 6 o'clock and the horizontal line represents 9 and 3 o'clock. The other numbers on the face of a clock are then placed appropriately. The location of the mass is drawn in the sketch. (Figure 12-8).

After palpating the breasts, the examiner palpates the areolae and nipples. The areolae and nipples are palpated between the thumb and forefinger. Nor-

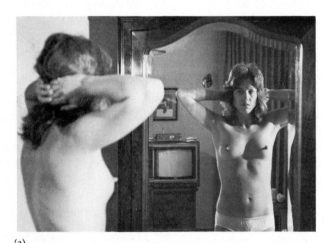

(a)

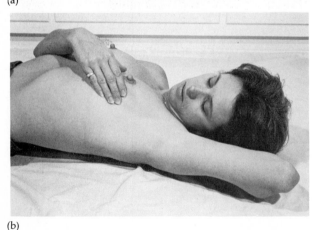

(b)

Figure 12-9. Breast self-examination: (a) inspection; (b) palpation.

mally there is no nipple discharge except during pregnancy and lactation. A discharge at any other time may be indicative of acquired disease; all areas of the breasts are palpated to determine from which lobe the discharge originates. It is also important to attempt to ascertain whether the discharge originates from one or more ducts.

Examination of the Male Breasts

This is a very brief and simple procedure but should not be omitted. As in the female, the breasts and axillae are inspected and palpated. The position for the male is generally sitting with arms at his sides. Since the breast is already flat and evenly distributed across the chest wall the supine position is not necessary. If a mass is palpated, the procedure and observations are the same as in the female. Most male breast tumors are in the areolar areas, so particular attention is paid here.

The color of the male areola and nipple varies with skin complexion, as it does in the female; dark-skinned males have more deeply pigmented areolae than fair-skinned males. Any change in color is related to altered hormonal levels.

If the breast is enlarged it is important to distinguish the enlargement from fat (soft and mushy) or breast tissue (firm and perhaps slightly nodular) called gynecomastia. Gynecomastia often occurs with puberty and is normal. It may be related to liver disease, side effects of drugs, or it may be idiopathic.

Breast Self-Examination

It must be stressed that most breast masses are discovered during self-examination. As with all cancer, early detection is paramount. Breast examination is done by the client in the same manner as the examiner performs it, although in self-examination, inspection is done in front of a mirror with the arms hanging and then raised onto the head (Figure 12-9). The American Cancer Society recommends that, in addition to palpating the breasts while supine, it also be done during a bath or shower while the breasts are soapy and wet. Because of the similarity in the procedure, it is most natural for the examiner to instruct clients about breast self-examination during the actual assessment. This encourages a relaxed, free-flowing exchange of questions and answers.

Breast self-examination is done at regular intervals, especially since the breasts normally change in character during various stages of the menstrual cycle. The best time for the examination is somewhere between day four through seven of the menstrual cycle.

This is when the breasts are their smallest since the glandular tissue is the least congested. If the client is nearing or has passed menopause, she is reminded that breast self-examination must still continue on a regular basis. Clients are advised to notify a health professional promptly if a change is noticed. This includes findings of a lump, change in appearance, and discharge.

Life Cycle Variations

Childhood

Many newborns have areolar and breast engorgement from transplacental estrogen. This may last up to two to three weeks. There is no difference between males and females until about the age of nine or ten. Both have small nipples with no evidence of glandular breast tissue. The size of the nipple and the areola grow in proportion to the size of the chest.

Adolescence

Between the ages of 9 and 15, breast budding begins in females; more often than not it proceeds unilaterally. The first area for "budding" is subareolar (Figure 12-10). The areolae and nipples become more pigmented and the breasts are often well developed by the time of menarche. Breast development before the age of 9 is considered precocious; total lack of development by the age of 17 is abnormal. Both are the result of disturbances of the endocrine system. In pubescent males the breasts generally remain flat; if not, the enlargement is self-limiting and usually disappears within four to six months. Gynecomastia has been reported in chronic use of marijuana.

Pregnancy and Lactation

In pregnancy the placenta produces estrogen and progesterone; these hormones stimulate the lobules to enlarge and multiply in number. Thus, the breasts are fuller, firmer, larger, and more tender. Depending on the rapidity of the growth and the elasticity of the breast skin, striae and venous engorgement may occur. Estrogen and progesterone also cause the nipple to be more erect, Montgomery's glands to be more prominent, and the nipples and areola to be pigmented more deeply. The color returns to normal after pregnancy in some women and remains darkened in others. During the last half of pregnancy there generally are clear, thin, yellowed secretions from the nipples that occur with sucking or manual manipulation of the breast. During lactation, and after lactation for several weeks or months, a creamy-white, relatively thick discharge occurs. Estrogen and progesterone medications cause breast changes similar to those of early pregnancy.

Nipple inversion does not interfere with the lactating function of the breasts. Often the baby's sucking everts the nipple. If the baby is unable to do this, the mother usually can evert the nipple by squeezing the areola at the nipple base between her thumb and index finger.

During lactation, breast appearance depends upon the amount of milk in the breast. Immediately after nursing, the breasts are generally soft and not engorged. After a few hours, the breasts begin to enlarge in size and become firmer and more lobular. It is common for breast lobes to be very distinct on inspection. If milk production exceeds the storing capacities of the breast, milk leakage occurs. Breast milk is creamy-white and relatively thick. Often leaking occurs if the mother thinks of her baby or hears a crying voice. This is a normal response from the secretion of oxytocin.

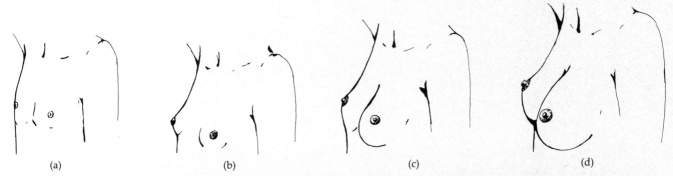

(a) (b) (c) (d)

Figure 12-10. *Female breast development: (a) undeveloped breast: (b) subareolar "budding"; (c) developing breast; (d) developed breast.*

After lactation, the appearance of the breasts approximates the pre-pregnant size and contour, although this may take many months to a year. The breasts in women who have been pregnant, whether they have nursed or not, are less dense, more nodular, and less protuberant.

Late Adulthood

After menopause there is an involution and atrophy of the glandular tissue, along with more fat deposits.

This gives rise to a slightly smaller, less dense, and less nodular breast. The breasts appear more pendulous, flabby, and flattened with dependent crests of thickened tissue. This is related not to past pregnancies or lactation, but to decreased estrogen production by the ovaries. The lower levels of estrogen also cause the nipples and areolae to lighten in color. The breasts appear lower on the chest since the rib cage shrinks as a normal process in aging.

Anatomy and Physiology

The abdomen contains the abdominal aorta, liver, gallbladder, kidneys, spleen, stomach, pancreas, small intestine, colon, and spermatic cords in males and ovaries in females. For ease of identification of underlying structures, the abdomen is divided into topographical areas. There are two methods of subdivision. The more widely used system divides the abdomen into four areas by extending two hypothetical lines through the umbilicus. One line is vertical and extends from the xiphoid process to the symphysis pubis. The other is horizontal and intersects the vertical at right angles at the umbilicus. These lines divide the abdomen into right upper, right lower, left upper, and left lower quadrants (Figure 13-1, Table 13-1).

Table 13-1. Topographical Mapping: Four Quadrants

Right Upper Quadrant	*Left Upper Quadrant*
Liver and gallbladder	Left lobe of liver
Duodenum	Spleen
Head of pancreas	Stomach
Portion of right kidney	Body and tail of pancreas
Hepatic flexure of colon	Portion of left kidney
	Splenic flexure of colon

Right Lower Quadrant	*Left Lower Quadrant*
Cecum	Sigmoid colon
Appendix	Lower pole of left kidney
Lower pole of right kidney	Portion of descending colon
Portion of ascending colon	Left ureter
Right ureter	Left spermatic cord
Right spermatic cord	Left ovary
Right ovary	

The other method of subdivision divides the abdomen into nine topographical areas. This is achieved by extending vertical lines from the right and left midclavicular areas downward to a midpoint on the right and left inquinal ligaments. These vertical lines are then intersected by two horizontal lines; one line joins the lower border of the costal margins while the other joins the crest of the right and left iliac bones. With the intersection of these lines, the abdomen is divided from top to bottom into right hypochondrium, epigastric, left hypochondrium, right lumbar (flank), umbilicus, left lumbar (flank), right inguinal, suprapubic (hypogastric), and left inguinal areas (Figure 13-2).

Chapter 13

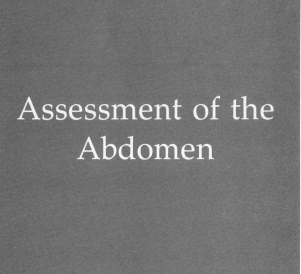

Assessment of the Abdomen

Objectives

The examiner will be able to do the following:

1. Inspect the abdomen
2. Auscultate the abdomen
3. Percuss the abdomen and locate the liver and spleen
4. Palpate the abdomen
5. Recognize abnormalities of the abdomen
6. Record the information obtained

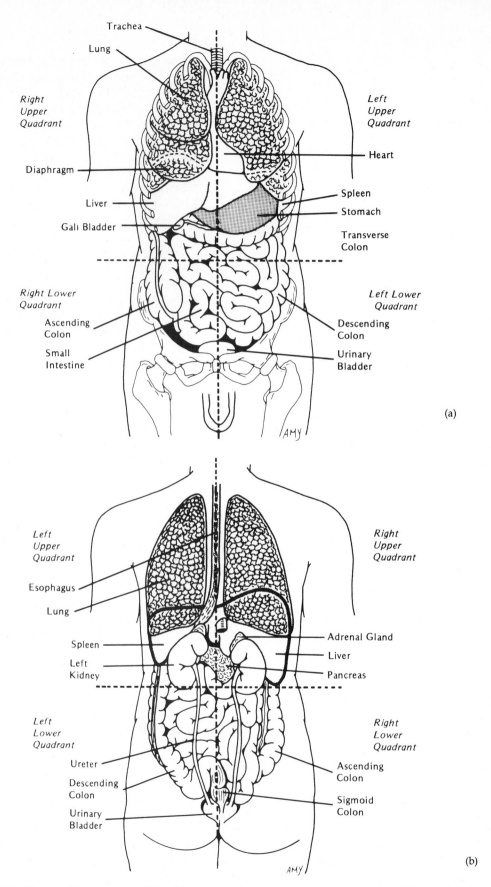

Figure 13-1. *Topographical mapping of the abdomen into four quadrants: (a) anterior view; (b) posterior view.*

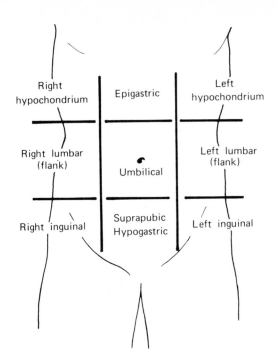

Figure 13-2. *Topographical mapping of the abdomen into nine subdivisions.*

The liver is a wedge-shaped organ located primarily in the right upper quadrant. It lies beneath the dome of the diaphragm behind the rib cage and is divided into two parts: the larger right lobe and the smaller left lobe. The left lobe extends into the left upper quadrant. The functions of the liver are numerous: conversion of glucose into glycogen, amino acids into carbohydrates, and carotene to vitamin A; detoxification of certain drugs, chemicals, and hormones; production of bile; metabolism of lipids and cholesterol; storage and filtration of blood from the gut; and storage of fat-soluble vitamins A, D, E, and K and water-soluble B-12.

The gallbladder, also located in the right upper quadrant, is a pear-shaped sac, which lies on the posterior surface of the right lobe of the liver lateral to the right midclavicular line. The gallbladder concentrates and stores bile.

The right and left kidneys are located in their respective right and left quadrants with their lower poles extending into the lower quadrants. The kidneys are located retroperitoneally on either side of the vertebral column with their upper poles at the level of the twelfth dorsal vertebra and lower poles at the level of the third lumbar spine. The right kidney lies somewhat lower than the left. The kidneys maintain the constancy of the internal environment by the excretion of nitrogenous waste products and by regulation of fluid, electrolyte, and acid-base balance via filtration, reabsorption, secretion, and excretion.

The spleen, located in the left upper quadrant, is a large, oblong, flattened organ. It lies below the vault of the left diaphragm under the anterior left costal margin. Its long axis follows the oblique position of the 10th rib; its short axis extends between the 9th and 11th ribs in the midaxillary line. It acts as a filter that recognizes and removes aging red blood cells, damaged red blood cells, and sensitized platelets that have been complexed with antibodies. The spleen also removes particulate inclusions from red blood cells without destroying them. It responds to antigenic stimulation and to overuse of its filtering function by cellular proliferation (similar to a lymph node—Chapter 19).

The stomach also lies in the left upper quadrant, although when full it can extend into the adjacent quadrants. The stomach stores, mixes, and propels ingested food. It mixes food with gastric juices containing hydrochloric acid and digestive enzymes (pepsin) until it becomes a semiliquid mixture called chyme and slowly propels the chyme forward to the small intestine.

Although the head of the pancreas lies in the curve of the duodenum in the right upper quadrant, the major portion of the pancreas is found in the left upper quadrant. It is a tongue-shaped organ, which lies transversely across the posterior abdominal wall behind the stomach. The pancreas produces pancreatic juices important in digestion and secretes two hormones, insulin and glucagon.

Each quadrant contains a portion of either the small or large intestine (Table 13-1). In the small intestine the major portion of the absorption of nutrients takes place. Digestion of these nutrients is aided by the secretion of bile and other pancreatic and intestinal secretions. That portion unable to be absorbed is propelled into the large intestine via the ileocecal valve. The large intestine has only a minor role in digestion; its primary function is the absorption of water and the continued propulsion of its contents toward the rectum for defecation.

The anatomy and tone of the abdominal musculature may affect the findings of physical assessment. The flat muscles and recti abdomini are the two groups of superficial abdominal muscles. The recti abdomini are two large muscles, found on either side of the midline. They extend from the anterior costal margin to the symphysis pubis. The flat muscles, including the internal and external oblique muscles and the transverse muscles, form the superficial covering of the abdomen and join to form the inguinal ligament.

Assessment Modalities

Preparation

Examination of the abdomen is best achieved with adequate exposure and proper positioning. Full exposure of the abdomen from the costal margins to the symphysis pubis is required. Protection of the client's modesty is accomplished by covering the genitals of both sexes and by draping the woman's breasts. Proper positioning is achieved by placing the client in a supine position with the head elevated on a pillow and knees slightly bent, which relaxes the abdominal musculature.

Prior to the examination, the client is given the opportunity to empty the bladder. A warm room is essential since shivering causes tensing of the superficial abdominal muscles, which decreases ease of examination. The examiner asks the client to identify areas of tenderness so that they can be examined last.

The equipment necessary includes a stethoscope, flexible tape measure, and watch with a second hand. Although all four examination techniques are utilized, the order is inspection, auscultation, percussion, and palpation. Auscultation precedes percussion and palpation to prevent distortion of auscultatory findings due to pressure on the abdominal wall. Percussion precedes palpation to screen for the presence of an enlarged spleen prior to deep palpation.

Inspection

Inspection includes assessment of skin characteristics, contour, movement, and symmetry. The skin is inspected for color and venous patterns. Normally the abdomen is the same color as the remainder of the body and is free of pigmentary changes. However, it may appear somewhat lighter in color since it is often protected from sun exposure. For this reason evidence of color variation or unusual pigmentation sometimes is first seen on the abdomen. Color changes are explored thoroughly to eliminate such extrinsic causative factors as suntanning, drugs, or other chemical substances (Table 13-2).

The normal venous pattern of the abdomen is inconspicuous but may appear prominent in thin or wasted individuals. Normally the direction of blood flow in superficial abdominal veins is away from the umbilicus; blood in abdominal veins superior to the umbilicus flows toward the head (cephalad) while blood in abdominal veins inferior to the umbilicus drains downward toward the feet.

Normally the contour of the abdomen is flat from the xiphoid process to the symphysis pubis with the umbilicus centrally located. Nutritional status, however, can alter these findings. The abdomen of an obese individual appears protuberant, and the umbilicus may be slightly inverted. Sometimes striae are seen. The abdomen of a malnourished or very thin individual may appear concave (scaphoid) with prominent bony landmarks (iliac crests).

Normally the abdomen rises slightly with inspiration and falls with expiration. On inspiration it is not unusual to see a slight protrusion of the abdomen; this is caused by the descent of the diaphragm. Peristalsis may be observed in thin individuals. Visible peristalsis appears as slow, undulating waves that move obliquely across the abdomen. Several minutes may be required to make this observation. Unusually active peristalsis may indicate intestinal obstruction.

Normally the abdomen is symmetrical. To inspect for symmetry the examiner stands and observes the abdomen from the side and from below. The examiner may also ask the client to perform a Valsalva maneuver (forced expiration with mouth closed) or lift the head off the pillow to tense the recti muscles.

Table 13-2. Selected Color Abnormalities of the Abdomen

Finding	Condition	Description
Yellow abdomen	Liver disease	Generalized yellow appearance to skin, often referred to as jaundice. Most noticeable on abdomen, sclerae, and mucous membranes. Due to deposition of bilirubin in skin.
Bluish-gray umbilicus (Cullen's sign)	Tubal pregnancy Hemorrhagic pancreatitis	Faint blue-gray discoloration in area of umbilicus. Indication of intraperitoneal bleeding.
Bluish-gray flanks (Grey Turner's sign)	Hemorrhagic pancreatitis Strangulated bowel	Bluish-grey, red, or purple discoloration in flanks and lower abdomen. Not the result of trauma. Indicates the presence of blood in extraperitoneal tissues.
Purple striations (stretch marks)	Cushing's disease	Purple stretch marks due to loss of connective tissue in skin.

In this way, areas of localized bulging may be detected. Sometimes it is necessary to have the client stand to bring out the bulges (Tables 13-3 and 13-4).

Auscultation

The abdomen is auscultated for bowel and vascular sounds. Auscultation is performed with both the diaphragm and bell of the stethoscope. The diaphragm is used to detect high-pitched intestinal and arterial sounds while the bell is used to hear the low-pitched sounds of murmurs and venous hums. The diaphragm is gently placed on the abdomen and may be held in place by light pressure of the middle and index fingers or simply laid upon the abdominal wall (Figure 13-3). When ausculatation of one area of the abdomen is completed, the stethoscope is carefully lifted and then gently replaced on another area of the abdominal wall. Normal bowel sounds are the result of peristaltic activity moving gas, solids, and liquids in the intestinal tract. These sounds vary among individuals and also in the same individual depending upon meal ingestion. Bowel sounds become quite loud when a meal is long overdue and increase in frequency immediately after a meal. The diversity of normal bowel sounds is great; they are generally low-pitched gurgling sounds heard every 3 to 5 seconds and lasting approximately 0.5 second (Table 13-5).

The abdomen is then auscultated for detection of vascular and peritoneal sounds (Table 13-6). Both the diaphragm and bell of the stethoscope are used. Areas examined include the epigastrium, the regions superior and lateral to the umbilicus, over the liver, spleen, kidneys, and femoral arteries. Normally there are no vascular or peritoneal sounds.

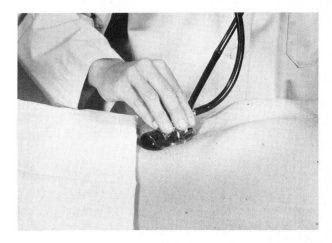

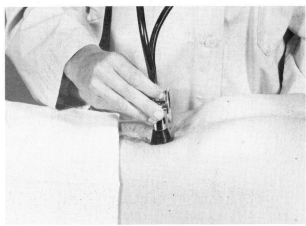

Figure 13-3. *Auscultation of the abdomen.*

Table 13-3. Localized Abdominal Bulging

Finding	Condition	Description
Bulging around incision	Incisional hernia	Abdominal scar may appear normal while client supine. Protrusion represents spreading apart of muscle defect beneath scar with a knuckle of mesentery at intestinal filling defect. Standing or Valsalva maneuver may be necessary.
Bulging in region of umbilicus	Umbilical hernia	Protrusion may appear while standing or supine. Results from incomplete formation of fascial ring. May appear following pregnancy, longstanding ascites, or obesity.
Small midline bulge in epigastrium	Epigastric hernia	May not be observed on inspection but detected by running pad of index finger along linea alba while client is standing. May present with epigastric pain. Due to protrusion of small amount of fat between fibers of linea alba.
Midline ridged bulging	Diastasis recti	Separation of the two rectus abdominal muscles. May be either congenital or acquired, as in pregnancy or obesity. Of no clinical significance.

Table 13-4. Symmetrical and Asymmetrical Abdominal Distention

Finding	Condition	Description
Distention-symmetrical	Obesity	Abdomen is protuberant giving appearance of distention. Umbilicus is inverted. Increase in adipose tissue observed on other body parts. Striae may be present.
	Cirrhosis Abdominal tumor Cardiac failure	Distention caused by accumulation of free fluid in peritoneal cavity (ascites). Flanks bulge. Umbilicus is flat or everted. Skin appears tight. Fluid wave and shifting dullness present.
	Gaseous distention	Distention caused by excessive accumulation of gas in intestine. May be found in malabsorption syndromes or small intestinal obstruction. Percussion is tympanitic.
	Constipation	Distention caused by excessive accumulation of feces in colon. May be palpated in left lower quadrant. Disappears with bowel movement or following enemas.
Distention-asymmetrical	Pregnancy	Distention caused by the presence of a fetus in last trimester of pregnancy. Umbilicus pushed upward. Skin may have striae and presence of linea nigra. Heart sounds of fetus and placental blood flow may be audible on auscultation.
	Benign tumors Malignant tumors	Soft to hard, regular to irregular masses due to abnormal tissue growth. Distention more apparent in lower half of abdomen due to presence of tumor arising out of pelvis. Dull to percussion as gas-filled intestine pushed to upper abdomen.

Percussion

Percussion provides the examiner with an orientation to the underlying structures of the abdomen and also establishes the presence of gas, fluid, or masses. Percussion is performed with the client in the supine position while the examiner stands to the right. Light, mediate percussion is the method of choice since it produces clear, recognizable tones. Three sounds are normally heard on abdominal percussion: tympany, hyperresonance, and dullness. Tympany is heard over the stomach; hyperresonance is heard over the intestines; and dullness is heard over the liver and spleen.

The abdomen is percussed in a thorough and systematic manner. Areas of dullness are best appreciated when the examiner approaches them from areas of resonance or tympany. Percussion is begun in the left midaxillary line. A resonant sound is initially heard over the underlying lung. As the examiner percusses inferiorly, a dull sound is noted posterior to the midaxillary line around the 10th rib from the mass of the underlying spleen. This sound may be obscured in the presence of gastric or colonic air and for this reason percussion of the normal spleen may be difficult.

Percussion in the right midaxillary and midclavicular lines is then performed. Beginning at the midaxillary line, the examiner percusses for the upper limit of liver dullness. This is normally noted somewhere between the fifth and seventh intercostal spaces. To obtain a more accurate assessment of liver

Table 13-5. Selected Abnormal Bowel Sounds

Finding	Condition	Description
Absence of bowel sounds	Peritonitis Paralytic ileus Postanesthesia	Bowel sounds are not heard for at least 5 minutes. Only complete absence of bowel sounds is significant. Indication of inhibited motility.
Increased bowel sounds	Diarrhea Intestinal obstruction	Loud, rushing, high-pitched tinkling sounds. Abdominal pain may be present. Indication of increase in motility of bowel. May indicate bowel obstruction with increase in motility proximal to site of obstruction.

Table 13-6. Selected Abnormal Abdominal Sounds

Finding	Condition	Description
Bruit	Aneurysm of abdominal aorta Renal artery stenosis Iliac artery stenosis Femoral artery stenosis	A bruit is a soft, high-pitched sound heard over a blood vessel. It is the result of interference of laminar blood flow through the vessels creating turbulence. Caused by atherosclerotic plaques, aneurysms, or congenital bands. Should be heard in same area even if client's position changes. May be continuous or heard only during systole.
Venous hum	Liver disease with portal hypertension Portal or splenic vein thrombosis	Continuous soft, humming sound heard over liver or upper abdomen. Caused by increase in collateral circulation of portal and systemic venous system or dialated periumbilical circulation. Rare finding.
Friction rub	Splenic infarction Primary or metastatic tumor of liver Peritonitis	Rough, grating sounds resembling two pieces of leather rubbing together. Occurs when there is irritation of peritoneal surface of an organ. Rare finding.

size, percussion is performed at the right midclavicular line (Figure 13-4). The examiner identifies the upper border of liver dullness by percussing inferiorly from lung resonance to liver dullness. The first note of liver dullness is lightly marked on the client's abdomen. The lower border of liver dullness is then identified by percussing from below the umbilicus superiorly toward the liver. The examiner notes the change from hyperresonance to dullness, which denotes the liver's lower border; it is normally located at the costal margin. By measuring the distance between the upper and lower borders, the vertical span of the liver is determined. The liver span normally measures 6 to 12 centimeters at the right midclavicular line. The liver span can also be percussed at the midsternal line. Normally the expanse of the liver in this area is 4 to 8 centimeters.

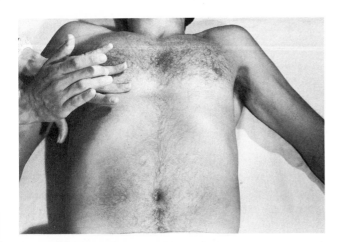

Figure 13-4. The examiner percusses the right upper quadrant to demarcate the superior liver border.

The examiner percusses the remainder of the abdomen following percussion of the liver and spleen. A tympanitic sound is normally heard in the epigastrium and left hypochondrium from the stomach, while a hyperresonant sound is heard in the remaining areas (Tables 13-7 and 13-8).

Palpation

There are two palpation techniques used when assessing the abdomen: light and deep palpation.

For both techniques the examiner stands to the right of the client, if right-handed, and to the left of the client if left-handed. Light palpation is performed for the purpose of determining the muscular tone of the abdomen, identifying organ enlargement and superficial masses, and detecting areas of abdominal tenderness. The gentle quality of light palpation is also of value in helping the client to relax.

Light palpation is performed with the client in the supine position. The client is assisted in relaxation by supporting the slightly flexed knees with a pillow. The examiner uses the closely approximated fingers of the right hand by placing the palmar surface of the pads of the fingertips upon the abdomen (Figure 13-5). The examiner exerts and increases pressure in a slow, gentle, yet deliberate manner and begins in the pubic area and proceeds superiorly toward the costal margin. The fingers depress the abdominal wall approximately 1 centimeter.

With a relaxed client, adequate explanation of the procedure, and proper examining technique, light palpation normally reveals little or no musclar resistance. The rectus abdominis muscles normally are relaxed during expiration.

Table 13-7. Selected Abnormal Percussion Findings

Finding	Condition	Description
Dullness above 9th interspace in left anterior axillary line	Enlarged spleen	One of the first signs of an enlarged spleen may be the change from tympany to dullness noted in this area. When spleen is normal size, percussion in this area is tympanitic. Splenic dullness may also be caused by fluid in the stomach or feces in the colon. Percussion of dullness requires careful palpation of the splenic area.
Absence of liver dullness	Presence of free air in abdominal cavity	Caused by perforation of hollow viscus. Must be distinguished from presence of hepatic flexure between diaphragm and liver, which is of no clinical significance.
Liver dullness greater than 12 cm. in the right midclavicular line	Liver disease	Normal border of liver dullness may be distorted in presence of liver enlargement, mass adjacent to liver, or downward displacement of liver. Measurement of liver descent and vertical span at right midclavicular and midsternal line important. Careful, thorough palpation of liver required.
Dullness in suprapubic area	Distended bladder Pregnancy Uterine or ovarian tumor	Percussion in this area should be tympanitic. Dullness may indicate that the client has not emptied bladder or may signify urinary retention. May also indicate pregnancy in female client. History and presenting signs and symptoms helpful in differentiating causes. Follow-up palpation necessary

Table 13-8. Percussion Tests for Abdominal Distention

Finding	Test	Description
Ascites	Fluid-wave	Client supine. Examiner places left hand against client's right flank. Ulnar edge of client's hand is lightly placed at midline. Examiner's right hand lightly taps left flank of client. In presence of ascites, examiner will feel sharp slap against left hand. Occurs only when large amounts of fluid have accumulated.
	Shifting dullness	Client supine. Starting at midline and moving laterally to each flank, examiner percusses abdomen until dullness heard. Areas of dullness are lightly marked on client's abdomen. Client is turned on side and percussion is performed from midline to flank; the points of dullness are marked. Procedure repeated with client turned on opposite side. Shift in line of dullness indicates presence of intraperitoneal fluid.
	Knee-chest position	Client placed in knee-chest position. Abdomen is percussed from flanks toward midline or most dependent area. When free fluid is present, it accumulates at the dependent area (often the periumbilical region). Finding of dullness in dependent area indicates presence of fluid. Test used to detect small amounts of fluid.

In the presence of voluntary guarding, the examiner may wish to use the stethoscope to perform light palpation. Because the client does not associate the stethoscope with pain, muscle resistance is usually minimal or nonexistent. Although the stethoscope does not have sensitivity like the pads of the fingertips, it does allow the examiner to accomplish light palpation to screen for organ enlargement and abdominal tenderness. If guarding is the result of ticklishness, the examiner can have the client's fingers placed over the fingers of the examiner's palpating hand.

Table 13-9. Muscular Resistance to Abdominal Palpation

Finding	Condition	Description
Voluntary guarding	Nervous or fearful client	Voluntary tightening of the abdominal muscles due to fear, anxiety, or ticklishness. Rigidity is often symmetrical. Client is encouraged to relax and examiner carefully explains procedure in an attempt to reduce guarding.
Involuntary guarding	Intra-abdominal lesion Generalized peritonitis Appendicitis Mesenteric infarction	Involuntary tightening of abdominal muscles due to increased muscle tonus. Rigidity is often unilateral. Client is unable to relax. Rectus abdominis muscles will remain rigid on expiration in presence of involuntary guarding.

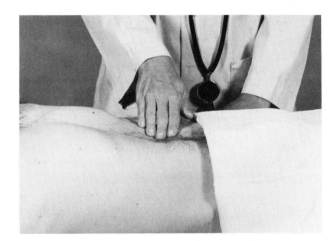

Figure 13-5. *Light palpation of the abdomen.*

The normal abdomen is free of enlarged organs and abdominal masses; there are no areas of tenderness. Areas of known tenderness are palpated last.

Deep palpation is performed to identify abdominal organs and masses. Although the examiner begins with the client supine with knees flexed, the client can be asked to turn onto the side, assume a knee-chest position or stand to enhance the examination. The client is encouraged to breathe deeply through the mouth during palpation maneuvers. Deep breathing not only facilitates relaxation but also helps the examiner delineate organs. With each successive expiration the examiner increases the depth of the probe until the organ or mass is identified. The examiner does not push into the organ with the fingers but rather lets the organ descend upon the fingers while concentrating on its characteristics. Methods of palpation differ depending upon examiner preference, organ being assessed and client presentation. They include single-handed palpation and two types of bimanual palpation.

In single-handed palpation the examiner places the palmar surface of one hand on the abdominal wall. With the fingers approximated, the examiner presses deep into the abdomen with a slow, gentle, deliberate manner. The examiner's fingers press downward and at the same time allow the abdominal wall to glide 4 to 5 centimeters over the underlying abdominal structures (Figure 13-6).

The examiner uses reinforced palpation, a bimanual technique, in the presence of obesity or muscular resistance or when deeper palpation is desired. The examiner positions one hand used as in single-handed palpation and uses the fingers of the other hand to apply pressure on the interphalangeal joints of the lower hand. The examiner exerts pressure with the upper hand while concentrating on the tactile sensations received by the lower hand (Figure 13-7).

Table 13-10. Abdominal Tenderness

Finding	Condition	Description
Tenderness to direct palpation	Appendicitis Intestinal obstruction Salpingitis Peptic ulcer Acute cholecystitis	Client relates sharp stab of pain while examiner palpates over affected area.
Rebound tenderness	Peritoneal inflammation	Client relates sharp stab of pain when examiner suddenly withdraws fingers after having applied pressure on abdominal wall. Due to inflammation of peritoneum overlying diseased viscus.

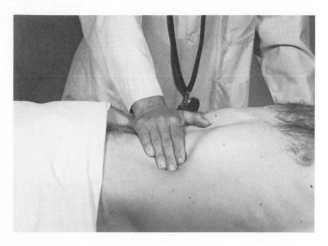

Figure 13-6. Singlehanded deep palpation of the abdomen.

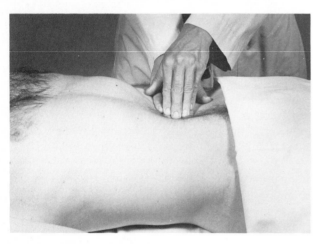

Figure 13-7. Reinforced palpation.

Another bimanual technique is used when assessing abdominal masses or individual organs. It involves placing one hand on the back and the other on the abdomen. For example, the left hand is placed on the back between the twelfth rib and iliac crest and presses upward while the right hand is placed on the abdomen and presses downward. The fingers of the right hand are used to identify the characteristics of the organ or mass palpated.

Deep palpation is used to assess the abdominal structures in all four quadrants and the midline. The sequence in which the quadrants are evaluated is arbitrary; however, a quadrant known to be tender is palpated last.

The left upper quadrant is normally free of masses or palpable organs. Although the spleen and left kidney are normally not palpable, the examiner attempts to locate these organs during deep palpation. Bimanual palpation is used to examine the splenic area. The spleen must be enlarged two to three times nor-

mal to be palpable. The examiner stands to the right of the client and places the left hand on the back with the fingers pressing upward at the twelfth rib. The right hand is placed inferior to the left anterior costal margin with the fingertips in the mid-clavicular line. The client is instructed to inhale slowly and deeply while the examiner lifts the posterior wall with the left hand. The right hand does not move during inspiration (Figure 13-8).

Since the spleen normally descends with inspiration, an enlarged spleen sometimes touches the fingers of the right hand during this maneuver.

As the client exhales and the abdominal muscles relax, the examiner probes slightly deeper and repeats the palpation process. If the spleen is not palpated, this maneuver is performed repeatedly, while the examining hand is moved about 2 centimeters laterally each time until the midaxillary line is reached. If the examiner questions the presence of an enlarged spleen, the client is turned slightly to the left, and the procedure is repeated. When it is suspected that the splenic capsule is distended, care is taken not to induce splenic rupture by too vigorous palpation.

Palpation of the left kidney is also attempted during bimanual palpation. The examiner uses the same maneuver as in examining the splenic area except that the right hand is positioned closer to the midline and pressed deeper into the abdominal wall. The left kidney is normally not palpable except in thin clients.

Deep palpation of the right upper quadrant generally reveals several structures. While the liver is normally not palpable, its edge may be palpated at or slightly below the right costal margin on deep inspiration. Any of the preceding methods can be used to palpate the liver. Using the single-handed method, the examiner places the right hand parallel to the rectus muscle with fingers pointing toward the right

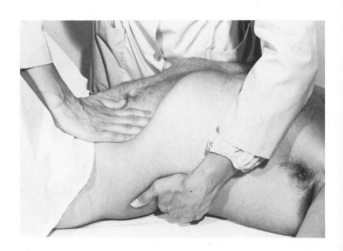

Figure 13-8. Bimanual palpation of the spleen.

costal margin. The hand is placed well below the lower border of the liver. The client is asked to breathe deeply. During inspiration the examiner's hand moves upward with the abdominal wall toward the costal margin. During expiration the examiner exerts pressure with the right hand in a downward and forward direction.

When the desired depth is reached the examiner maintains the position and requests that the client again take a deep breath. On inspiration the diaphragm pushes the liver inferiorly 2 to 4 centimeters and the examiner may be able to palpate the liver's edge. The liver's edge is firm, sharp, and smooth. Palpation of the liver's edge 1 or more centimeters below the costal margin is usually considered an abnormal finding. Exceptions are congenitally enlarged livers or livers displaced due to chronic obstructive pulmonary disease. In both cases, however, liver span is within normal limits.

It is not unusual for the examiner to feel the lower pole of the right kidney during deep palpation of the right upper quadrant. This is especially true when the client is thin. Palpation for the right kidney is performed in the same manner used for palpating the left. Other abdominal organs located in the right upper quadrant are normally not palpable. A palpable gallbladder or pancreas occurs only in the presence of disease.

The abdominal aorta is normally palpable in the midepigastric region as a soft, pulsatile tube. Using single-handed palpation, the examiner locates the abdominal aorta by pressing firmly and deeply to the left of the midline. After identifying the aortic pulsation, the examiner palpates the expansion of the abdominal aorta (Figure 13-9). The examiner feels for expansion either by placing the thumb on one side of the aorta and fingers on the other or by placing one hand on either side of the aorta (Figure 13-9). The examiner normally feels no lateral expansion as pulsations in the normal abdominal aorta are transmitted forward rather than laterally.

Portions of the sigmoid colon and cecum may be identified upon deep palpation of the lower quadrants. The sigmoid colon, a ropelike structure that extends vertically into the left iliac fossa, may be felt on deep palpation of the left lower quadrant. It is palpated as a slightly tender, freely movable mass. At times firm stool may be palpated in this area. The cecum, located in the right lower quadrant, may be palpated as a soft, slightly tender, fluctuant mass. Palpation of other structures or masses in the lower quadrants or suprapubic area is abnormal (Table 13-11).

Life Cycle Variations

Childhood

Assessment of the abdomen in the infant and young child may be performed early in the physical examination. Similar to the abdominal assessment of the adult, the abdomen must be visible, the client comfortable, and the hands of the examiner warm. The infant and toddler may feel more secure lying longitudinally on an adult's lap with feet on the knees of the examiner (Figure 13-10). The older child, however, is examined while supine on the examining table.

Inspection of the umbilicus is an important part of the newborn abdominal examination. Three umbilical

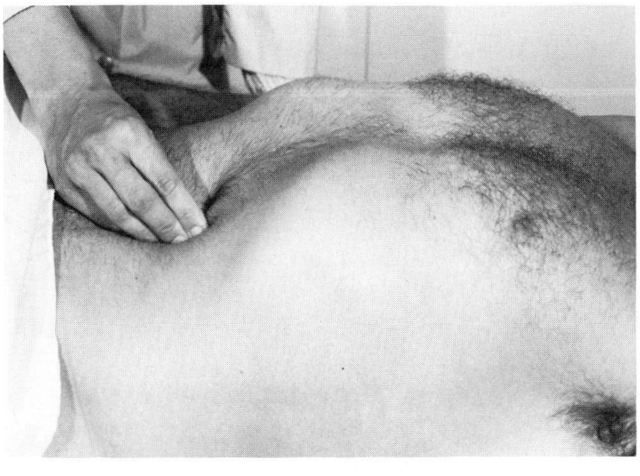

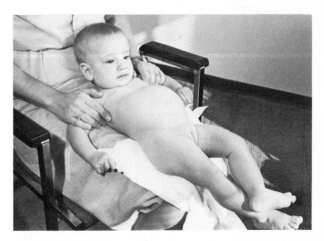

Figure 13-9. *Palpation of the abdominal aorta for lateral expansions.*

Figure 13-10. *Positioning of infant during abdominal assessment.*

Table 13-11.   Selected Causes of Organomegaly (Enlarged abdominal organs)

Finding	Condition	Explanation
Splenomegaly	Lymphoma Leukemia	Infiltration by malignant cells
	Congestive heart failure	Vascular congestion
	Cirrhosis of the liver	Portal hypertension
	Infectious mononucleosis	Reactive hyperplasia
Hepatomegaly	Cirrhosis	Portal hypertension and hepatotoxin
	Hepatitis	Inflammation
	Neoplasm	Infiltration by malignant cells

Enlarged
  kidney
	Hydronephrosis	Obstructed urine
		  outflow

	Neoplasm	Infiltration by malignant cells
Enlarged gallbladder	Acute cholecystitis	Inflammation
Enlarged pancreas	Pancreatitis	Inflammation

Pulsatile mass
  in epigastrium
	Abdominal
	  aortic aneurysm
		Dilation at point of
		  weakness in vessel
		  wall

vessels are normally observed. The umbilicus is usually dry by the 5th day and the stump sloughs by the 14th. At this time the skin retracts so that the umbilicus appears flush with the abdominal wall. A superficial venous pattern, normally observed until puberty, may appear more prominent in the premature or normal small infant.

The abdomen of the infant and young child is relatively larger than the chest. The abdomen is also protuberant. This is a normal finding, and is due to the poorly developed abdominal musculature. This "pot-bellied" appearance is present both in the upright and supine positions in the young child and disappears by age 5 (Figure 13-11). In the older child the abdomen is protuberant on standing but disappears upon lying down.

Inspection for abdominal movement normally reveals a visible epigastric impulse. The abdomen also moves with respiration in the young child, who until age seven is primarily an abdominal breather.

Auscultation of the abdomen is performed prior to palpation. The examiner delays auscultation in the event of crying. Under normal circumstances the characteristics of the bowel sounds are similar to those heard in an adult.

Abdominal palpation in the young child is similar to that performed in the adult. The examiner may find it easier to palpate the infant's abdomen while the infant lies on an adult's lap. The examiner can flex the infant's knees and hips with one hand while palpating with the other. Light palpation always precedes deep palpation. Because the infant and young child are unable to pinpoint areas of tenderness, the

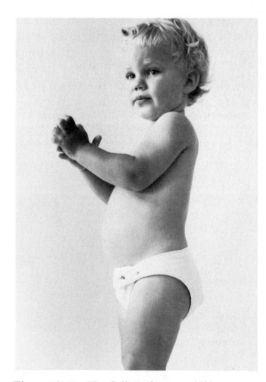

Figure 13-11. *"Pot-belly" of young child.*

examiner must be alert to changes in facial expressions or crying patterns during palpation.

Findings on abdominal palpation change with the age of the child being examined. Throughout infancy and childhood the liver is palpable 1 to 2 centimeters below the right costal margin; its edge is smooth, soft, and sharp. The tip of the spleen, palpable in the newborn along the lateral aspect of the left upper quadrant, is normally smooth, soft, and freely movable. The kidneys are normally palpated bilaterally until puberty, at which time only the pole of the right kidney may be felt in some individuals. Except for portions of the small and large intestines, no other structures are palpable and the presence of such findings is considered abnormal.

In infants, an increased amount of air may be percussed over the stomach and intestines. This is a normal finding, and it is caused by air swallowed during feeding and crying.

Pregnancy

Visible signs of pregnancy become evident during the second trimester. Inspection may reveal the presence of striae gravidarum. Striae normally appear pink; in the multiparous the silvery white striae of past pregnancies are a common finding. Darkening of the linea alba is frequently seen and is called the linea nigra. As the pregnancy advances the abdomen appears more protuberant. At the twentieth week the fundus is at or slightly above the umbilicus, causing the umbilicus to be pushed outward. During the 8th month the uterus is observed to be slightly below the xiphosternum, and by the 9th month it drops slightly below this level in primiparas. Late in pregnancy fetal movements are visible.

Fetal heart tones are normally auscultated after the twentieth week of gestation with a fetuscope, but may be heard as early as the ninth week with a doppler. They vary between 120 to 160 beats per minute. During the early months they are heard best above the symphysis pubis. Toward the end of pregnancy, the location of fetal heart tones depends upon the position of the fetus. Another sound heard in the pregnant abdomen is the uterine souffle, the sound of blood coursing through the placental blood vessels.

The pregnant uterus is normally palpable after the twelfth week of gestation. Uterine palpation in the nulliparous woman may be more difficult than in the multiparous woman as the abdominal wall is more likely to be tense and firm. In the multipara, the abdominal wall is often lax, making uterine palpation easier. With excessive loss of muscle tone, the uterus sags forward and downward and gives the abdomen a pendulous appearance.

Late Adulthood

Physical findings on inspection of the elderly client's abdomen are similar to those found in the younger adult. Striae may be more prevalent, and scars from past surgeries and trauma may be seen. An increase in the amount of truncal body fat is observed.

Palpation of the abdomen may be easier in some clients due to a decreased abdominal muscle tone but may be more difficult in others due to obesity. The edge of the liver is often palpable slightly below the right costal margin but this is a normal finding in the presence of chronic obstructive pulmonary disease, a frequent disease entity in the elderly.

Anatomy and Physiology

The rectum and anus are the terminal portions of the gastrointestinal tract and have the primary function of defecation. The rectum is anterior to the sacrum and extends from the sigmoid colon at the third sacral vertebra to the anal canal. The rectum is a canal of varying diameter and is approximately 12 to 15 centimeters long. The upper portion is the same diameter as the sigmoid colon, but the lower third dilates and forms the rectal ampulla which narrows abruptly at the anal canal (Figure 14-1).

While empty, the rectal lining has several longitudinal folds that disappear when the rectum is distended from feces or flatus. The rectum also has two to four semilunar transverse folds (valves of Houston), which aid in supporting the weight of fecal material.

The anal canal is the terminal portion of the gastrointestinal tract. It extends in an oblique downward and backward line for 2 to 4 centimeters from the narrowed portion of the rectal ampulla to the anus. The anal canal is lined with mucosal tissue and blood vessels that form 6 to 10 longitudinal folds or columns (columns of Morgagni). The blood vessels form the elevations in the columns, and the depressions between the columns are called anal sinuses. At the anorectal junction the columns end as anal valves, which form a serrated line called the pectinate or dentate line (Figure 14-1).

The anus is at the perineum, where the skin changes from dry and hairy to moist and hairless. It is maintained in a closed position by two concentric layers of sphincter muscles: the voluntary external muscles and the involuntary internal muscles. The mucosal lining of the lumen continues to the outside of the sphincter muscles, which causes exposure of the mucocutaneous junction for inspection.

The function of the rectum, anal canal, and anus is defecation. Feces are generally stored in the sigmoid colon or higher until immediately prior to defecation. At this time the fecal material enters the rectum and distends it. The distension relaxes the anal sphinctors and combined with contraction of the diaphragm, pelvic muscles, and abdominal muscles, the bowels are evacuated.

Defecation is largely a reflex of habit. Some people defecate according to the time of day, while others according to location. It is normal for some individuals to defecate several times a day and others once or twice a week.

Chapter 14

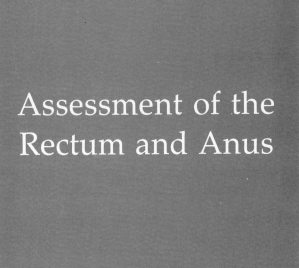

Assessment of the Rectum and Anus

Objectives

The examiner will be able to do the following:

1. Inspect the anus
2. Palpate the anus and rectum (including prostate gland in male clients)
3. Recognize abnormalities
4. Record the information obtained

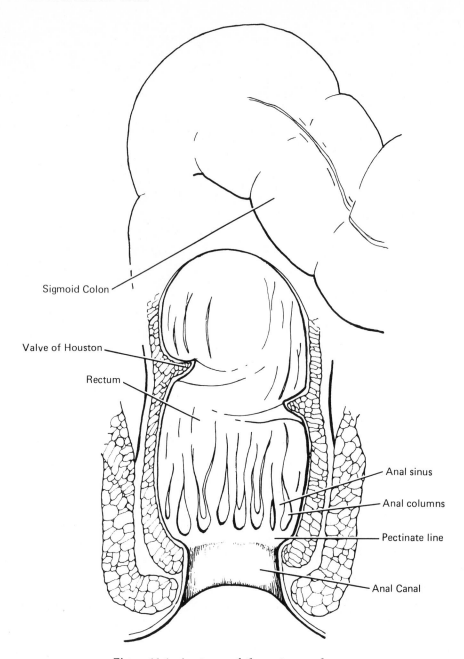

Sigmoid Colon

Valve of Houston

Rectum

Anal sinus

Anal columns

Pectinate line

Anal Canal

Figure 14-1. Anatomy of the rectum and anus.

Prostate Gland and Seminal Vesicles

The prostate gland and seminal vesicles are accessory structures in the male reproductive system, but they are assessed during the rectal examination. The prostate is a combination of glandular and fibromuscular tissue located below the urinary bladder. The size of the prostate varies considerably, but it is approximately 3 centimeters long and 4 centimeters wide. The apex of the gland points downward; the base points superiorly and is adjacent to the urinary blad-

der at the urethra. The prostate has five lobes: the median, anterior, posterior, and two lateral lobes. Only the median and two lateral lobes are clinically significant. The median lobe is separated by the ejaculatory duct and urethra. The two lateral lobes are separated by the urethra and median sulcus (Figure 14-2).

The prostate produces a secretion to help neutralize the acidity of the male urethra. This secretion also helps neutralize vaginal acidity, which decreases acidic damage to the semen following ejaculation.

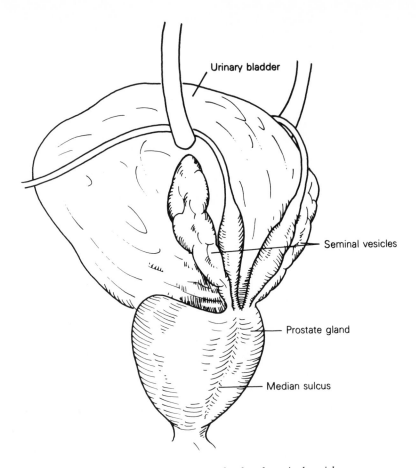

Figure 14-2. *The prostate gland and seminal vesicles.*

The two seminal vesicles lie along the lower posterior portion of the bladder and are above and lateral to the prostate gland. They are approximately 2.5 centimeters long and store semen (Figure 14-2).

Assessment Modalities

Preparation

Inspection and palpation are the examination modalities used in the assessment of the rectum and anus. If the examination is done carefully, the client experiences little discomfort.

The four most commonly used client positions are (1) standing, (2) knee-chest, (3) left lateral, and (4) dorsolithotomy positions (Figure 14-3). In the standing position the client bends the upper torso over an examining table that is approximately waist high. This position is effective for palpating the prostate gland and is the position used most commonly for men.

In the knee-chest position the client sits on his knees with his shoulders and head on the examining table. This position is also very good for palpating the prostate gland.

The left lateral or Sim's position is used for deblilated clients who are unable to stand. The client lies on the left side with hips and knees flexed, and buttocks close to the edge of the examining table. This position reduces the valves of Houston by gravity and causes the rectal ampulla to be pushed inferiorly and posteriorly; therefore, it is helpful in detecting rectal masses.

The dorsolithotomy position is used most often on females since the rectal examination is done after the pelvic examination. In this position the client's buttocks are at the bottom of the examining table with legs abducted, knees flexed, and feet in stirrups or drawn up as close to the buttocks as possible.

For an effective examination the client's rectum and anal canal need to be free of feces. If the client is unable to defecate and the rectum is packed with feces, a cleansing enema is often given.

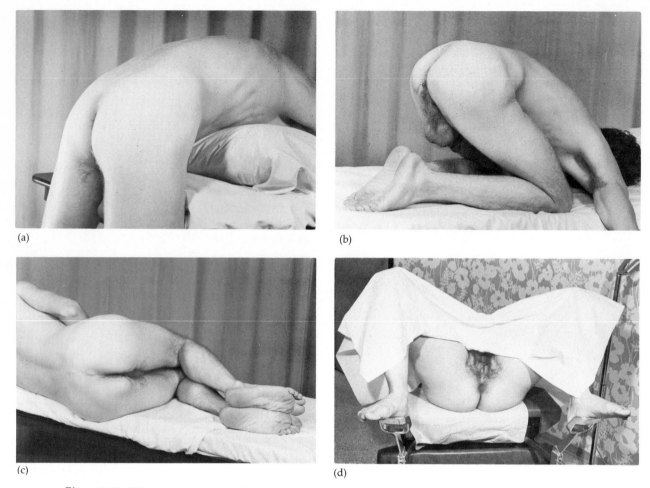

(a)

(b)

(c)

(d)

Figure 14-3. Client positions for rectal examination: (a) standing; (b) knee-chest; (c) left lateral; (d) dorsolithotomy.

Other equipment needed for the examination include a glove or finger cot, lubricant, an adjustable light, and filter paper for the guaiac examination for occult blood.

Inspection

The examiner inspects the anus by separating the buttocks with both hands and looking at the area under a bright light. The anus and perianal area are coarser and more pigmented than the surrounding skin. Often there is sparse circumanal pubic-type hair.

While the buttocks are separated, the client is instructed to take a deep breath and bear down as if having a bowel movement (the Valsalva maneuver). During this procedure the anus opens slightly and the moist mucosal lining of the anal canal is exposed (Figure 14-4, Table 14-1).

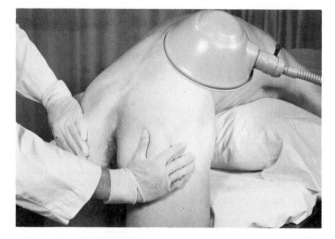

Figure 14-4. Inspection of the anus.

Table 14-1.   Selected Abnormalities of the Anus and Anal Canal

Finding	Condition	Description
Pain	Hemorrhoids Anal fissure Perianal laceration Cancer of the anus Anal abscess	Client experiences pain in anal canal during palpation. Pain becomes more intense with bowel movements, sitting or straining.
Bulges or lumps outside anal orifice	External hemorrhoids	Purplish bulges below the anorectal junction that are covered with anal skin. Unless thrombosed, the bulges are easily compressed by finger palpation.
	Thrombosed hemorrhoids	Firm, tender, purplish bulges below the anorectal junction.
	Internal hemorrhoids	Soft, irregular swellings above the anorectal junction that are covered by mucous membranes. These swellings are not generally palpable but become visible when they prolapse through the anus.
Skin tags	Hemorrhoids	Painless, flabby flaps of purplish skin from previously thrombosed or inflamed hemorrhoids.
Annular protrusion of moist red mucosa	Rectal prolapse	Protrusion of rectal mucosa or rectal mucosa and wall through the anus. Occurs during bowel movements, cough, or sneeze but may extrude permanently from the rectum.
Skin excoriation	Pruritis ani Poor hygiene	Ranges from mild erythema to severe inflammation with maceration and fissuring of the anal and perianal areas. Characterized by persistent itching of the involved area and is often associated with a burning sensation.
Tight anal sphincter		Upon inserting the index finger into the anus, the sphincter tightens and interferes with insertion. The client is instructed to bear down while the index finger is gently inserted. Insertion of the finger is stopped during any pain and advanced when the sphincter is more relaxed.
	Anxiety	In response to a previously painful examination, the client contracts the anal spincter.
	Anal fissure	An anal fissure often causes an anal spasm and stenosis of the anal canal. Sometimes the fissure may be seen during the Valsalva maneuver. It is usually in the posterior midline of the anal mucosa.
	Cancer of the anus	The cancerous mass causes narrowing of the anus.
Relaxed anal sphincter	Perianal laceration (childbirth, surgery) Neurologic deficit (spinal cord lesions)	Little or no resistance is felt by the examiner during insertion of the index finger; the anal sphincter lacks muscle tone.
Mass	Cancer of anus Abscess	Possibly ulcerated, hard mass palpated on anus. Tender, soft mass palpated in anal canal.

Palpation

The client is informed that palpation of the anus and rectum need not be painful, but it may be uncomfortable; the sensation is similar to that of defecation. The client is instructed to perform the Valsalva maneuver, which aids in insertion of the examining finger.

The examiner separates the buttocks with the ungloved hand and palpates with the gloved hand. The pad of the gloved, liberally lubricated index finger is gently but firmly placed over the anus. During the Valsalva maneuver the anal sphinter relaxes and the curve of the pad enters the anal canal.

Normally the anus tightens when the palpating finger is placed on it, then relaxes sufficiently to allow insertion of the finger. After the index finger is in-

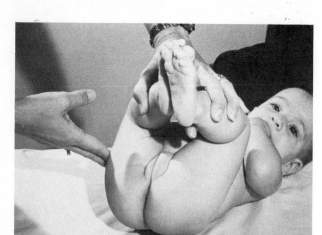

***Figure 14-5.** Inspection of an infant's anus.*

Table 14-2. Selected Abnormalities of the Rectum

Finding	Condition	Description
Mass	Fecal impaction	Hard, dry masses of feces palpated inside rectal lumen.
	Malignant tumor	Hard, nodular mass with an irregular surface is palpated on the walls of the rectum.
	Polyps	Soft mass that is smooth or irregular is palpated on the walls of the rectum.

serted, the client takes very slow, deep breaths through the mouth to aid in relaxation and lessen any discomfort. While the finger is in the anus, the client is instructed to tighten the anal sphincter around the examining finger for an assessment of muscle tone. The examiner feels muscular pressure equally around the index finger. With the index finger still in the anal canal, the examiner places the thumb externally over the perineum. The entire circumference of the anus is palpated between the thumb and index finger. The anus feels soft with no masses or swellings.

After examining the anus, the finger is rotated into the axis of the canal and inserted as far as possible in an oblique line pointing toward the umbilicus. With the pad of the index finger, the lateral and posterior walls of the anal canal and rectum are palpated in sequence. They feel smooth with no irregularities or tenderness. The finger is able to reach the lower 6 to 10 centimeters of the rectum, and sometimes the first two valves of Houston. The client is instructed to perform the Valsalva maneuver since this pushes 5 to 8 centimeters of the rectum in contact with the examining finger (Table 14-2).

The anterior wall of the rectum is examined last. In the female client the cervix is felt as a small, round mass (Chapter 15).

In the male client the prostate gland and seminal vesicles are palpated in the anterior wall of the rectum. The size, shape, and consistency of the prostate are evaluated. The prostate protrudes into the rectal lumen less than 1 centimeter and is sometimes described as shaped like a chestnut with an apex pointing down. The prostate is felt as a symmetrical, bilobed gland with a median sulcus. It is firm, rubbery,

smooth, and slightly movable. When the prostate is palpated with light pressure, the client experiences no tenderness and no secretions are produced through the urethra. The seminal vesicles are slightly corrugated structures that are generally too soft to be palpated. They are located lateral to and above the prostate (Table 14-3).

After the anterior wall of the rectum is examined, the finger is removed and inspected for any fecal material. The feces are normally dark brown and soft, with no mucus or blood. A smear for occult blood is normally negative. (Table 14-4).

Life Cycle Variations

Childhood

In examining the anus or rectum, children are placed in a supine position on the examining table. The examiner uses one hand to hold the feet together with the knees and hips flexed onto the abdomen, while the other hand is free for palpation (Figure 14-5).

The anal area is routinely inspected, but a rectal examination is performed only when there are lower gastrointestinal symptoms such as severe constipation, pain, or bleeding. The procedure for inserting the finger and examining the rectum is the same as that for adults. Although the index finger is more flexible and has better tactile sensitivity, the fifth finger is often used since it is less uncomfortable for the child.

In boys the prostate feels like a flat mass on the anterior wall of the rectum. In girls the uterus is palpable on the anterior wall of the rectum and feels like a small oval mass (1 to 2 centimeters in diameter). Sometimes the ovaries are palpated as very small masses (0.5 to 1.0 centimeter in diameter) 2 to 3 centimeters lateral to and immediately above the uterus.

Table 14-3.   Selected Abnormalities of the Prostate

Finding	Condition	Description
Enlarged prostate		Is often associated with an obliterated median sulcus. Recorded according to how far the gland bulges into the rectal lumen. Grades: I—bulges less than 1 cm.; II—1 to 2 cm.; III—2 to 3 cm.; IV—greater than 3 cm.
	Benign prostatic hypertrophy	Prostate palpated as a symmetrical nontender, soft, smooth mass. Associated with complaints of nocturia and decreased force of stream.
	Prostatitis	Prostate palpated as a slightly asymmetrical, sometimes tender, soft, fluctuant mass. Palpation or massage of the gland produces secretions through the urethra. With chronic prostatitis the gland may feel normal with some areas of fibrosis.
	Abscess	Prostate palpated as a very soft, fluctuant, tender mass that is often associated with a fever. A laboratory analysis of the secretions determines if they are bacterial or cellular contents. Prostatic abscess is usually from gonorrhea.
	Cancer	Prostate palpated as an asymmetrical very hard, fixed gland. Single or multiple irregularities may be felt as firm nodules or ridges in an otherwise normal gland.

Pregnancy

It is common for hemorrhoids to develop during pregnancy since the enlarged uterus may interfere with venous circulation and constipation is common. If hemorrhoids are present before the pregnancy, they often worsen.

Late Adulthood

Research has not been able to prove any age-related anatomic or physiologic changes in the gastrointestinal tract until after the ninth decade (such as decreased colonic peristalsis). Although constipation is a frequent symptom during late adulthood, its occurrence has not been proven. The normal range of bowel habits does not change with age but continues to vary from several times each day to perhaps once or twice each week.

Constipation or infrequent, hard, dry bowel movements are the result of an insufficient intake of bulk-producing foods, medications, overuse of laxatives, or a sedentary life. These causes have an equal effect on all age groups. Generally the constipation that occurs in late adulthood is a result of a change in life style and diet that is often self-treated with laxatives.

During palpation, loss of anal sphincter tone may be apparent. Also, older people may have difficulty being able to distinguish between feces or gas in the rectum. These factors may cause fecal incontinence. Also noted on inspection and palpation are hemorrhoids. It is estimated that over 70 percent of people over 40 years old have hemorrhoids.

In most males over 50 years old the prostate is often enlarged and is palpated as a firm, smooth, symmetrical, slightly elastic enlargement. If the prostate is atrophied from the treatment of prostatic cancer, it is palpated as a very soft mass.

Table 14-4. Selected Variations in Feces

Finding	Condition	Description
Black	Gastrointestinal bleeding from small intestine or above (gastric ulcer)	Feces are black from partially digested blood, hematest positive.
	Iron or bismuth ingestion	Preparations darken feces to a black color, hematest negative.
Red Blood	Rectal bleeding (hemorrhoids, rectal cancer)	Red blood is streaked on the surface of the feces.
	Colonic bleeding (ulcerative colitis, cancer of the colon)	Red blood is mixed in with the feces.
Light gray	Obstructive jaundice	Feces are light gray in color from the absence of bile pigments.
Milky white	Barium ingestion	Barium mixes with the feces and lightens its color to almost white.
Mucus streaks	Inflammation of large intestines (ulcerative colitis, regional enteritis)	Feces are streaked with mucus as a result of the desquamation of the colonic epithelium from the inflammatory process.
	Constipation	Glands in the colon secrete mucus in response to fecal masses.
Greasy, pale, foamy diarrhea with a foul odor	Malabsorption syndromes (steatorrhea, sprue)	Diarrhea or frequent loose bowel movements with a high fat content occur since the small intestine loses absorptive surface area from the disease process.
Diarrhea	Infections (dysentery, food poisoning). Disease of the large intestines (colitis, enteritis)	Loose, semisolid bowel movements.
	Medications (laxatives, antibiotics)	Watery bowel movements with no form.
	Disease of the small intestines (sprue, steatorrhea)	
Constipation	Medications (morphine), lead poisoning, cancer of the colon, lack of exercise, lack of bulk and liquids in diet	Hard, dry bowel movements that sometimes have mucus streaks.
Greenish	Excessive spinach ingestion	Consistency of feces is normal, but they have a greenish hue.
Reddish	Excessive carrot or beet ingestion	Consistency of feces is normal, but they have a reddish hue.

Anatomy and Physiology

The female genitalia comprise organs and tissues involved in seven interrelated physiologic functions: micturation, defecation, menstruation, ovulation, copulation, pregnancy, and parturition. The genitalia consist of parts located on the exterior surface of the body—the external genitalia—and parts located internally—the internal genitalia.

External Genitalia

The external genitalia are also known as the vulva or pudendum. The vulva consists of the mons pubis, labia, clitoris, vestibule, urethral orifice, vaginal introitus, perineum, and fourchette (Figure 15-1).

The mons pubis or mons veneris is a hair-covered mound of fat covering the symphysis pubis. The hair is dense and curly and forms an inverted triangular pattern with the base parallel to the symphysis pubis (Figure 15-2). The skin color is consistent with or darker than the remainder of the body.

There are two pairs of labia or genital lips: the labia majora and the labia minora. The labia majora are hair-covered, rounded folds of adipose tissue. Their color is consistent with or darker than that of the rest of the body. They extend from the mons pubis to the perineum. The labia minora are thinner, hairless, and resemble the vaginal mucosa in their deep pink color and moistness. The labia minora are located within the labia majora and extend from the clitoris to the fourchette. At the clitoris the labia minora form the prepuce or hood and the frenulum. The prepuce is the superior covering of the clitoris; the frenulum is the inferior surface or base of the clitoris.

The clitoris is comprised of highly sensitive erectile tissue and is the female genital organ primarily responsive to sexual stimulation.

The vestibule is a boat-shaped area between the labia minora that contains the urethral orifice and vaginal introitus. The urethral orifice is inferior to the clitoris and is an irregularly shaped opening. Within the urethra on the posterolateral aspect of its floor are the paraurethral or Skene's glands. They are normally not visible although the openings of their ducts are sometimes visible immediately posterolateral to the urethral orifice.

The vaginal introitus is the vaginal opening and is located inferior to the urethral orifice.

Beneath the vestibule on the posterolateral aspects of the vagina are the Bartholin's glands. These two pea-to-bean sized glands secrete mucus, which lubricates the vagina, a particularly important function

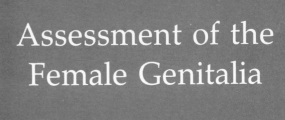

Chapter 15

Assessment of the Female Genitalia

Objectives

The examiner will be able to do the following:

1. Inspect the external genitalia
2. Evaluate the pelvic musculature
3. Inspect the vagina and cervix
4. Obtain cervical smears for cytologic examination
5. Perform bimanual pelvic and rectovaginal examinations
6. Obtain vaginal discharge, prepare slides, and inspect them under the microscope
7. Obtain specimen for gonorrheal culture
8. Obtain specimen for urinalysis and urine culture and sensitivity
9. Recognize abnormalities
10. Record the information obtained

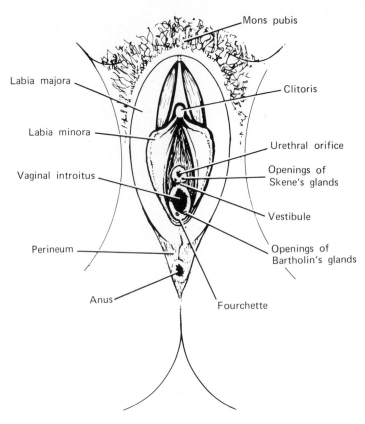

Figure 15-1. External genitalia of the adult female.

during coitus. Usually neither the openings of the glands nor the glands themselves are visible.

The perineum and fourchette are structures inferior to the introitus. The perineum comprises the skin and underlying tissues between the vaginal introitus and anus. The fourchette is a membranous fold that connects the posterior aspects of the labia minora.

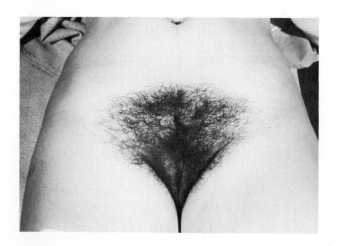

Figure 15-2. Inverted triangular pubic hair pattern.

Internal Genitalia

The internal genitalia comprise the vagina, uterus, Fallopian tubes, and ovaries, all of which are located between the urinary bladder and rectum (Figure 15-3).

The vagina is a muscular, collapsed, and distensible canal. It consists of pink mucosa with many rugae or folds, which facilitate its tremendous distensibility. It is the female organ of copulation, the outlet for menstruation, and the outlet for birth at parturition. The vagina extends posteriorly between the urethra and rectum and terminates in a cup-shaped area known as the fornix. The fornix is anatomically divided by the uterine cervix into an anterior, a posterior, and two lateral fornices.

The uterus is a fibromuscular, pear-shaped organ that contains and nourishes the embryo and fetus from the time of implantation to parturition. It lies at about a 90-degree angle from the vagina and has three main parts: the body, the isthmus, and the cervix. The body comprises the bulk of uterine tissue and is the portion above the isthmus. The uppermost aspect of the body of the uterus is the fundus. The isthmus is the short, constricted middle portion connecting the

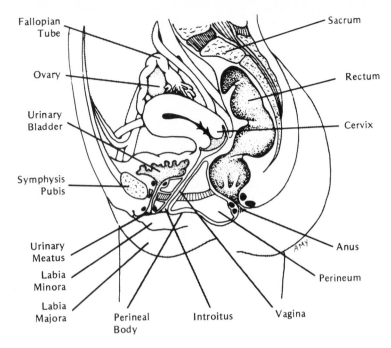

Figure 15-3. Internal genitalia of the adult female.

body to the cervix. The cervix is the lowermost portion of the uterus and extends from the isthmus into the vagina.

The cervix is the opening through which the menses flow, the fetus passes into the vagina during parturition, and the sperm travel from the vagina into the uterus. It protrudes into the vagina anteriorly and superiorly and is covered by pink, easily shed, squamous cell epithelium. The cervical os, located in the center of the cervix, is a small, circular opening in nulliparous clients. In parous clients it is usually enlarged and slitlike, elliptical, or irregularly shaped.

The ovaries are two almond-shaped organs that produce female sex hormones and ova in response to cyclical variations of anterior pituitary hormones. They are located deep within the pelvis, lateral and slightly posterior to the uterus at about the level of the anterosuperior iliac crest near the lateral pelvic walls.

Two Fallopian tubes or oviducts extend from the uterine fundus bilaterally toward the ovaries, where they end in a cuplike shape of fingerlike projections called fimbrae. The fimbrae direct ova from the pelvic cavity to the interior of the tubes, where fertilization occurs.

The term *adnexa* refers to the ovaries, tubes, and supporting structures. The uterus, ovaries, and tubes are supported by the muscles of the pelvic floor and four pairs of ligaments.

The pelvic floor is a hammocklike muscle layer attached to the front and back of the pelvis. This muscle layer consists of five pairs of muscles: the bulbocavernosus, ischiocavernosus, transverse perineal, levator ani, and gluteus maximus muscles (Figure 15-4). Besides providing passive support, they are involved in voluntary contraction of the vaginal introitus and anus and in micturation. The four pairs of ligaments are the broad, cardinal, round, and uterosacral (Figure 15-5).

Menstruation

The uterine cavity is lined by glandular epithelium called the endometrium. The endometrium undergoes a periodic series of changes related to hormonal influences. These changes occur within three stages of the menstrual cycle: the premenstrual phase (immediately following ovulation), the menstrual phase, and the postmenstrual phase. During the 12- to 14-day premenstrual (secretory) phase, the secretion of progesterone predominates and the endometrium nearly doubles in thickness in preparation for nourishment of an implanted embryo. In the absence of implantation, the endometrium is shed during the 5 to 6-day menstrual phase. Following this desquamation of the endometrium, the postmenstrual (proliferative) phase occurs for the next 9 to 11 days. During this stage estrogen secretion causes a re-epithelialization of the endometrium.

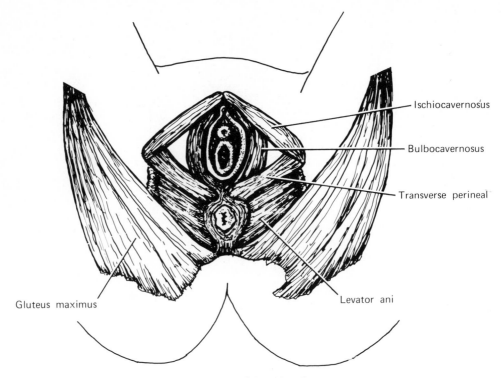

Figure 15-4. Muscles of the pelvic floor.

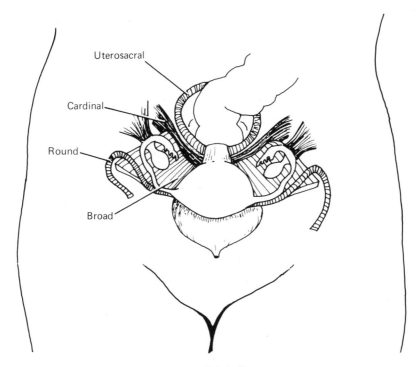

Figure 15-5. Pelvic ligaments.

The average interval between menstrual periods is 29.5 ± 2 days. The average duration of flow is 5 ± 2 days. Generally the interval between ovulation and menstruation is 14 days. Variations in the length of the menstrual cycle occur in the interval preceding ovulation. Cycles from 18 to 40 days are considered normal when they are the established pattern and occur consistently. Menstrual discharge consists of endometrium, blood, mucus, and vaginal cells; it is dark red in color and does not contain clots.

Sexuality

Although the genitalia are responsible for the sensory and motor aspects of sexual function, the central nervous system integrates and directs the drive for sexual expression. This drive occurs in response to androgen secretion by the adrenal cortex. Psychic factors integrated in the limbic and hypothalamic centers also play an important role in sexuality. During early arousal, anticipation of physical contact makes the woman psychologically receptive to later stages of sexual response.

Masters and Johnson identified four stages of female sexual response: excitement, plateau, orgasm, and resolution. The excitement phase includes changes resulting from direct or indirect clitoral stimulation. These are genital vasocongestion including mottling of the skin, myotonia, vaginal lubrication, vasocongestion of the clitoris, uterine elevation within the pelvis, and the beginning of ballooning of the vaginal barrel. Direct clitoral stimulation results from manual or oral contact. Indirect stimulation occurs as a result of traction on the prepuce during penile penetration. During the plateau stage increased mottling occurs, the labia minora swell, the lumen of the anterior one-third of the vagina constricts, the orgasmic platform forms in the lower vagina, and the clitoris retracts immediately prior to orgasm. The orgasmic platform refers to the vaginal and perivaginal muscles that contract during orgasm. During orgasm, reflex rhythmic contractions of the vaginal and perineal muscles occur at intervals of 0.8 seconds. Women are capable of multiple orgasms within seconds after the first orgasm. During resolution the genital organs return to normal. Most abnormalities of sexual function are discovered during history taking (Tables 1-3 and 15-1).

Table 15-1. Selected Abnormalities of Sexual Function

Finding	Condition	Explanation
Lack of libido (disinterest in sex)	Fatigue	Situational; frequently occurs in first trimester of pregnancy and postpartum while infant requires night feedings.
	Boredom with partner Marital difficulty or interpersonal conflict with partner	Usually is functional; woman who previously had active interest in sex and was orgasmic experiences disinterest in sex.
	Endocrine pathology (hypothyroidism)	Decreased BMR and decreased energy for most activities of daily life.
Dyspareunia (painful intercourse)	Vulvitis (usually monilialis or herpes progenitalis)	Inflamed or excoriated vulva is painful, inhibiting genital contact.
	Postpartum Lactation Postmenopause	Decreased estrogen results in dry vagina.
	Depression Interpersonal conflict with partner Sexual conflict	Often is secondary to ineffective sexual preparation (foreplay), or psychic inhibition preventing sexual arousal.
	Pelvic pathology (endometriosis, pelvic inflammatory disease)	Pain causes psychic inhibition of arousal.
Painful involuntary spasm of introitus during coitus and pelvic examination	Vaginismus	May be late sequela of rape or molestation, or result from fear of mutilation during vaginal penetration.
Orgasmic disability	Depression Interpersonal conflict with partner Sexual conflict	Most frequently secondary to ineffective sexual preparation (foreplay).
	Pelvic pathology (endometriosis, pelvic inflammatory disease)	Pain inhibits progression of sexual arousal to orgasm.

Assessment Modalities

Preparation

Assessment of the genitalia evokes considerable anxiety in some women. This anxiety may be due to embarrassment over exposure of the sexual organs, fear about painful procedures, or fear of the results of the examination. Some measures that minimize discomfort and anxiety and facilitate relaxation are the following: having all the necessary equipment readily available; assuring privacy by screening and draping; performing the assessment in a warm room; providing pillows for support of the head and back; and explaining the procedures, probable sensations, and findings.

The equipment necessary includes the following (Figure 15-6):

Examining table,
pillows and drapes

Adjustable light source (gooseneck lamp)	Large cotton-tipped applicator
Gloves	Cytology fixative
Specula of different sizes	Culture plates for gonorrhea screening
Glass slides	Mirror
Glass coverslips	Stool for examiner
Ayer spatula	Footstool

Sterile cotton tipped
applicators

Lubricant on a piece of
paper

Although not necessary, an examining table is preferable to a bed because it has variable backrest positions and stirrups for support of the feet. Since metal stirrups are cold and hard, they can be covered with knit mittens or socks for greater comfort. The client is encouraged to keep her shoes or socks on if stirrup covers are unavailable.

Male examiners sometimes prefer to have a female attendant present during the pelvic examination. This may reduce client embarrassment but sometimes causes client reluctance to talk openly because of the presence of a third person. Female and male examiners should have an assistant if the client is emotionally disturbed.

Immediately prior to assessment, the client is instructed to empty her bladder. Assessment is enhanced if the client has had a bowel movement prior to the examination. Clients should receive instructions not to douche within 24 hours prior to pelvic examination since douching can remove some of the cervical epithelial cells necessary in the Papanicolaou cytological examination. It also removes normal vaginal discharge, which may make the examination more uncomfortable, and removes evidence of abnormal discharge, which may delay recognition and management.

The examiner provides a sheet for draping and instructs the client to disrobe from the waist down. Draping is illustrated in Figure 15-7. The examiner assists the client in assuming the dorsolithotomy position on the examining table. The client's thighs are flexed and abducted, feet are in the stirrups, and buttocks extend slightly over the edge of the table. The examiner provides a pillow for head support and elevates the head of the table to 30 degrees or more. Some professionals and clients prefer the head of the table to approximate 90 degrees, enabling clients to sit. This facilitates eye contact during the exam-

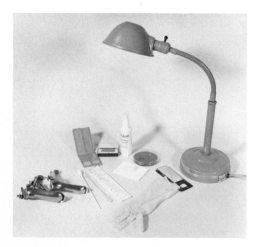

Figure 15-6. Equipment necessary for assessment of the female genitalia.

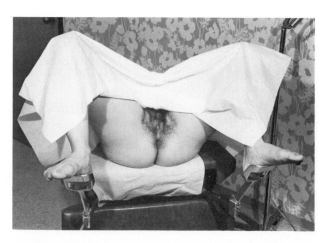

Figure 15-7. Draping during assessment of the female genitalia.

ination, enables the woman to observe the assessment, and enables the examiner to monitor the woman's responses. The examiner provides a hand-held mirror to clients interested in observing the pelvic examination.

Although the dorsolithotomy position is optimal for assessment of the female genitalia, the left lateral or Sim's position is an alternate position for debilitated clients. The client's buttocks are close to the table edge while the knees are bent and abducted and the examiner stands to the left of the client (Figure 15-8).

Some examiners wear a glove on each hand throughout the assessment while others prefer one glove. The examiner dons a new glove for the examining hand prior to performing the rectal examination. This practice is important in order to minimize the spread of infection from the vagina to the rectum, particularly of gonorrhea, which is frequently an asymptomatic condition in women.

Conventionally one hand is used for separation of the labia during inspection, the digital portion of the bimanual examination, and insertion of the speculum. The other hand is used for the abdominal portion of the bimanual examination, separating the labia during insertion of the speculum, and handling other equipment.

Most examiners sit for inspection of the external and internal genitalia and obtaining the Papanicolaou smear and stand for bimanual palpation. When sitting, the examiner adjusts the seat to a position where the cervix and other internal structures are easily visualized. (Figure 15-9). While standing, it is helpful for the examiner to place one foot on a footstool using the knee as a fulcrum for the arm of the examining hand to rotate upon. In this way the arm and hand are used as a unit (Figure 15-10).

The modalities used in assessment of the female genitalia are inspection, palpation, and selected diagnostic screening tests.

Inspection and Palpation of the External Genitalia

The examiner directs the adjustable light onto the vulva and inspects the external genitalia. The skin of the normal mons pubis and labia contain no lesions. The labia are separated for inspection of the clitoris, vestibule, urethral orifice, vaginal introitus, perineum, and fourchette. The labia move freely and are nontender. The clitoris is normally less than 2 centimeters in length, and the vestibule is pink and smooth. The urethral orifice is moist and free of dis-

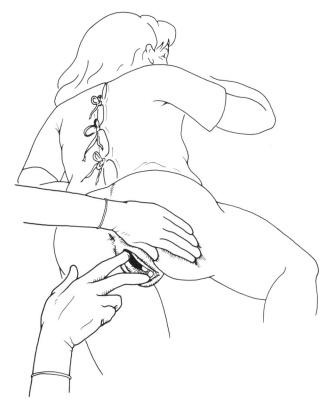

Figure 15-8. Left lateral (Sim's) position for debilitated women.

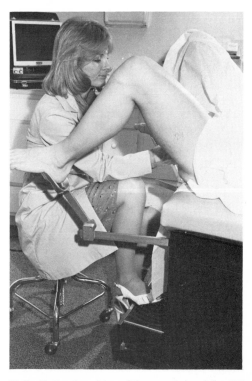

Figure 15-9. Optimal position of the examiner while sitting during cervical inspection.

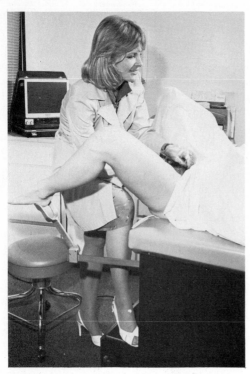

Figure 15-10. *Optimal position of the examiner while standing during bimanual palpation.*

charge. The appearance of the vaginal introitus depends upon the condition of the hymen and parity. When the hymen is intact, it appears as a continuous circular or a crescent-shaped band of membranous tissues just within the vaginal introitus (Figure 15-11). The introitus in virginal females is usually circular or ovoid. After hymenal penetration it assumes an irregular or vertical slitlike appearance bordered by hymenal fragments called hymenal caruncles (Figure 15-12). The introitus of multiparous women may gape in varying degrees (Figure 15-13).

The perineum and fourchette are pink and moist and may show evidence of scarring from lacerations or episiotomy during parturition. Occasionally these lacerations or episiotomies extend through the perineum to the anus.

After inspection of the external genitalia, the examiner further assesses the introitus and Bartholin's and Skene's glands. After inserting one or two fingers into the vagina, the tissue between the urethra and introitus is milked in an anterior direction. With this maneuver there is no tenderness or discharge from the urethral orifice or Skene's glands. (Figure 15-14).

Moving the fingers in a posterolateral direction in the vaginal introitus enables the examiner to assess the Bartholin's glands. During this maneuver the

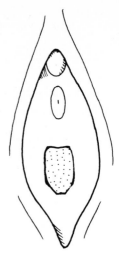

Figure 15-11. *Vaginal introitus with an intact hymen.*

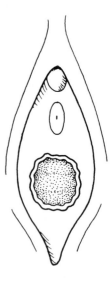

Figure 15-12. *Vaginal introitus after hymenal penetration.*

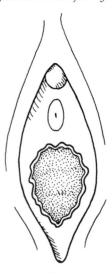

Figure 15-13. *Vaginal introitus of multiparous woman.*

Table 15-2. Selected Abnormalities of the External Genitalia

Finding	Condition	Description
Vulvar inflammation.	Moniliasis	Infection with Candida albicans (yeast organism) causes red, tender, and swollen vulva. Occurs frequently during antibiotic therapy. When normal bacterial flora of vagina is destroyed, yeast proliferates. Yeast grows best in a warm, moist, and dark environment; clients often relate that they wear synthetic underwear.
Vulvar inflammation.	Contact dermatitis	Vulvar irritation results from sensitivity to soap, detergent, feminine hygiene spray, or a synthetic undergarment.
One or more vesicular or ulcerative lesions 1.0 to 5.0 mm. in size on an erythematous base.	Herpes progenitalis	Usually results from infection with Herpes simplex virus type 2. The primary occurrence is frequently painful and tender. Usually recurs, but subsequent infections usually clear faster and are not as painful. Sometimes associated with pelvic lymphadenopathy and dysuria.
Vulvar papules, vesicles, and burrows.	Scabies (infestation by Sarcoptes scabiei)	Occurs concomitantly with scabies in other body regions, causes severe itching. Mites deposit eggs and feces in burrows in the skin. Spread by genital and other close physical contact, for example, sleeping on contaminated bed linen.
Small inflamed maculopapules with or without crusts with ova and tiny parasites. Found on hair-covered vulvar regions.	Pediculosis pubis (infestation by crab lice—Phthirius pubis)	Commonly causes severe itching. Clients often present with itching and are unaware of skin changes or parasites. Looks like flakes of dandruff on pubic hair, but after removal from skin and observed closely looks like tiny flat transparent spiders with moving legs. Spread in the same manner as Sarcoptes scabiei.
Verrucous lesions on the vulva and perianal region 0.5 to 2.0 cm. in size, occurring singly or in clusters.	Condylomata acuminata (venereal warts)	Asymptomatic lesions, which can also occur in the vagina. Grow larger during pregnancy and may prevent vaginal delivery if extremely large.
Expression of purulent drainage from urethral orifice during maneuver of milking Skene's glands.	Inflamed Skene's glands	Results from occlusion of duct due to infection by Neisseria gonorrhea. Accompanied by exquisite tenderness and/or dysuria.
Unilateral swelling and inflammation of labia from 2.0 to 6.0 cm. in size.	Bartholin's abscess	Results from infection of Bartholin's duct. When duct is occluded, continued secretion of the gland results in distended duct and cyst formation. Accompanied by exquisite pain and tenderness. Usually attributed to gonorrheal infection.
Small, firm, cystic lesion less than 2.0 cm. in size on inner aspect of labia majora and minora.	Sebaceous cyst	Usually are asymptomatic, result from obstruction of the duct of a sebaceous gland. When lanced, they yield a cheesy, sebaceous exudate. Secondary infection can result in abscess formation.
Eroded papule with raised indurated border on vulva.	Chancre of primary syphilis (Table 15-4)	Usually painless, accompanied by inguinal lymphadenopathy. Occurs within 10 to 90 days (average—three weeks) after invasion of mucous membrane by the spirochete Treponema pallidum. Lesions can also appear in vagina, on the cervix, fingers, lips, tongue, and nipples.
Large maculopapules that coalesce to form plaques on anogenital region.	Condylomata lata	Highly contagious lesions of secondary syphilis, which occur one to several months after primary syphilis. They also occur in the axillae. Associated with systemic symptoms including generalized lymphadenopathy, malaise, anorexia, headache, low-grade fever, and vague joint pains. Sometimes accompanied by loss of hair on eyebrows and eyelashes. (Table 15-4)
Red, fleshy several mm. to 1.0 cm. protrusion in posterior urethral mucosa.	Urethral caruncle	Asymptomatic, usually results from ectropion of the posterior urethral wall secondary to postmenopausal shrinkage of the genital tissues.

thumb of the palpating hand is placed on the lateral aspect of each side of the labia minora in turn while the vaginal fingers palpate the medial aspects (Figure 15-15). The labia minora feel smooth and nontender, and there is no discharge (Table 15-2).

Assessment of the Pelvic Musculature

The examiner separates the labia with the middle and index fingers, observes the vaginal introitus, and asks the patient to bear down or strain as if having a bowel movement. Normally the muscles of the pelvic floor maintain the anatomic separation of urethra, vagina, and rectum during straining. After observation, the examiner inserts two fingers into the vagina and assesses the competence of the pelvic muscles by palpation. When the client strains or bears down, there is normally no bulging (Table 15-3).

Speculum Examination and Collection of Specimens

A vaginal speculum is necessary for viewing the vagina and cervix and for collecting cytologic and other specimens. There are two types of vaginal specula available: the Pederson and the Graves specula (Figure 15-16).

The Pederson speculum is narrower and flatter than the Graves and is used with clients who have small vaginal orifices. The Graves speculum comes in

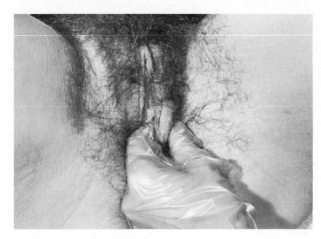

Figure 15-15. Palpation of Bartholin's glands.

a variety of sizes ranging from 8.75 to 12.5 centimeters long and 1.75 to 3.75 centimeters wide. Transparent plastic disposable speculums are available in the most common sizes but are more difficult to use for beginners.

Metal specula are warmed prior to insertion. Some facilities keep their specula on heated pads; however, the most commonly used method of warming is by passing the speculum under a faucet with warm running water. The water also serves as a lubricant.

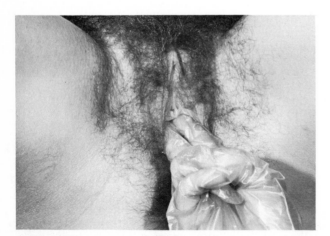

Figure 15-14. Palpation of Skene's glands.

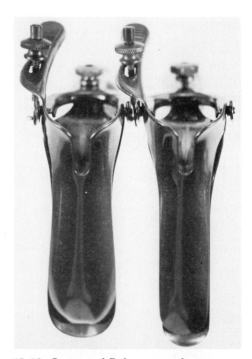

Figure 15-16. Graves and Pederson specula.

Table 15-3. Selected Abnormalities of the Pelvic Muscles

Finding	Condition	Explanation
Bladder prolapse. During straining, the anterior vaginal wall bulges downward and is visible at the introitus and palpable against the examining fingers.	Cystocele	Loss of pelvic muscle support results in relaxation of the anteriol vaginal wall. Often accompanied by stress incontinence and inability to empty the bladder fully during urination. Frequently represents long-term sequela of difficult delivery.
Rectal prolapse. During straining, the posterior vaginal wall is visible at the introitus and palpable against the examining fingers.	Rectocele	Loss of pelvic muscle support results in relaxation of the posterior vaginal wall. Often accompanied by constipation. Occurs as result of previous injury to the perineum, for example, perineal laceration during delivery.
During straining, the cervix or part of the entire uterine fundus is visible at the introitus.	Uterine prolapse Degrees of uterine prolapse: 1st degree—cervix is visible at the introitus 2nd degree—cervix extrudes from the introitus 3rd dgree—fundus extrudes from the introitus	Disruption of pelvic muscle support allows varying degrees of descent of the uterus. May be accompanied by incontinence or constipation.

Table 15-4. Laboratory Procedures Useful in Diagnosing Syphilis

Test	Description	Disadvantages
VDRL (Venereal Disease Research Laboratory)	Reflects serum titre of nonspecific antibodies against the antigen of the Treponema or the antigen formed by the reaction of the host to the Treponema. Most widely used non-Treponemal test. Easy, inexpensive serologic test. Excellent screening test. Positive within one to two weeks after primary lesion (4-5 weeks initial infection). Positive reaction may be delayed if client has undergone antibiotic therapy (particularly penicillin).	3 to 40% false-positive rate (hepatitis, infectious mononucleosus, viral pneumonia, malaria, chicken pox, measles, pregnancy, drug abuse, collagen diseases, pneumococcal pneumonia)
RPR	Newer, inexpensive, technically easier serologic screening test, which reflects nonspecific antibodies against the Treponema. Positive within same time frame as VDRL and positive reaction may be delayed under the same circumstances.	
FTA-ABS (Fluorescent Treponema antibody absorption test)	Most sensitive clinical test, which diagnoses all stages of syphilis because it is a serologic test that measures specific Treponemal antibodies.	Too expensive for screening
Dark field examination	Visualization of Treponema pallidum under microscope, which gives absolute and immediate diagnosis of syphilis (except in oral lesions, as spirochetes can be found in the mouth normally).	Rarely used because it is technically difficult, requires an expensive microscope, and results are not necessarily conclusive, that is, nonvisualization of the Treponema does not guarantee that Treponema is not present.

Lubricant jelly is never applied to the speculum since it distorts cells on the cytologic smear and is bacteriostatic.

Prior to insertion of the speculum, the examiner relaxes the perineal muscles and opens the introitus using the following maneuver: The pads of the index and middle fingers are placed in the vagina against the posterior vaginal wall, and slight pressure is exerted in a downward direction. The speculum is grasped between the index and middle fingers of the other hand and the blades are inserted obliquely at approximately a 45-degree angle. When a third of the length of the speculum is in the vagina, the examiner withdraws the fingers from the vagina and rotates the speculum to a transverse position. The speculum is advanced in an inferior direction at a 45-degree angle from the table until it contacts the end of the vagina. Ideally as the speculum blades are opened, the cervix appears. Occasionally the cervix is not visible. In this case the speculum is withdrawn about a third of the way and redirected at a different angle. When the cervix is in full view, the thumb screw is tightened, which maintains the open position of the blades (Figure 15-17).

The cervix is observed for its color, position, size, discharge, surface characteristics, and characteristics of the os. The color is normally pink, and its position depends upon the position of the uterus in the pelvis (Table 15-5). Most commonly the cervix penetrates the vagina in a superior and anterior direction for about 2 to 3 centimeters. It is usually 2 to 3 centimeters in diameter and exhibits an odorless discharge, which varies in appearance during the menstrual cycle. Throughout most of the menstrual cycle, cervical discharge is thin to thick and cloudy to white. Immediately prior to ovulation and during ovulation it is clearer and thinner, characteristics which encourage rather than impede the migration of sperm.

The surface of the cervix is normally smooth and free of lesions. The shape of the os varies with parity. The nulliparous woman usually has a circularly-shaped os, while the parous woman has an elliptical or slitlike os. Varying degrees of scarring are possible after traumatic delivery. (Table 15-5).

The client with an intrauterine device generally has one or two strings visible protruding from the os.

After inspection of the cervix, the examiner obtains the Papanicolaou (Pap) smear for cytologic study and other specimens as indicated. The Papanicolaou smear is a slide prepared from scraped epithelium of the cervix, which can detect abnormalities that indicate the presence of cancer. Prior to obtaining the Pap smear specimens, it is sometimes necessary to use a large cotton-tipped applicator to remove some of the cervical mucous. Dabbing the cervix lightly and twist-

Table 15-5. Common Cervical Abnormalities

Finding	Condition	Explanation
Red, swollen, edematous cervix with purulent discharge exuding from the os. Client may have backache, bearing down feeling in the pelvis, dull abdominal pain, urinary frequency, urgency, and dyspareunia.	Acute cervicitis	May be due to gonococci, streptococci, Staphylococci, or enterococci. Cervical smears and cultures identify the offending pathogen.
Usually asymptomatic client with zone of tissue around os, which looks granular and beefy red. Accompanied by a yellow, mucopurulent cervical discharge. Client may have postcoital spotting.	Chronic cervicitis (cervical erosion)	Loss of squamous epithelium on ectocervix results in overgrowth of infected endocervical epithelium (columnar type).
Area of endocervix exposed—appears as a beefy red area on cervix.	Ectropion	Laceration or dilatation of os during childbirth exposes portion of endocervix to vaginal acidity and bacterial flora.
Yellow, round translucent nodules several mm. to 1 cm. in diameter on cervix.	Nabothian cysts (retention cysts)	Endocervical glands blocked by secretions from inflammatory process of cervicitis.

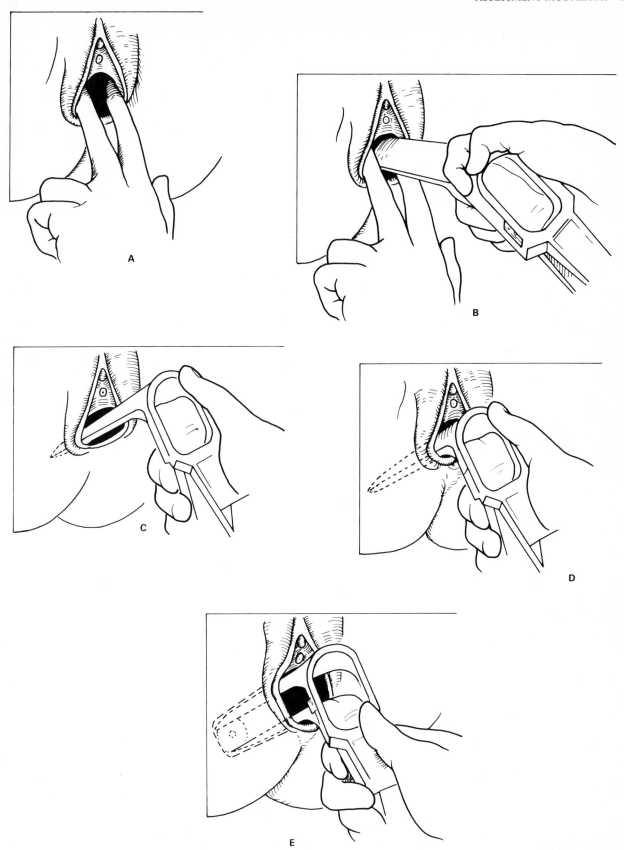

Figure 15-17. *Sequence of insertion of the vaginal speculum.*

ing the applicator as it is withdrawn removes some of the tenacious mucous, which sometimes prevents the examiner from obtaining a representative specimen. The Pap smear is usually deferred to a later time during the menses and when an infection is present.

The Pap smear comprises one to three types of specimens: the endocervical swab, the cervical scrape, and the vaginal pool. The cervical scrape is never omitted, although one or both of the other two specimens frequently are.

To obtain the endocervical swab the examiner moistens a cotton-tipped applicator with saline and inserts it into the os. The applicator is rolled clockwise and counterclockwise a full 360° within the os for 30 seconds (Figure 15-18). After removal from the os the applicator is rolled across a slide marked with an E (Figure 15-19). The slide is fixed immediately by spraying it with cytologic spray or by inserting it in a bottle containing ether-alcohol fixative.

For the cervical scrape the examiner places the larger humped end of the Ayre spatula within the endocervical canal and the smaller humped end against the cervix. This assures contact between the spatula groove and cervical lip. The spatula is rotated 360 degrees while slight, steady pressure is maintained against the cervical lip. The examiner withdraws the spatula, applies both sides of the spatula to a slide marked C, and immediately fixes it (Figure 15-20).

The vaginal pool specimen is obtained from the posterior fornix. The opposite end of the Ayre spatula is used to scrape the posterior fornix, the specimen is

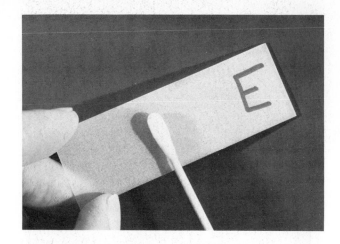

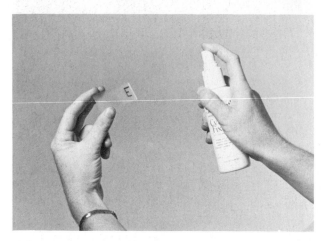

Figure 15-19. *Preparation of slide for Pap smear. The examiner uses clear slides only; frosted slides are used for photographic purposes.*

applied to the slide marked V, and the slide is immediately sprayed with fixative or placed in a fixative solution (Figure 15-21).

Although the Pap smear is an excellent screening test for cervical carcinoma, it is not always 100 percent accurate. Any suspicious lesions should be brought to the attention of a physician skilled in colposcopy. In posthysterectomy clients the Pap smear is obtained from the vaginal pool and cuff (the area of scarring). Suspicious clinical findings are brought to the attention of the cytologist by a notation on the lab requistion (Table 15-6).

Before removing the speculum, the examiner determines whether other specimens are indicated (Table 15-7).

The examiner slowly withdraws the speculum and releases the thumb screw closing the blades after clearing the cervix. To minimize discomfort while removing the speculum the examiner exerts downward pressure and avoids pinching the vaginal mucosa.

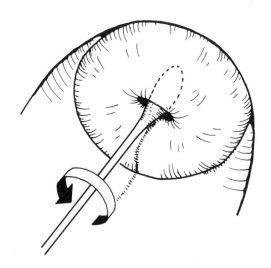

Figure 15-18. *Endocervical specimen—Pap smear.*

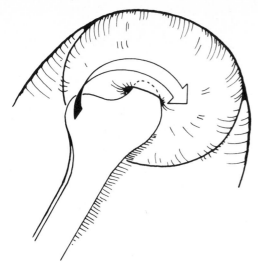

Figure 15-20. Cervical specimen—Pap smear.

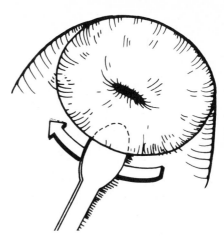

Figure 15-21. Vaginal pool specimen—Pap smear.

During withdrawal the vagina is inspected. It is moist, dark pink in color and rugated; it contains a thin clear to white, nonoffensive discharge.

Bimanual Examination

The bimanual examination provides information about the position, mobility, and structural characteristics of the uterus and adnexa, and identifies any abnormalities (Table 15-8). It consists of two parts: the vaginal examination and the rectovaginal examination.

From a standing position with one foot resting on the footstool, the examiner spreads the labia with the thumb and index finger of one hand. The gloved index and middle fingers of the other hand are lubricated with lubricant jelly and introduced into the vagina in a posterior direction with the palmar surfaces upward. The thumb is abducted; the ring and little fingers are flexed onto the palm and remain outside of the vagina (Figure 15-26).

The examiner places the other hand on the abdomen above the symphysis pubis and presses downward until the cervix is palpated by the fingers in the vagina. The cervix is palpated and assessed for size, surface characteristics, position, mobility, and the patency of the os. It is normally 2 to 3 centimeters in diameter and protrudes 2 to 3 centimeters into the vagina. It feels smooth and firm; its consistency is described as that of the tip of the nose. Most frequently the cervix is midline and points downward from its location on the anterior vaginal wall. The examiner's fingers completely encircle the cervix and palpate the fornices. With one finger in each lateral fornix the cervix is moved laterally. The normal cervix moves freely and without tenderness 1 to 2 centimeters laterally and is open and admits the examiner's finger approximately 0.5 centimeters.

The uterus is palpated to determine its position, size, shape, consistency, mobility, and surface characteristics. There are three major positions of the uterus: anteposition, midposition, and retroposition. There are two types of ante and retroposition: anteversion and anteflexion, retroversion and retro-

Table 15-6. Papanicolaou Results

Class I	Absence of atypical or abnormal cells
Class II	Atypical cytologic picture, but no evidence of malignancy
Class III	Cytologic picture suggestive, but not diagnostic of malignancy
Class IV	Cytologic picture strongly suggestive of malignancy
Class V	Cytologic picture diagnostic of malignancy

Table 15-7. Indications and Procedures for Cervical and Vaginal Specimens

Indications	Procedures
1. History of sexual intercourse with infected partner 2. Copious foul-smelling gray, homogeneous vaginal discharge.	Wet smear for Hemophilus vaginalis 1. A specimen of vaginal discharge is applied to a glass slide. 2. One drop of normal saline is applied to the slide. 3. The slide is covered with a cover slip and viewed under high power. 4. Characteristic "clue" cells are visible. They are heavily stippled epithelial cells (Figure 15-22).
1. Pruritus 2. White, curd-like vaginal discharge adherent to vaginal walls	Wet smear for moniliasis (Candida albicans) 1. A specimen of vaginal discharge is applied to a glass slide. 2. One drop of potassium hydroxide solution is applied to the slide. 3. The slide is covered with a cover slip and viewed under low power. 4. If Candida are present, hyphae and spores are visible (Figure 15-23).
1. History of sexual intercourse with infected partner 2. Yellow frothy vaginal discharge 3. "Strawberry spots" on vaginal surface—red punctate lesions on vaginal epithelium	Wet smear for trichomoniasis 1. A specimen of vaginal discharge is applied to a glass slide. 2. One drop of normal saline is applied to the slide. 3. The slide is covered with a cover slip and viewed under high power. 4. Trichomonads are flaggelated, moving organisms about the size of white blood cells (Figure 15-24).
1. Exposure to gonorrhea or other venereal disease. Some agencies recommend routine culture for gonorrhea in all women since it is frequently asymptomatic. Others culture all women with vaginitis. 2. History of pelvic pain 3. Green purulent discharge from cervical os	Gonorrheal culture 1. The examiner inserts a cotton-tipped applicator moistened with saline into the endocervical canal. 2. The applicator is rotated 360° in clockwise and counter-clockwise directions for 1 minute. 3. The applicator tip is rolled across the Thayer-Martin medium in a Z-shaped pattern (Figure 15-25). 4. The specimen is taken to a laboratory immediately or placed upside down in a candle jar with the candle lit. 5. The oropharynx and anus are similarly cultured when there is a history of oral or anal intercourse.

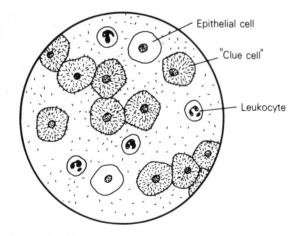

Figure 15-22. *"Clue" cells of hemophilus vaginalis.*

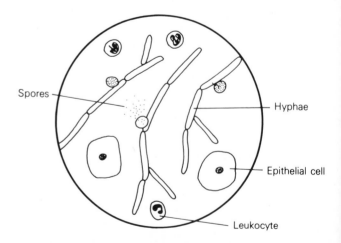

Figure 15-23. *Hyphae and spores of Candida albicans.*

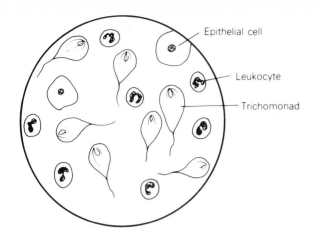

Figure 15-24. Trichomonads.

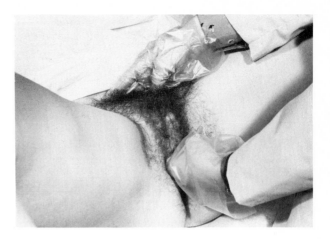

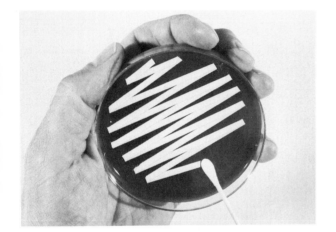

Figure 15-25. Procedure for smearing Thayer-Martin medium.

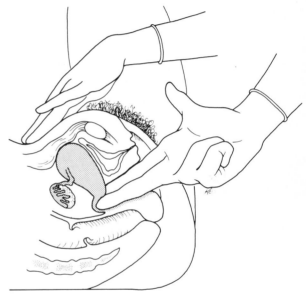

Figure 15-26. Bimanual palpation

flexion. In anteversion and retroversion the angulation of the isthmus is slight. In both flexion positions the angulation of the isthmus is more pronounced. In a uterus that is in midposition the angulation of the isthmus is slight. The fundus of a uterus in anteposition is palpable by the hand on the abdomen. The fundus of a uterus in midposition is not palpable by the hand on the abdomen, and may not be palpable by the finger in the rectum in the rectovaginal examination. The fundus of a uterus in retroposition is palpable by the finger in the rectum in the rectovaginal examination (Table 15-8).

Since most uteri are in anteposition, uterine size can be estimated as the distance between the hand on the abdomen and the fingers in the vagina. The abdominal hand presses downward from its position midway between the symphysis pubis and the umbilicus. The intravaginal fingers are positioned in the anterior fornix and lift upward against the abdominal

hand. Normally the uterus is approximately 5.5 to 8.0 centimeters long, 3.5 to 4.0 centimeters wide, and 2.0 to 2.5 centimeters in thickness and resembles an inverted pear in shape. It is firm in consistency, similar to the cervix. The uterus ballottes freely between the examining hands; that is, the examiner can easily move it between the abdominal and intravaginal hands.

While stabilizing the uterus in the pelvis with the abdominal hand, the examiner assesses its surface characteristics by palpating it on all surfaces with the intravaginal fingers. Normally it is smooth.

If the uterus is in midposition or retroposition, the examiner may not be able to assess its position, size, shape, consistency, mobility, and surface characteristics until the retrovaginal examination.

Table 15-8. Findings in Bimanual Vaginal and Rectovaginal Examination

| | Bimanual | | |
Position of Uterus	Direction of Cervical Os	Body and Fundus	Illustration
Anteverted	Posterior	Palpable by one hand on the abdomen and the fingers of the other hand in the vagina	
Midposition	In the same plane as the vagina	May not be palpable	
Retroverted	Anterior	Not palpable	
Anteflexed	Anterior or midposition; the axis of the cervix is different from the axis of the body of uterus; angulation of isthmus may be felt in the anterior fornix	Easily palpable	
Retroflexed	Anterior, midposition, or posterior	Not palpable	

From Malasanos, Lois; Barkauskas, Violet; Moss, Muriel; and Stollenberg-Allen, Kathryn; *Health Assessment*, 2nd ed.

Following palpation of the uterus the examiner assesses the adnexa beginning on one side and then repeating the assessment sequence for the other side. The intravaginal fingers are placed in one lateral fornix, and the abdominal hand is placed on the ipsilateral iliac crest. As the hands are brought together, the abdominal hand stabilizes the adnexa and the intravaginal fingers palpate the adnexal organs. Frequently the examiner is unable to palpate any organs in this maneuver. Sometimes the ovaries are palpable and are assessed for size, shape, consistency, and mobility. The ovaries vary considerably in size among individuals but average 3 to 3.5 centimeters in length, 2 centimeters in width, and 1 to 1.5 centimeters in thickness. They are generally no larger than 4 to 6 centimeters in their greatest dimension. The ovaries are almond-shaped, firm, freely movable, sensitive to touch, but nontender. The Fallopian tubes are normally not palpable. Occasionally the round ligaments are palpable, and feel like cordlike structures. After completion of the examination of the adnexa, the examiner withdraws the fingers from the vagina, discards the glove, dons a new glove, and lubricates the middle and index fingers in preparation for the rectovaginal examination.

Rectovaginal Examination

The rectovaginal examination confirms the findings of the bimanual vaginal examination and assesses the size, position, consistency, mobility, and surface

Table 15-8 *(continued)*

| | Rectovaginal | | |
Anterior and Posterior Portion of Uterus	Cervix	Body and Fundus	Illustration
Palpable as the uterus is rotated even more anteriorly	Palpable through the rectovaginal septum	Not palpable by the finger in the rectum	
May not be palpable	Posterior portion felt through the rectovaginal septem	May not be palpable	
Posterior portion may be palpable by fingers in the posterior fornix	May not be palpable by finger in the rectum	Body easily palpable by the fingers in the rectum; fundus may not be palpable	
Easily palpable	Same as anteverted	Same as anteverted	
Not palpable	Palpable through the rectovaginal septum	Angulation of isthmus palpable, body and fundus easily palpable	

(St. Louis: The C. V. Mosby Co., 1981).

characteristics of uteri in retroposition. The client is asked to bear down while the examiner presses the pad of the middle finger against the anus. The examining finger is directed into the rectum with the palmar surface downward. After passing the internal anal sphincter (Chapter 14), the hand is rotated to bring the palmar surface upward. The index finger is directed into the vagina with the palmar surface upward. The maneuvers for assessing the uterus in retroposition are the same as those for the uterus in anteposition. The examiner places the finger in the vagina on the surface of the cervix as a point of reference and palpates the uterus between the hand on the abdomen and the finger in the rectum (Figure 15-27).

The rectovaginal septum is palpated and is normally thin, smooth, firm, pliable, and intact. The cul-de-sac is palpated, and is a potential space through which the pelvic organs are palpable (Table 15-9).

The vaginal finger is withdrawn, and the rectal examination is completed as discussed in Chapter 14. The examiner withdraws the rectal finger, wipes any lubricating jelly from the vulva and anus, removes the glove, and assists the client to a sitting position.

Assessment of the Urinary Tract

Because of the proximity of the urinary tract to the genital structures, there are two noninvasive testing methods commonly utilized during assessment of the female genitalia: urinalysis (Appendix 9) and urine culture. Normally there is an insignificant number of bacteria present in the urine after a clean catch mid-stream, voided specimen; therefore, urine culture is negative.

The client is instructed to separate the labia with the fingers of one hand. The other hand cleanses the vestibule with antiseptic solution wiping once with each swab from forward to back. The client begins to void into the toilet and places the specimen cup under the vulva, catching the middle of the urinary stream (Table 15-10).

Life Cycle Variations

Childhood

Some of the genitalia assessment techniques and findings differ in prepubescent girls. Although inspection and palpation of the external genitalia are never omitted, rarely are the speculum and bimanual examinations performed. In rare instances when these techniques are indicated—for example, the presence of a foreign body in the vagina—the client is referred to a specialist, preferably a gynecologist who has expertise with pediatric clients.

Frequently at birth the vulva is edematous and the clitoris is prominent due to maternal hormone stimulation. This edema subsides during the first two weeks. However, marked or persistent clitoromegaly may signal the existence of an adrenogenital syndrome. A small number of newborn girls have a scant bloody vaginal discharge lasting for a few days up to a month of age. This results from the absorption of sex hormones from the mother during pregnancy.

Prior to puberty the mons and labia are hairless and the genitalia are small in proportion to the rest of the body.

During the preschool years it is not uncommon for young children to insert foreign bodies into the vagina. Common examples are lipsticks, crayons, chalk, raisins, and toilet paper. Usually a parent notices a foul smelling vaginal discharge and brings the child to the attention of a health care provider.

Occasionally children traumatize the external genitalia during masturbation with a hard or sharp object. It is important for the examiner to assume a matter-of-fact attitude toward masturbation and elicit the parent's and child's feelings toward this practice. Sometimes the parent's discomfort with the child's genital manipulation while unclothed for the physical examination provides an excellent opportunity for discussion of early sexuality.

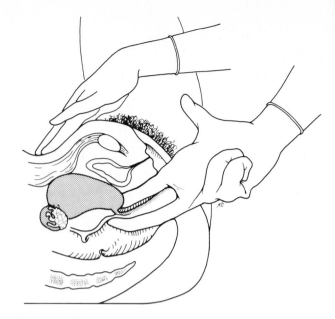

Figure 15-27. *Rectovaginal examination.*

Prior to puberty the child is normally curious about the genitalia of both sexes but limits sexual expression to self-stimulation.

The examiner maintains an inquisitive approach to any signs of genital trauma. Vulvar edema or hematoma may suggest sexual molestation. The parent and child are questioned separately regarding these findings, and the examiner bears in mind the possibility of contact with sexually deviant friends or relatives.

A common cause of nonbacterial urethritis is chemical irritation from bubble baths. The most common urinary tract pathogen is Escherichia coli, which enters the urethra from fecal contamination when the child or parent wipes from the anal area forward after defecation.

The most frequent cause of pediatric vulvar pruritis is pinworms. The examiner observes the anal area for the presence of pinworms. Usually they migrate out of the anus in darkened conditions; therefore, they are usually not present during the genital examination. The examiner instructs the parent in the scotch tape test. About 30 minutes after the child is in bed at night or in the morning before the child is out of bed, the parent removes the clothing, exposing the genitalia, and presses a piece of scotch tape against the anus. After pulling the tape away, eggs from pinworms are seen adherent to the tape. The scotch tape is applied to a glass slide for further evaluation.

Table 15-9. Selected Abnormalities of the Bimanual Vaginal Examination

Finding	Condition	Description
Tender adnexa	Mittelschmerz Endometriosis Intrauterine contraceptive device (IUCD)	Client experiences vague discomfort to dull pain during palpation of the adnexa.
Tender cervix	Acute pelvic inflammatory disease (PID)(acute salpingitis)	Exquisite tenderness results when the cervix is moved between the examiner's fingers. Most frequently results from infection with Neisseria gonorrhoeae, streptococci staphylococci, or Chlamydia trachomadis.
Bilateral tender, irregular and fixed adnexal masses	Chronic pelvic inflammatory disease (PID)	Late sequelae of infection with Neisseria gonorrhoeae. Results from untreated or inadequately treated gonorrhea.
Tender, adnexal mass	Ectopic pregnancy	Refers to implantation outside of the uterus, most frequently in a Fallopian tube. Symptoms vary depending on when the patient is seen: before, during, or after rupture. Accompanied by a variety of menstrual abnormalities, usually postponed or prolonged menses. Before rupture, patient presents with vague pain and frequently no masses are palpable yet. During rupture patients experience severe unilateral pain; pain may exacerbate and subside; cervix is exquisitely sensitive to movement; fever and leukocytosis may be present; tense, exquisitely tender adnexal mass palpable. After rupture patient has severe unilateral pain; signs of shock—rapid, thready pulse, cold sweat, pallor, restlessness, anxiety, air hunger; affected abdominal side boardlike in rigidity; radiation of pain to shoulder from diaphragmatic irritation.
Firm, irregular nodules on uterine surface	Leiomyomata (fibroids)	Common, benign uterine tumors; may be single or multiple, varying in size.
Enterocele, bulging of upper posterior vagina behind cervix	Herniation of the cul-de-sac	Some are congenital hernias in which the posterior vaginal wall lined with peritoneum protrudes into the rectovaginal septum from above. Others are acquired after surgery (correction of uterine malposition and abdominal or vaginal hysterectomy). It may contain omentum, ascitic fluid, or sigmoid.
Unilateral adnexal mass (sometimes bilateral)	Functional cysts Benign tumors Malignant tumors	Cystic dilation of graafian follicles on corpus luteum, usually less than 6-8 cm. in diameter. May cause delayed menses, unilateral pelvic pain, deep dyspareunia, or low back pain.

Adolescence

Adolescence begins with puberty. Puberty is the time when the secondary sex characteristics appear and the reproductive organs begin to function. Sexual functioning usually occurs later in adolescence. In females puberty begins between the ages of 9 and 14 (usually between 10 and 12) when secretion of estrogen assumes a cyclic pattern. The developmental changes of puberty occur over a period of 3 to 5 years (Chapters 5 and 12). This results in the growth of pubic and axillary hair and precedes menarche by about 2 years. The other changes resulting from estrogen secretion are enlargement of the uterus and ovaries, development of the labia minora and Fallopian tubes, increase in vaginal acidity, and cornification of the vaginal epithelial cells.

Menarche usually occurs between the ages of 11 and 16. The average age is 12. The usual adolescent menstrual cycle is anovulatory and irregular for the

Table 15-10.   Common Urinary Tract Abnormalities

Finding	Condition	Explanation
Urinalysis reagent strip positive for protein; microscopic examination reveals bacteruria or pyuria.	Urinary tract infection (cystitis or urethritis)	Usually accompanied by dysuria, urinary frequency, and urgency. Most commonly due to fecal contamination because of transmission of perianal organisms to urethra from incorrect hygiene after defecation or during coitus. Culture usually reveals Escherichia coli. When Skene's glands are involved—that is, a discharge is expressed—infection with Neisseria gonorrhea is most likely, and appropriate cultures are indicated.
Sterile urine in client who reports dysuria, frequency, and urgency.	Trigonitis (honeymoon cystitis)	Occurs primarily in females who suddenly become sexually active and results from inflammation of the trigone (the triangular space at the base of the bladder) caused by frequent and forceful penile penetration.
	Nongonococcal urethritis	Infection with chlamydia trachomadis

first 2 years. Wide ranges in cycle length (18 to 45 days) are common; although bleeding usually lasts 5 days, a duration from 3 to 8 days is normal. In questioning an adolescent about menstruation, it is often helpful to compare the last period with several preceding it. Frequently the pregnant adolescent misinterprets vaginal spotting as menstruation.

A major developmental goal during adolescence is the establishment of a sexual identity. Sexual feelings, drives, and fantasies increase at this time. Early in adolescence sexual interest is evident; curiosity about sex, seeking of sexual information, frequent sexual innuendos in conversation, sexual daydreaming, fantasies about heterosexual relationships, and masturbation are common. Homosexual interest may predominate while the individual adjusts to temporarily discomforting unfamiliar sexual urges. Examples of homosexual practices are handholding, kissing, breast fondling, and mutual masturbation.

The age at which heterosexual expression begins is highly variable. Although the pelvic examination is usually not performed prior to age 18, the sexually active adolescent requires the same thorough assessment of the genitalia as the adult.

A discussion of sexuality and contraception is of paramount importance in this age group. Examiners can begin by asking if the client has a steady boyfriend. Sometimes providing an explanation of normal behavior assures the client that the examiner is open-minded and interested. For example, the examiner can say, "Frequently after people go steady, they become closer and begin to explore each other's bod-

ies. This is usually a good time to make a decision about whether or not they are ready for sex or going all the way'." Although some adolescents are actually looking for permission to request contraception, others are seeking permission to remain virginal and limit sexual expression.

As with the adult client, examiners should maintain a high level of suspicion regarding venereal disease. Treatment of minors for venereal disease, contraception, pregnancy, and abortion without parental consent varies among states. Even in states where parental consent is required, adolescents deserve a private interview with the examiner during which these topics can be discussed.

Pregnancy

The most frequent symptom of pregnancy is amenorrhea. Other symptoms are breast fullness and tenderness, nausea or vomiting ("morning sickness"), fatigue, lethargy, and urinary frequency. As early as the fifth week after the first day of the previous menstrual period, urine tests for pregnancy can be positive. Usually they are positive in the eighth week. Urine tests reflect the presence of chorionic gonadotropin, a placental hormone excreted in the urine. The two-minute slide test is practical for most offices, although the two-hour tube test performed by clinical laboratories is more sensitive. Home urine tests are available, but are not always accurate if used incorrectly. It is recommended that clients reporting amenorrhea beyond six weeks past the last menses have a pelvic examination to rule out pregnancy. Radioimmunoassay of serum for chorionic gonadotropin is positive two weeks after conception.

During the initial interview with the pregnant woman it is important for the examiner to elicit her and her partner's feelings about the pregnancy. If abortion is contemplated, it is easiest and most safely accomplished prior to the tenth week of gestation.

Pregnancy is a time of considerable physiologic change (Table 15-11). These changes suggest approximations of gestational age; however, gestational age is more accurately estimated by ultrasonography preferably performed between the 20th and 28th weeks.

Pregnant women frequently experience emotional lability. It is a time of anticipation interspersed with anxiety about the health of the baby and the ability of the woman to parent. Ambivalent feelings about being female and sexuality emerge as the client contemplates a role change. While some women are proud of their changing bodies, others have difficulty adjusting to a new body image.

The normal pelvic vasocongestion of pregnancy elevates the baseline of sexual tension throughout pregnancy; many pregnant women note an increase in sexual interest, anticipation, and fantasy especially in the midtrimester. As a result, the achievement of orgasm is easier; some women become orgasmic or multiorgasmic for the first time while pregnant. The resolution stage occurring after orgasm is slower and the period of postorgasmic satiation is shorter. Coital frequency is not necessarily increased, as many women fear harm to the baby or miscarriage and prefer to refrain from coitus. The examiner encourages the woman to include her partner in prenatal visits, and attempts to provide an open forum for discussion of sexual practices and alternatives. Some research suggests that coitus during pregnancy predisposes toward intrauterine infection of the fetus. The decision to have or refrain from coitus requires careful consideration by the pregnant woman and her partner. Coitus is contraindicated if discomfort occurs, although a change in position often helps. Coitus is also contraindicated when vaginal bleeding occurs. Vaginal spotting occurs in 30 percent of pregnant women during the first trimester, although the exact cause is unknown.

The pregnant client is susceptible to venereal disease as well as vaginal infections like other adult women; therefore, evidence of these conditions is sought throughout pregnancy. Passage of the fetus through a birth canal infected with gonorrhea or herpes simplex can result in blindness, severe neurologic impairment and severe liver disease. Congenital syphilis can result in lesions of the skin, mucous membranes, hematologic system, bones and viscera.

Late Adulthood

Menopause is the time when menstruation ceases. It usually occurs between the ages of 45 and 55 years. Considerable variation in cessation of menses exists. Some women have anovulatory cycles for a period of time, others gradually begin to skip menstrual periods, while others experience a sudden cessation of the menses. Ovulation ceases sometime prior to the last menstrual period. Individual reactions to menopause vary. Some women welcome it as a time when the fear of pregnancy no longer exists. Others fear a loss of sexual desire and desirability and the associated symptoms of hormonal disequilibrium.

Since the genital structures are estrogen dependent, the cessation of estrogen production by the ovaries during menopause results in considerable changes. The vulva atrophies, pubic hair thins, labia majora and minora become flatter, and introitus gradually constricts. The vagina shortens and narrows, and its rugae disappear. It appears pale due to decreased vascularity and becomes drier and more friable due to a decrease in the number of epithelial cell layers. Because the vagina loses elasticity and tone, frequently cystocele, rectocele, and uterine prolapse appear or worsen after menopause. The uterus becomes smaller, the fundus decreasing to the size of the cervix. Relaxation of the uterosacral ligaments lessens the normal uterine anteflexion so that it becomes midposition. The ovaries become smaller and are usually not palpable (Table 15-12).

Sexual interest reflects previous ideas toward sexuality. Women with regular partners generally have regular sexual activity although the frequency is often decreased. Women without partners often maintain sexual activity through masturbation. The capacity for orgasm is often decreased or dyspareunia is experienced when atrophic vaginal changes or decreased lubrication occur. Women continue to be capable of multiple orgasms throughout life although the number of contractions during orgasm decreases from five to six at age 30 to two to three at age 70.

Table 15-11.   Changes in the Female Genitalia During Pregnancy

Change	Time Change Becomes Apparent
Ladin's Sign—soft spot at the midline of the isthmus.	4th to 5th week
Hegar's Sign—softening of the isthmus compared to cervical firmness.	6th week
Braun von Fernwald's Sign—uterus feels asymmetrical; site of implantation is enlarged and softened.	6th week
Softening of cervix—resembles consistency of lips instead of nose.	8th week
Leukorrhea—increased vaginal secretion from increased production of cervical mucus, increased vaginal transudation secondary to pelvic vasocongestion, and increased exfoliation of vaginal epithelium stimulated by estrogen.	8th week
Chadwick's Sign—purplish coloration of vaginal mucosa and cervix.	9th to 12th week
Auscultation of fetal heartbeat with doppler.	9th to 12th week
Palpation of fundus at symphysis pubis. McDonald's Sign—increased anteflexion of uterus because of softening of the isthmus.	12th week
Palpation of fundus midway between the symphysis pubis and umbilicus.	16th week
The fundus is at the umbilicus. Fetal heartbeat heard with fetoscope. Quickening (client feels life).	17th to 20th week
Fundus above umbilicus.	21st to 24th week
Fetal movements palpable.	21st to 24th week
Linea nigra—increased deposition of melenin results in darkening of the linea alba from the umbilicus to the symphysis pubis.	21st to 24th week
Fundus is three finger breadths above the umbilicus.	25th to 28th week
Fundus is three finger breadths below the xiphosternum.	29th to 32nd week
Fundus is two-finger breadths below the xiphosternum.	33rd to 36th week
Fundus drops below previous level as presenting part settles in the pelvis—lightening.	37th to 40th week
Cervix may begin to shorten—efface.	37th to 40th week
Cervix may begin to open—dilate.	37th to 40th week

Table 15-12. Selected Genital Abnormalities of Late Adulthood

Finding	Condition	Description
White spots or patches on the vulva	Leukoplakia	Hypertrophic skin lesion, often asymptomatic. May cause pruritus and tenderness. May be malignant.
Dry and shiny mucosa of vestibule, urethral orifice inner aspects of labia majora and the vagina	Kraurosis	Atrophic mucous membrane becomes painful. May be inflamed.

Anatomy and Physiology

The male genitalia comprise structures involved in micturation and reproduction. The external male genitalia consist of the penis and scrotum (Figures 16-1, 16-2). The penis, a cylindrical structure suspended from the anterior portion of the perineum, is composed primarily of three columns of erectile tissue: two dorsolateral columns (corpora cavernosa) and one ventromedial column (corpus spongiosum). These columns are bound together by heavy fibrous tissue that forms the shape of the penile shaft. The penis is part of the urinary system since the corpus spongiosum contains the terminal portion of urethra. The penis is also part of the male reproductive system. In this function the penis is the male organ of copulation and deposits the spermatozoa into the vagina.

At the distal end of the shaft are the glans penis, corona, and, in some males, the foreskin and frenulum. The glans is a cone-shaped extension of the corpus spongiosum. The corona, an annular expansion of the glans, is at the junction of the glans and shaft. In the uncircumcised male there is a flap of skin—the foreskin or prepuce—that arises from the corona and covers most of the glans. The frenulum is a fold of the foreskin that extends ventrally from the urethral meatus to the corona. During circumcision, the foreskin is removed. At the tip of the glans penis is the urethral meatus.

The scrotum is a pouch that hangs from the posterior base of the penis. It is covered with sparse hair and deeply pigmented rugous skin overlying a layer of dartos muscle. A medial ridge extends from the root of the penis to the anus and separates the scro-

Chapter 16

Assessment of the Male Genitalia

Objectives

The examiner will be able to do the following:

1. Inspect and palpate the penis and scrotum
2. Palpate the femoral canals
3. Health teach self-examination of the testes
4. Auscultate the scrotum
5. Obtain specimen for gonorrheal culture
6. Obtain specimen for urinalysis and urine culture and sensitivity
7. Recognize abnormalities
8. Record the information obtained

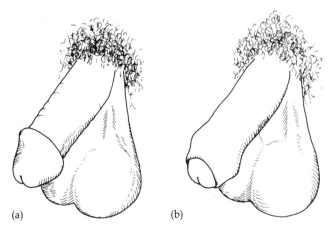

(a) (b)

Figure 16-1. External male genitalia: (a) circumsized; (b) uncircumcised.

tum into two halves. Internally the two scrotal halves are separated by a septal fold of the dartos muscle. Each half of the scrotum contains a testis, epididymis, and part of the spermatic cord.

The scrotum functions as a thermal regulator to keep the testes 1 to 2° cooler than body temperature. In cold environmental temperatures or with exercise, the walls of the scrotum contract, the skin becomes more wrinkled, and the scrotum becomes smaller. In warm environmental temperatures the walls relax and the scrotum becomes larger and more pendulous.

The testes are a pair of nearly symmetrical oval bodies surrounded by a serous membrane, the tunica vaginalis, and are suspended vertically in the scrotum. They are approximately 4 centimeters long, 3 centimeters wide, and 2.5 centimeters in diameter. The testes produce the male sex cells (spermatozoa) and testosterone. The testes must be in the scrotal sac to maintain a temperature cooler than the body. If the

testes are in the abdominal cavity, the higher temperature inhibits spermatogenesis.

On the posterolateral surface of each testis is the epididymis, a comma-shaped, convoluted structure that suspends the testes and stores the spermatozoa. The head of the epididymis is on the top of the testis with the body along the posterolateral surface and the tail on the lower portion.

Arising from the epididymis is the vas deferens, a duct that delivers the spermatozoa from the epididymis to the ejaculatory duct. The spermatic fascia surrounds the vas deferens, arteries, veins, nerves, and lymph vessels that form the spermatic cord.

The ejaculatory duct is a short, straight duct formed by the vas deferens and the duct from the seminal vesicle. The ejaculatory duct pierces the prostate gland and empties into the urethra.

The two seminal vesicles store semen and are small saclike structures approximately 2.5 centimeters long. They lie along the lower posterior portion of the bladder and superior and lateral to the prostate gland (Chapter 14).

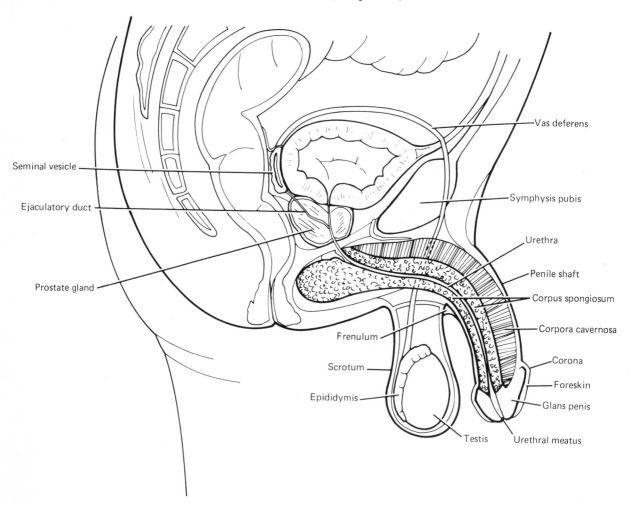

Figure 16-2. Internal male genitalia.

The inguinal canal is a 4- to 6-centimeter long oblique tunnel in the abdominal wall through which the vas deferens and other contents of the spermatic cord travel (Figure 16-3). At either end of the tunnel is a triangular, slitlike opening: the external and internal inguinal rings. The external inguinal ring is superior and lateral to the pubic tubercle. The internal inguinal ring is approximately 1.5 centimeters above the inguinal ligament and midway between the anterior superior iliac spine and the pubic symphysis. The spermatic cord passes through the external inguinal ring, inguinal canal, and internal inguinal ring into the abdominal cavity, where its contents disperse.

The femoral canal is a potential space approximately 4 centimeters long and is medial and parallel to the femoral artery, just below the inguinal ligament (Figure 16-3). The femoral canal contains fat, a few lymph vessels, and possibly lymph nodes. The canal is covered with periteneum; sometimes abdominal contents slip into it.

Sexuality

Human sexuality is governed by the central nervous system, the endocrine system, and the autonomic nervous system. The central nervous system serves as an integrating force in the drive for sexual fulfillment, while adequate levels of androgens, especially testosterone, are needed to sustain an interest in sexual feelings and activities. The autonomic nervous system affects the extragenital responses during sexual activity, such as perspiration, an elevated blood pressure, heart rate, and respiratory rate.

Masters and Johnson identified four stages of adult sexual activity: excitement, plateau, orgasmic, and resolution. The excitement phase is triggered by psychogenic and tactile stimuli. This produces penile erection, plus the scrotal sac tenses and thickens and the spermatic cord shortens, which causes the testes to rise toward the perineum. During the second phase of sexual response, the plateau phase, the penis engorges with more blood and the penis and testes enlarge. A few drops of a clear mucoid material is often released from the urethral meatus at this time. During the orgasmic phase there are expulsive contractions from the epididymis, vas deferens, seminal vesicles, prostatic urethra, and penile portion of the urethra. These contractions force the expulsion of semen and are referred to as an ejaculation. In the final phase, the resolution phase, the penis becomes flaccid and refractory to stimulation. Also, the scrotum relaxes and the testes descend to their pre-excitement location (Table 16-1).

Assessment Modalities

Preparation

Inspection and palpation are the examination modalities used in the assessment of the male genitalia.

The equipment needed for the examination includes gloves, a penlight, and a low stool. The gloves are indicated for the examiner only when there are open lesions and drainage with the potential for cross infection. A penlight is used to transilluminate scrotal contents and the examiner sits on the stool.

On rare occasions a stethoscope is used to auscultate scrotal contents for bowel sounds when an inguinal hernia is suspected in a very obese man. If a discharge is present, or if there is a history of venereal disease (VD) exposure, slides are needed to obtain a smear for a culture.

The client's chest and abdomen may be covered with a short gown while the genitalia and groin area are exposed. For the examination the client stands and faces the examiner, who sits on a low stool. Sometimes the client is instructed to place a foot on a low stool. If the client is unable to stand, he lies on a flat surface.

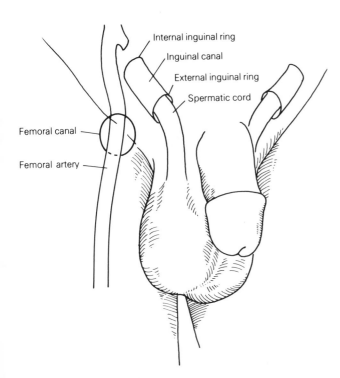

Figure 16-3. Location of inguinal and femoral canals.

Table 16-1.   Selected Abnormalities of Male Sexual Function

Finding	Condition	Description
Inability to attain or maintain an erection	Impotence	May progress insidiously from the inability to attain an erection firm enough for coitus to the inability to have an erection for masturbation. Most frequently is caused by psychologic problems. Impotence is often associated with endocrine, vascular, neurologic diseases, and ingestion of many drugs including alcohol, sedatives, narcotics, antihypertensives, antiandrogenic and dopamine blocking agents.
Prolonged penile erection	Priapism	Sustained, painful erection that often occurs with high spinal cord lesions, leukemia, or sickle cell anemia. It is rarely caused by excessive sexual stimulation.
Difficulty with orgasm	Premature ejaculation	Premature emission of seminal fluid; loss of control of ejaculation which is generally associated with psychological difficulties.
	Ejaculatory incompetence	Erection occurs but there is no emission or a retarded emission of seminal fluid. This condition is generally associated with psychological difficulties.
Painful intercourse	Penile ulceration, (herpes progenitais or intrauterine device in woman)	Penile thrusting during coitus causes irritation of the ulcerated area. The cord from the intrauterine device or part of the device itself irritates the glans penis and produces an ulcerated area.
	Improper placement of a diaphragm	The ring of the diaphragm irritates the glans penis.
Lack of libido	Sexual drive or urge is decreased or absent which may produce a transient impotence	Commonly caused by fatigue, psychological stress, boredom with partner or marital difficulty. May be caused by endocrine disease, ingestion of antiandrogenic drugs.

Inspection

The examiner inspects the pubic hair, penis, and scrotum. The amount and distribution of pubic hair varies greatly among individuals and has little clinical significance. In general, it is darker and coarser than other body hair and often forms a diamond-shaped pattern extending up to the umbilicus and down to the upper thighs.

The penis is inspected for appearance, presence of foreskin, location and size of the urethral meatus, and any abnormalities (Table 16-2). The penile skin is thin, freely movable, and free of hair except near the pubis. The size of the penis is proportionate to body size; in the uncircumcised male the foreskin is easily retracted. The client is instructed to retract the foreskin, which exposes the glans penis. The foreskin retracts easily; no smegma should be present. Smegma, a whitish, cheesy secretion of the sebaceous glands, collects under the foreskin and is a sign of uncleanliness. The client is instructed to exert slight pressure at the tip of the glans. This opens the urinary meatus, which enables the examiner to observe for any abnormal discharge or scarring. If a discharge is present, a smear is obtained for culture. If the client reports a discharge from his penis during the history, he is instructed to milk the penis from the base to the glans; a smear of the drainage is obtained for culture. (Table 15-4). (Laboratory Procedures Useful in Diagnosing Syphilis).

The normal scrotum has deeply pigmented rugous skin with sparse pubic-type hair and a diffuse venous pattern. The client is instructed to hold the penis away from the scrotum; the examiner inspects the skin by spreading the layers of skin between the fingers. The scrotum is manipulated to expose the posterior and posterolateral surfaces for inspection. The scrotum is a slightly asymmetrical structure with the left side usually lower than the right. All surfaces of the scrotal sac are observed for skin appearance, hair distribution, and venous pattern (Table 16-3).

Palpation

The examiner palpates the penis and scrotum. The entire shaft of the penis is palpated between the thumb and first two fingers of one hand (Figure 16-4). Gloves are used if there is any drainage, open lesion, or chance of cross infection. The nonerect penis feels

Table 16-2. Selected Acquired Abnormalities of the Penis

Finding	Description	Possible Conditions
Discharge through urinary meatus	Yellow-green purulent discharge present, especially after "milking" the penis.	Gonorrhea
	Thin mucoid discharge.	Nonspecific urethritis
Meatal stenosis	Thin membrane at urinary meatus narrows the opening.	Trauma, local infection
Vesicle	One or more vesicular or ulcerative lesions 1.0 to 5.0 mm. in size on an erythematous base.	Herpes progenitalis
Ulcer	First seen as a single small red papule behind the glans or on the foreskin. After several days the papule enlarges, breaks, and forms a watery, painless, indurated ulcer with a relatively clear base and well defined borders. Appears 2 to 4 weeks after contact. Associated with palpable inguinal lymph nodes.	Syphilitic chancre
	First seen as a small red papule that enlarges into a pustule and opens into a painful, draining ulcer. Occurs in multiples.	Chancroid
Abnormally small penis (infantilism)	Extremely small external genitalia. Often occurs with no pubic hair and a lack of libido.	Hypopituitarism
Abnormally large penis (virilism)	Abnormally large external genitalia. Sometimes seen as precocious puberty.	Hyperadrenalism
Inflammation of the glans penis	Mucosa of glans erythematous, swollen, painful, and sometimes associated with a purulent discharge at the corona. Occurs more often in uncircumcised males after recurrent infections of the prepuce and glans.	Balanitis
Multiple warts	Multiple, friable, moist, red papules on glans and shaft that sometimes extend to the scrotum.	Condylomata acuminata (venereal warts)
Inability to retract foreskin	Adhesions present that join the foreskin with glans penis. Often the adhesions separate spontaneously, and if not, they are broken by a probe inserted under the foreskin. Often associated with smegma, bacteria or urine under the foreskin.	Phimosis
Inability to return retracted foreskin to its normal position	Foreskin retracted behind glans penis. Glans penis inflamed, swollen, and painful.	Paraphymosis
Mass	Small ulcer or wart that grows very slowly into a painless, sometimes bleeding mass that does not heal. Generally seen on the coronal area.	Epidermoid or squamous cell cancer
Palpable plaques on penile shaft	Palpable plaques on the dorsum of the penile shaft. Associated with a fibrotic thickening of the corpora cavernosa, which produces a curvature of the shaft on erection; erection is often painful.	Peyronies disease

soft and rubbery with no masses, tenderness, or induration (Table 16-2). Any masses are palpated for tenderness, induration, size, contour, and consistency. If the client did not milk the penis during inspection, the examiner does so by palpating the penis from the base to the glans penis. This expresses any discharge accumulated in the urethra; a smear is obtained on a slide and examined under a microscope for identification.

The testes, epididymis, and vas deferens are palpated in the scrotal sac simultaneously or separately (Figure 16-5). In simultaneous palpation each testis is palpated with one hand between the thumb and first two fingers. The thumb is in front of the scrotum with the fingers behind it. The two testes are compared for size, shape, consistency, mobility, and tenderness. Small variations in testicular size are not abnormal. The testes are ovoid in shape; feel firm, smooth, and rubbery; and are freely movable in the scrotal sac. Moderate pressure on the testes produces tenderness.

In palpating the testes separately, a bimanual method is used. The right hand is held perpendicular to the floor with the index and middle fingers separated.

Table 16-3. Selected Acquired Abnormalities of the Scrotum and Scrotal Contents

Finding	Description	Possible Conditions
Enlarged scrotum	Dilated, engorged veins in scrotum that feel like a "bag of worms." Often disappears when client lies down. Scrotal contents do not transilluminate, or they transilluminate a bluish glow.	Varicocele
	Fluctuant painless mass, scrotal skin is shiny and stretched tightly. Scrotal contents transilluminate a red glow.	Hydrocele Spermatocele
	Edematous scrotum reaching several times the normal size. Often the scrotal skin is very tight and shiny.	Ascites, Nephritis Congestive heart failure
	Swollen, tender, and very painful testes. Occurs frequently with mumps.	Orchitis
Scrotal mass	Painful, firm mass in scrotum. Skin overlying the epididymis is red and warm. Pain decreases when the testis is elevated. With repeated episodes the epididymis becomes enlarged and indurated.	Epididymitis
	Single or multiple small nodules along epididymis. Occurs commonly after a vasectomy.	Nodules on epididymis
	Painful mass in scrotum that increases in severity when the testis is elevated. Occurs most often in prepubescent boys.	Torsion of spermatic cord
	Painless mass in testis that is not translucent.	Testicular tumor
	During palpation pressure is felt on examining fingertip when the client bears down. On inspection a bulge may be seen over the inguinal area when the client bears down. If a loop of bowel descends into the scrotum, bowel sounds can be auscultated. Scrotal contents will not transilluminate.	Inguinal hernia
Cysts	Epithelial white cysts that generally occur in multiples. Most often there are no associated symptoms.	Sebaceous cysts

These two fingers are placed on the scrotum at the medial ridge. By closing the fingers in a scissorlike fashion the left and right testes are separated, with the right testis in the right hand. The fingertips on the left hand gently palpate the right testis. To palpate the left testicle, the procedure is the same, except that the

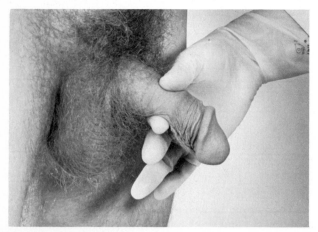

Figure 16-4. *Palpation of the penis.*

left index and middle finger separate the two testes and the fingertips of the right hand gently palpate the testis.

The examiner palpates the epididymis, vas deferens, and inguinal canal with the index finger (the right side is palpated with the right index finger, and the left side with the left finger). The index finger is directed along the posterolateral surface of the testis into the loose scrotal skin. The finger moves along the epididymis and spermatic cord until the fingertip stops at the internal inguinal ring (Figure 16-6). The epididymis is palpated for shape, position, and tenderness. It is felt as a bulging, nontender, comma-shaped ridge with soft nodules that extend from the top of the testes to the bottom. In 93% of the male population the epididymis is palpated along the posterolateral border of the testes. The epididymis in the other 7% is located along the anterolateral or anterior surface of the testis.

The vas deferens is the most distinctly felt structure in the spermatic cord. It is felt as a hard, smooth, movable cord that extends from the epididymis to the external inguinal ring. The arteries, veins, lymph ves-

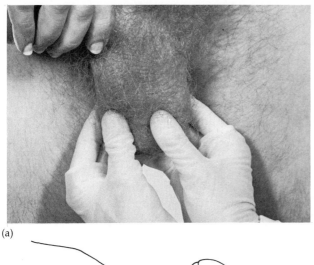

(a)

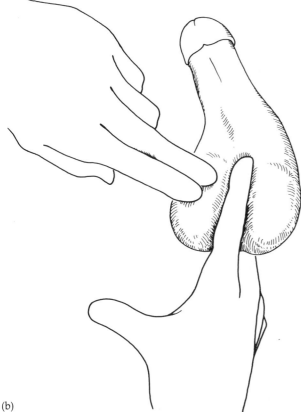

(b)

Figure 16-5. *Palpation of the testis: (a) simultaneous palpation; (b) bimanual palpation.*

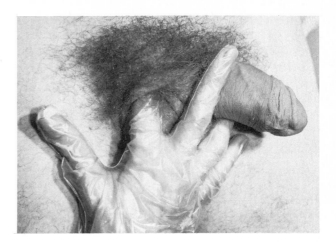

Figure 16-6. *Palpation of the inguinal canal.*

is then instructed to take a deep breath and bear down or cough. This exerts abdominal pressure with the diaphragm and abdominal muscles. If no hernia is present, no masses, swelling, or bulges are felt on the index finger or seen over the inguinal area on the abdomen.

Any mass, swelling, or other abnormality palpated in the scrotal sac is transilluminated to determine if the contents are solid or fluid-filled. The room is darkened and a small light source is placed behind the scrotum. The light source is directed towards the anterior scrotum and through the mass. Solid tissue, most hernial contents, and blood do not transilluminate. Serous fluid accumulation as in a hydrocele transilluminates a red glow (Figure 16-7, Table 16-3).

The femoral canals are also palpated for a potential hernia. The examiner's index and middle fingers are placed parallel to and over the femoral canal. The

sels, and nerves in the spermatic cord are felt as nondistinct threads on either side of the vas deferens. If there is difficulty in palpating the vas deferens, one hand exerts a gentle downward pressure on the testis, while the other hand palpates the vas deferens between the thumb and forefinger or thumb and first two fingers.

The examiner's fingertip is in the inguinal canal when the finger can no longer be advanced. The client

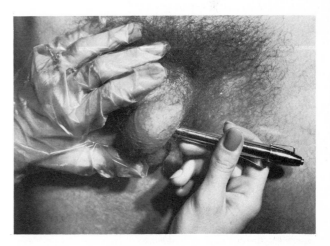

Figure 16-7. *Transillumination of the scrotum.*

client is instructed to take a deep breath and then cough or bear down. In the absence of a hernia, no masses or bulges are felt (Figure 16-8).

The prostate examination is discussed in Chapter 14.

Testicular Self-Examination

Ideally the testicles are self-examined monthly. An often convenient time and place are during a shower or bath. At this time the client is already disrobed and the hands are warm.

To perform the examination the client holds one testis in the palm of his hand and gently palpates it between his thumb and fingers (Figure 16-9). The testis feels smooth, rubbery, and free of any lumps. The epididymis is palpated as a bulging, nontender, comma-shaped ridge with soft nodules that extend from the top of the testis to the bottom. The spermatic cord is the firm, smooth, tubular structure that extends from the epididymis.

The client repeats the procedure for the other testis and reports any lumps or other changes to a health professional.

Auscultation

Auscultation of the scrotal contents is helpful in assessing an obese client for peristaltic sounds. The diaphragm of the stethoscope is placed on the scrotum and, if a loop of bowel is present, a gurgling sound may be heard.

Assessment of the Urinary Tract

In addition to the history and physical examination of the male genitalia, the examiner assesses the urinary tract through laboratory studies. The most common and important studies performed are the urinalysis and urine culture (Appendix 9). Normally no bacteria are present in the urine, therefore the urine culture is negative.

The best method for obtaining a urine specimen is a midstream-voided specimen. In the uncircumcised male, the foreskin is retracted. In all males the glans penis is cleansed with an antiseptic solution. The client is provided with one to three specimen containers. When one container is used, the client is instructed to void into the toilet and then place the specimen cup into the stream to catch the middle of the voiding. With two cups, the client begins to void in the first cup and uses the second cup after voiding the first 20 to 30 milliliters of urine. With this technique the first specimen contains bladder and renal urine plus urethral washings. The second specimen contains only urine from the bladder, ureters, and kidneys. In a three-cup specimen the client is instructed to interrupt voiding just before he has finished urinating. At this point the examiner massages the prostate and the client finishes urinating in the third cup. With this method the third cup has urine similar in content to the second cup, but it also has prostatic fluid (Table 16-4).

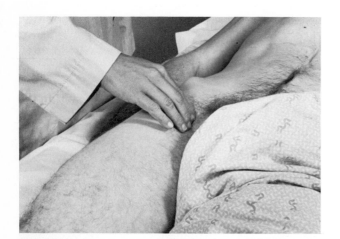

Figure 16-8. *Palpation of the femoral canal.*

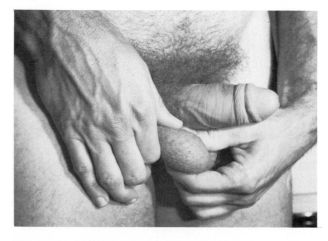

Figure 16-9. *Self-examination of the testicles.*

Table 16-4. Selected Urinary Abnormalities

Finding	Description	Possible Conditions
Incontinence	Involuntary loss of urine (dribbling) while straining, coughing, or sneezing.	Stress incontinence
	Continual urinary leakage. The bladder is unable to hold any amount of urine from damage to the external sphincter or neurologic deficit.	Total incontinence
	Continuous involuntary loss of urine (dribbling) that is not associated with straining, coughing, or sneezing.	Post prostatectomy with damage to the bladder sphincters
Nocturia	Client complains of awakening several times during his sleep to urinate.	Benign prostatic hypertrophy Urinary tract infection Diabetes mellitus Renal insufficiency
Dysuria	Difficult, painful urination. Sometimes described as a burning sensation along the urethra to the tip of the penis.	Urinary tract infection Foreign body Tumor
Polyuria	An abnormally increased volume of dilute urine.	Renal failure Diabetes mellitus Increased fluid intake
Oliguria	Less than 30 ml of urine output per hour.	Renal failure Shock Hypovolemia
Anuria	Total suppression of urine production and output.	Renal failure
Hematuria	Microscopic or gross blood in the urine. Blood may be noted at the beginning, end, or throughout urination.	Tumors Calculi Trauma Acute glomerulonephritis
Pyuria	Urine is grossly purulent and appears turbid.	Urinary tract infection Calculi Tumors Urinary obstruction
Pneumaturia	Small air bubbles in the urine.	Urinary tract infection Fistula
Proteinuria	Presence of any protein in the urine found during a urinalysis or dip stick assessment.	Acute and chronic renal disease Cardiac disease
Foul odor	Urine may develop a fecal or sulfurous odor from an underlying infection.	Urinary tract infection

Life Cycle Variations

Childhood

In the newborn the size of the external genitalia often appears out of proportion to the rest of the body. The nonerect penis is approximately 2 to 3 centimeters long and continues to grow in proportion to body size until puberty.

The foreskin in the newborn is very tight and completely covers the glans penis. The urinary meatus is seen as a tiny orifice centered at the distal end. The foreskin is not retracted, not even for cleaning, until the child is several months old because the foreskin is very friable. Retraction may tear the foreskin and result in adhesions.

The scrotal sac ranges from a small size with a tightly covering skin to a hanging appearance with loosely folded skin. The testes are palpated and feel soft and rubbery. Their size is approximately 1 to 2 centimeters long from birth until puberty.

In utero the testes develop in the abdominal cavity of the fetus. They descend aong the inguinal canal and into the scrotal sac by birth or shortly afterward. Often the testes are in the inguinal canal at birth and can be milked down into the scrotal sac.

When the scrotum is palpated, the cremasteric reflex is activated. This causes the testes to ascend high into the scrotum, inguinal canal, or abdomen. This reflex is blocked by placing an index finger in the inguinal canal and exerting upward pressure from behind the scrotum. At this point the testes are palpated between the index finger and thumb of the other hand. In an older child the cremasteric reflex is inhibited by instructing the child to sit crosslegged or with his knees flexed on his chest with his feet on the chair. Sitting in either position increases abdominal pressure, which forces the testes into the scrotum. If the testes are not palpable, the procedure for blocking the cremasteric reflex is repeated. Often the cremasteric reflex is absent in boys under 6 months and over 12 years old. Besides palpation, the cremasteric reflex is also activated by stroking the inner aspect of the thigh, cold environmental conditions, and psychological stress (Table 16-5).

Adolescence

The first genital change in puberty is accelerated growth of the testes, which become larger and less firm. Concurrent with the larger testes is an increase in the size of the scrotal sac. The next change is a lengthening and increased diameter of the penis from an enlargement of the corpora cavernosa. Pubic hair growth begins after the testes and penis have begun enlarging (Chapter 5).

In examining young males a sensitive, open approach is needed. Parents are not present for the history or physical examination. With the client's consent the parent may be invited into the examining room after the assessment. Many sexual changes take place during adolescence; health teaching is important to the client and his parents is important. They need information about the physical changes that take place, in addition to the psychological changes.

It is natural for adolescent boys to have frequent erections and nocturnal emissions (wet dreams) and to be interested in masturbation. Generally, boys begin masturbation in the middle teenage years. Multiple research studies indicate that over 90 percent of the male population engages in active masturbation. This may range in frequency from several times a month to several times a day. There is no definition for excessive masturbation. Masturbation often takes place in private or as a group experience with other young men. Also, the adolescent is interested in sexuality, not only his own, but also that of others, both male and female.

A discussion on contraception and venereal disease is indicated. This subject may be approached by inquiring about the client's girlfriend: Is she a steady one or does he have several? From this information, additional information regarding contraceptive practices and venereal disease is sought.

The examination techniques in an adolescent boy are the same as those for an adult man. It is essential that the testes be located in the scrotal sac. If undescended testes are not surgically repaired, sterility results since the sperm cannot survive at normal body temperature. There also seems to be increased evidence of malignant tumors in the cryptorchial testis.

Late Adulthood

In late adulthood testosterone production gradually declines. This decline causes a decrease in testicular size and firmness. These physiological changes affect male sexuality by prolonging the four stages of adult sexual activity. In the excitement phase, the penis takes longer to become erect, and the erect penis is not as full or firm as it had been. Although the man is able to ejaculate, the time between an erection and orgasm increases (plateau phase). The ejaculation is

Table 16-5. Selected Congenital Abnormalities of the Penis and Scrotum

Finding	Condition	Description
Urinary meatus on ventral surface of penis	Hypospadias	Urinary meatus located ventrally on the glans, penile shaft, scrotum, or perineum. Often associated with Chordee, a fibrosis in the area of the malformed urethra, and causes a downward curvature of the erect penis. Foreskin incomplete on ventral surface with an excessive amount on the dorsal surface.
Urinary meatus on upper surface of penis	Episapadias	Urinary meatus located dorsally on the glans or penile shaft. Often associated with exostrophy of the bladder and urinary incontinence.
Nonpalpable testes	Undescended testicles (cryptorchism)	Scrotal sac soft with no firm structure palpable.

not as forceful, lasts for a shorter time, and has less volume (orgasmic phase). After ejaculation, the penis becomes flaccid more rapidly and the refractory period of the resolution phase lasts longer.

In late adulthood sexual activity often decreases for a variety of reasons. Often there is a feeling of boredom and monotony with the sexual partner. If the man is preoccupied with his career, economic stability, or adjusting to a new retirement lifestyle, sexual activity may decrease. A major factor in loss of sexual interest is mental and physical fatigue. In the American culture, overindulgence in food and drink is common, and this, too, may lessen sexual activity. As men age, acute or chronic physical illnesses can occur. These illnesses may affect sexual activity directly or the medications used in the treatment may produce impotence.

Once a man experiences failure in sexual expression, he often fears it will happen again. The fear of inadequate sexual performance may cause the man to avoid sexual expression.

Not all aging men experience a decline in sexual activity. If the man has a high level of sexual activity during his early and middle years, a similar pattern of sexual activity usually continues throughout life. Men with regular partners generally have regular sexual activity, although the frequency may decrease. Men without sexual partners often maintain sexual activity through masturbation.

Anatomy and Physiology

The structures of the skeletal system include bones, cartilage, and the joints between bones. The muscular system comprises muscles, tendons, and ligaments. Together, the two systems are responsible for body movement, support, and stability. In addition, the skeletal system has a major function in hematopoiesis, protecting vital internal structures, and acting as a reservoir for ions.

The Skeletal System

Bones. There are 206 bones comprising the framework of the skeleton; 80 bones form the axial skeleton (the upright axis of the body); 126 bones make up the appendicular skeleton. These bones form the appendages to the axial skeleton. The most common classification of bones categorizes them according to their shape (Table 17-1, Figure 17-1).

Table 17-1. Classification of Bones

Class	Description
Long bones	Bones of the upper and lower extremities. They include the humerus, ulna, femur, tibia, and fibula. They also include the small, miniature bones of the fingers and toes (phalanges).
Short bones	Bones of the wrists and ankles. They include the carpals and tarsals.
Flat bones	These bones are actually thin rather than flat and can usually be identified by a slight curvature. Bones of the skull vault (e.g., frontal and parietal), shoulder blade (scapula), and ribs.
Irregular bones	Bones of the spinal column and certain bones of the skull. They include the vertebrae, sacrum, coccyx, sphenoid, ethmoid, and mandible.
Pneumatic bones	These bones are filled with air-containing sacs. Bones of the paranasal sinuses and mastoid process.

The structure of long bones includes a diaphysis, epiphyses, articular cartilage, periosteum, osteoblasts, blood vessels, medullary cavity, and endosteum (Figure 17-2). The diaphysis is the bone shaft. It is a hollow cylinder composed of thick, compact bone.

Chapter 17

Assessment of the Musculoskeletal System

Objectives

The examiner will be able to do the following:

1. Inspect posture and gait
2. Inspect and palpate the bones, muscles, and joints
3. Measure the length of the extremities
4. Measure muscle circumference in each extremity
5. Screen overall muscle strength
6. Measure active and passive range of motion of joints with goniometer
7. Test muscle strength against resistance
8. Recognize abnormalities of musculoskeletal system
9. Record the information obtained

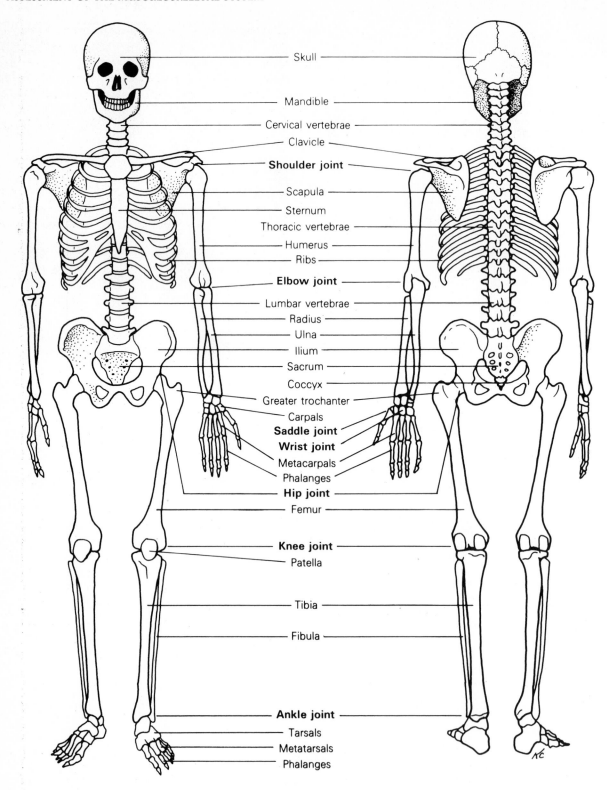

Figure 17-1. The skeletal system.

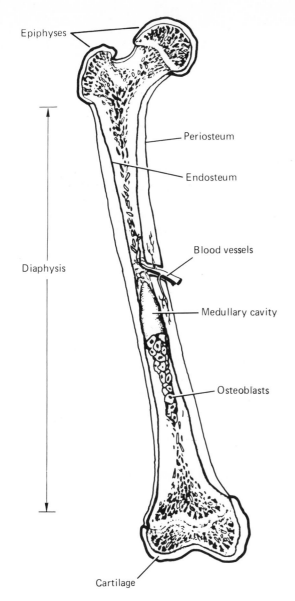

Epiphyses

Periosteum

Endosteum

Diaphysis

Blood vessels

Medullary cavity

Osteoblasts

Cartilage

Figure 17-2. Structure of the long bones.

This structure gives bone support without additional weight.

The epiphyses are the ends of the long bones. Bulbous in shape, they are made up of spongy or cancellous bone covered by a thin layer of dense, compact bone. The shape of the epiphyses provides a large area for the attachment of muscles and gives joints greater stability. The porous nature of cancellous bone makes the epiphyses lightweight.

Articular cartilage is a hyaline-type cartilage. A thin layer of hyaline cartilage covers the articular surface to the epiphyses. Hyaline cartilage is extremely resilient, smooth, and slippery; it acts as a cushion whenever a joint is jarred.

The periosteum is the tough, membranous layer that covers all portions of the bone except for the articular surfaces. It consists of an outer, fibrous, connective tissue layer and a deeper, more cellular layer directly on the bone's surface. The periosteum adheres to the bone by the penetration of fibrous bundles into the bone itself. Fibers from muscles, tendons, and ligaments blend with the periostial fibers and are continuous with them, thus firmly attaching these structures to the bone.

Osteoblasts are the specialized bone-forming cells found in the deeper cellular layer of the periosteum. These cells are responsible for the formation and repair of bone. They eventually become incorporated into the developing bone and are known as osteocytes.

The blood vessels of bone originate in the periosteal layer closest to the bone and pass into the bone proper as well as the bone marrow. These blood vessels provide essential nutrients to the bone cells.

The medullary cavity (marrow cavity) is the center, hollow portion in the diaphysis of long bone that contains the bone marrow. The marrow is the source of red and white blood cell production. The inner lining of the medullary cavity is the endosteum. It is a fine, connective tissue membrane that protects the marrow.

Short bones, flat bones, irregular bones, and pneumatic bones are basically cancellous bone on the inside with an outer covering of compact bone. This structure gives these bones flexibility as well as strength.

Bone is a living organ composed of an organic protein matrix impregnated with inorganic mineral substances. This composition of bone allows it to resist both tension and compression while retaining considerable flexibility. The primary minerals found in bone are calcium and magnesium salts. Calcium phosphates are the main substances that contribute to the hardness of bone. The combination of mineral salts and fibrous tissue plus the concentric tubular structure of bone give it both strength and adaptability.

The bones are connected to muscle tissue by ligaments, tendons, and fascia. These structures help support the bones and apply necessary stresses that affect the maturation and structure of bones. As bone is subjected to various mechanical stressors throughout life, it is constantly being remodeled. This continuous modification of the size and shape of bone in response to changing stress gives bone an adaptive quality that allows it to function optimally as the body's main support system.

Bone has five major functions: movement, support, protection, hemopoiesis, and reservoir. The primary function of bone is mechanical movement. Bones and their articulated joints act as levers. They are attached to muscles whose specialized function is contraction. When muscles contract, the levers are pulled and the end result is movement.

Bones are the skeletal framework of the body. Their anatomical structure gives the body stability by providing a framework of maximum strength with minimum bulk and weight.

Bones also protect vital internal structures. Bones surround structures like the heart and lungs (ribs), the brain (skull), and the spinal cord (vertebrae). The interior of bones also protects developing blood cells since it holds the bone marrow.

A fourth function of bone is hemopoiesis (the formation of blood cells). Specialized connective (myeloid) tissue is responsible for red and white blood cell production. This tissue is the marrow of bones.

Finally, bone functions as a reservoir for ions and has the ability to rapidly exchange ions as necessary. Bone acts as a storehouse for calcium and phosphates that can be withdrawn by the body as needed. It also stores and releases hydrogen ions, which give bone a buffering capacity.

Cartilage. Cartilage is a substance that differs from bone in two important ways. First, the collagenous fibers of cartilage are imbedded in a gel-like substance. Thus, cartilage is more flexible. Second, cartilage has no vascular system. Nutrients reach cartilage cells (chondrocytes) by diffusion through the gel matrix from capillaries found in the outer cartilage covering (perichondrium).

There are three types of cartilage: elastic, fibrous, and hyaline. Elastic cartilage contains both elastic and collagenous fibers. This gives it an elastic but firm quality. An example of elastic cartilage is the cartilage found in the nose. Fibrous cartilage is mostly collagenous fibers, which give it extensive tensile strength. The vertebral discs are an example of fibrous cartilage. Hyaline cartilage is a tough, smooth, slippery membrane found on the articular surfaces of bones. It is the most common cartilage found in the body and serves as a mechanical cushion for the joints between bones.

Joints. Joints are the structural and functional units of the musculoskeletal system. Joints are defined as articulations between two adjacent bones. They hold bones together and, at the same time, permit some degree of movement.

Joints are classified according to their characteristic features: fibrous, cartilaginous, and synovial. They are also classified according to the degree of movement: synarthroses, amphiarthroses, and diarthroses.

Fibrous joints are held closely together by connective tissue bands. The articular surfaces of the adjacent bones of this type of joint are in direct contact with each other and are bound together by fibrous bands. Essentially, no movement occurs at these joints: therefore, they are known as synarthrodial joints (immovable). Examples of fibrous or synarthrodial joints are the articulations between skull bones.

Cartilaginous joints are articulations in which two bones are joined by cartilage. Only slight movement occurs at this type of joint, which is also known as an amphiarthrodial joint (slightly movable). Examples of cartilaginous or amphiarthrodial joints include the articulations between the ribs and sternum, and the joints between the vertebrae.

Synovial joints are articulations characterized by a joint capsule, synovial membrane, articular cartilage, joint cavity, and ligaments. These are the most common and the most mobile joints in the body. They are also the most frequently afflicted by pathology. Synovial joints are also known as diarthrotic joints (freely movable).

A dense, fibrous joint capsule extends from the periosteum and completely covers the articulating ends of the diarthrotic joint. This capsule binds the ends of the bones to each other and is strengthened by ligaments between the bones of the joint.

The joint capsule is lined by a synovial membrane, which attaches at the margins of the articular cartilage. The membrane secretes synovial fluid, which acts as a lubricant for the inner joint surfaces. The amount of synovial fluid produced varies from joint to joint. It normally ranges from a very slight viscous layer to 3.5 milliliters of fluid.

The articular cartilage that covers the ends of the bones is normally smooth and resilient. It allows for smooth movement and acts as a cushion between the articulating ends of the bones.

The joint cavity is the space between the two ends of the bones. This space allows the joint to move freely. Strong ligaments grow between the articulating ends of the bones, securely holding them together.

The diarthrotic or synovial joint permits the joint motions of flexion, extension, abduction, adduction, internal rotation, external rotation, circumduction, pronation, supination, inversion, and eversion (Table 17-2).

In addition to their various characteristic features and degrees of movement, joints are also classified by their structural type (Figure 17-1). A ball-and-socket joint consists of a concave socket in the end of one bone which holds the "ball" end of the adjacent bone.

Table 17-2. Joint Movements

Movement	Description
Flexion	A bending movement, which increases the angle of the joint.
Extension	A straightening movement, which increases the angle of the joint. This movement returns the part from a flexed position to the anatomical position. Hyperextension is extension beyond the anatomical position.
Abduction	The movement of a body part away from the median plane of the body.
Adduction	The movement of a body part toward the median plane of the body.
Internal rotation	The pivoting or turning inward of a body part toward the median plane of the body.
External rotation	The pivoting or turning outward of a body part away from the median plane of the body.
Circumduction	The movement of a distal body part so that it performs a circular motion. This movement involves the motions of flexion, abduction, extension, and adduction.
Pronation	Turning the forearm so the palm of the hand is facing downward.
Supination	Turning the forearm so the palm of the hand is facing upward.
Inversion	Turning the sole of the foot inward, toward the medial plane of the body.
Eversion	Turning the sole of the foot outward, away from the medial plane of the body.

This type of joint structure is very stable and movement is possible in all directions. The hip and shoulder joints are both ball-and-socket type joints.

A ginglymus or hinge joint consists of two or three articulations between adjacent bones that are stabilized by sets of ligaments. Flexion and extension are the two major movements of this type of joint. Examples of hinge joints include the knee, elbow, and ankle.

A condyloid or ellipsoidal joint consists of an elliptical-shaped socket that surrounds an oval-shaped condyle. This joint is formed by many parts and is stabilized by both long and short ligaments. The specific structure of this joint permits a wide range of movements including flexion, extension, abduction, and adduction. An example of an ellipsoidal joint is the wrist or carpal joint.

A pivot joint consists of an arch of one bone into which a small part of another bone pivots. This arrangement allows the joint to rotate. The articulations between C1 and C2 in the vertebral column and be- tween the proximal ends of the ulna and radius are pivot joints.

A gliding joint consists of bones with facets that articulate with facets above and below. This joint permits a slight gliding motion back and forth and sideways. The joints between the vertebral segments are gliding joints.

A saddle joint consists of two saddle-shaped surfaces that fit into each other. The joint capsule is thickened and acts as a ligament. Short muscle groups stabilize this joint. The only saddle joint in the body is at the base of the thumb. The structure of this joint allows for flexion, extension, abduction, adduction, circumduction, and opposition—a unique motion that permits the thumb and fingers to grasp and hold objects.

Wherever there are bony prominences or pressure over moving parts, particularly around joints, bursae are found. These are small, disc-shaped sacs composed of connective tissue lined with a synovial membrane. The synovial membrane secretes synovial fluid, which acts as a lubricant. Bursae exist between points of potential friction particularly where ligaments, tendons, muscles, or skin move over prominent bony parts. The fluid-filled sacs act as cushions, preventing friction and pressure. If there is continual irritation in an area where bursae are not normally found, they may develop spontaneously (Figure 17-3).

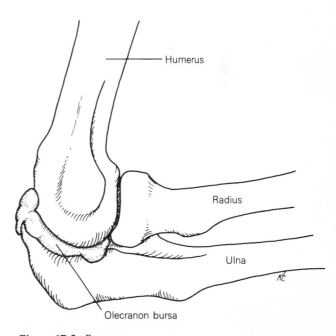

Figure 17-3. Bursa.

The Muscular System

Muscles. The specialized function of a muscle cell is contraction. Contraction of groups of muscle cells is the force behind body movements. Without muscles, bones and joints would be powerless. Every movement an individual makes is a result of the contraction of a muscle. Thus, the primary function of the muscular system is to produce movement.

Another important function of the muscular system is to maintain the body's posture in space. It is possible for an individual to assume a variety of positions, such as standing straight or lying supine, and maintain those positions for an indefinite period of time. This is made possible by the continuous contraction of various skeletal muscles.

There are approximately 600 muscles in the body. Information on how muscles are named and classified is helpful in identifying the various muscle groups. The nomenclature system for muscles is based on a description of some of the basic characteristics of muscles. Each muscle name is derived, in part, from the characteristics outlined in Table 17-3.

Muscles are classified according to their specific action such as flexors, extensors, rotators, abductors, and adductors. Muscles are also categorized according to their location in the body and are referred to as muscles of the neck, back, thigh, or hand.

Table 17-3. Muscle Nomenclature Characteristics

Characteristic	Example
Action	Flexion or extension
	Flexor or extensor
Location	Near the tibia
	Tibialis
Shape	Square or triangle
	Quadratus or deltoid
Points of attachment	At the sternum and mastoid
	Sternocleidomastoid
Fiber direction	Transverse
	Transversus
Number of divisions	Two or three
	Biceps or triceps

Skeletal muscles are always attached to bones but vary widely in their action, location, shape, points of attachment, fiber direction, and number of divisions. Skeletal muscle is also known as striated muscle because microscopically it is composed of thick and thin filaments (sarcomeres), which make up bundles of thin fibers (myofibrils). The thick and thin filaments appear as dark and light stripes, which contribute to the striated appearance.

Skeletal muscle contracts whenever it receives a stimulus from a motor nerve that innervates it. Once stimulated, an impulse is conducted over the muscle cell which causes the release of calcium ions. Calcium ions bind with troponin molecules to form calcium-bound troponin. Calcium-bound troponin stimulates the thin filaments of the sarcomeres, which in turn causes shortening or contraction of the myofibrils. The relaxation of muscle fibers is caused by the absence of calcium-bound troponin so the contraction mechanism is inhibited.

Whenever a skeletal muscle fiber contracts, it does so completely or not at all. This is known as the "all or none" principle. However, skeletal muscles themselves contract with varying strengths, depending on their surrounding conditions. The force of contraction of a skeletal muscle is influenced by several factors: the size of the load, the number of muscle fibers stimulated, the initial length of the muscle fibers, and the metabolic condition of the muscle fibers.

So that the entire muscle does not have to contract unless necessary, just enough fibers are stimulated to achieve the necessary force. The contraction of a muscle is matched to the size of the load, thus preventing the expenditure of useless energy. Muscle tissue has built-in reserve power, but only the force of contraction needed to get the job done is utilized. Usually, the heavier the load, the greater the force of contraction.

The number of muscle fibers stimulated at any one time also affects muscle contraction. The number of motor nerves activated by any given stimulus is a function of the frequency and intensity of the stimulation. In general, the more frequent and intense the stimulation, the greater the number of motor nerves activiated. As a result, more muscle fibers are stimulated and the contraction is stronger.

Another factor that influences the strength of muscle contraction is the metabolic condition of the fibers. Muscle function depends on an adquate oxygen and nutrient supply. If there is inadequate oxygen or nutrients to muscle fibers, their force of contraction diminishes significantly. There are several types of skeletal muscle contraction (Table 17-4).

Assessment Modalities

Preparation

The musculoskeletal system is assessed primarily by inspection and palpation. Percussion and auscultation are used only when necessary. The instruments needed to carry out a complete health assess-

Table 17-4. Types of Muscle Contraction

Muscle Contraction	Description
Tonic contraction	A continuous partial contraction. Characteristic of muscles responsible for posture when an individual is awake.
Istonic contraction	A continuous contraction in which the tension of the muscles remains the same. Characteristic of muscles doing work.
Isometric contraction	A contraction in which muscle tension increases; muscle action against resistance. Characteristic of muscles pushing against a stable object.
Twitch contraction	A very quick, slightly jerky contraction. Characteristic of muscles that have been overstrained.
Tetanic contraction	A series of contractions occurring in rapid succession; more sustained than a twitch. Characteristic of muscles exposed to abnormal metabolic conditions.
Fibrillation	A synchronous contraction of muscle fibers. Characteristic of an abnormal condition.
Convulsions	Uncoordinated contractions of different muscle groups; tetanic in nature. Characteristic of an abnormal condition.

ment of this system include the following: tape measure, goniometer, safety pin, and reflex hammer.

Moving from head to toe in an orderly method of assessing joints, bones, and muscles, tends to put the client at ease and prevents the examiner from "missing" an essential part of the examination. As the examiner proceeds with the examination, the client is continually repositioned in the most stable positions to provide for safety. The client is repositioned throughout the examination as follows: lying flat, sitting on the side of the examining table, and finally standing. The examiner stands facing the client and when necessary moves to the client's right.

For a thorough physical examination of the client, the extremities and spine are exposed so that the examiner can inspect and palpate the muscles, bones and joints of both extremities and back. A thorough examination cannot be done through clothing. The client's modesty is maintained by utilizing a gown or appropriate underwear.

The structure and function of each extremity is compared with the structure and function of its symmetrical part. The extensiveness of the examination depends upon the general condition of the client and the chief complaint or symptoms.

Health assessment of the musculoskeletal system begins when the examiner meets the client. The examiner observes the strength, speed, and coordination of all movements. Normal body movements are smooth, efficient, and coordinated. Upon greeting the client, the examiner evaluates the character of the client's handshake and pays special attention to the size and shape of the hand and the firmness of the grasp. A normal handshake is firm and strong. The examiner observes the client's general appearance, posture, and gait. The client is observed walking and changing positions from standing to sitting to lying.

The normal gait has two phases. The stance phase is when the foot is on the ground and includes the movements of heel strike, foot flat, midstance, and push-off. The second phase is called the swing phase. This is when the foot moves forward. Swing phase includes the movements of acceleration, midswing, and deceleration (Tables 17-5 and 17-6).

The average step is approximaely 15 inches in length; the average client takes approximately 90 to 120 steps per minute. The healthy client walks with a base of 2 to 4 inches from heel to heel; the knee remains flexed during foot flat, midstance, and push-off.

Table 17-5. Normal Gait

Phase	Description
I. Stance phase	
A. Heel strike	The heel is brought to the floor. The knee is normally extended.
B. Foot flat	The foot is placed flat on the floor. The knee is slightly flexed.
C. Midstance	The foot remains on the floor with knee flexed. Weight is evenly distributed on all aspects of foot.
D. Push-off	The heel rises from the floor. The knee flexes to approximately 40°. The toes hyperextend.
II. Swing phase	
A. Acceleration	The extremity begins to swing forward from push-off. The quadriceps contract. The knee is at maximum flexion. The extremity shortens to clear the ground.
B. Midswing	The extremity remains shortened and the knee flexes to approximately 65°. The foot moves smoothly past the opposite extremity.
C. Deceleration	The extremity swings forward. The hamstring muscles contract preparing the foot for heel strike.

Table 17-6. Selected Abnormalities of Posture and Gait

Finding	Condition	Description
Stooped forward	Kyphosis	Increased forward concavity of the thoracic spine; hunchback posture. Caused by faulty posture, Paget's disease, and senile osteoporosis.
Lateral bending	Scoliosis	S-shaped, complex curvature of the thoracic spine. May be compensatory due to shortened lower extremity or congenital dislocated hip. May be structural, due to congenital deformities of the spine.
Backward curvature	Lordosis	Accentuated concave curve of the lower lumbar spine. May be compensatory for an enlarged abdomen, congenital spinal deformities, or a contractured or dislocated hip.
Instability	Peripheral neuropathy Cerebellar disease	Client walks with a widened base usually greater than 4 inches. May be due to loss of sensation on bottoms of feet or decreased ability to maintain balance. Frequently looks at feet while walking to orient self.
Pain	Osteoarthritis of knee or hip Poorly fitted shoes	Pain occurs during all parts of the stance phase. Client limits time spent on affected extremity or avoids weightbearing altogether (antalgic gait).
	Heel spurs	Sharp pain occurs during the heel strike position of the stance phase. Client frequently hops on the affected foot to avoid bringing heel down on the floor.

Inspection and Palpation of the Bones, Muscles, and Joints

Bones are initially assessed for symmetry. Then each extremity is inspected and palpated individually. On inspection normal extremities appear smooth and symmetrical without bony protrusions or masses. Normal bone feels smooth and hard and is nontender when palpated (Table 17-7, Figure 17-4).

A tape measure is used to measure the length of the upper and lower extremities. The client is asked to lie down on the examination table with the legs extended and arms straight at the sides. The length of the upper extremity is measured from the acromion process to the end of the middle finger (Figure 17-5). The measurements of both upper extremities are then compared. The length of the lower extremity is measured from the lower edge of the superior iliac spine to the tibial malleolus. The measurements of the lower extremities are compared bilaterally. A slight asymmetry up to 1 centimeter in length is considered normal.

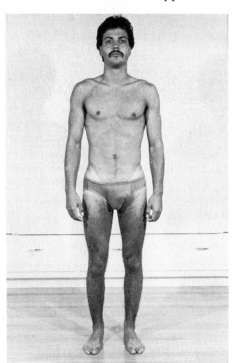

Figure 17-4. *Inspection of the musculoskeletal system.*

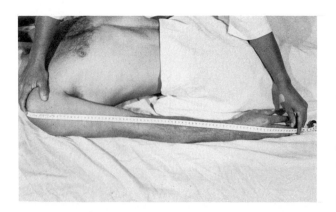

Figure 17-5. *Measurement of the length of the upper extremity.*

Table 17-7. Selected Bone Abnormalities

Finding	Condition	Description
Acute bone pain	Fracture	Often accompanied by localized tenderness, swelling, redness, and increased warmth. Pain intensified by movement or weightbearing; increased at night. Abnormal mobility, loss of function of the body part, and bony crepitus are usually present. May be associated with trauma or injury.
Chronic bone pain	Osteoporosis	Bone pain only symptom. No other physical signs. Especially affects vertebral and pelvic bones. Incidence increases with age. Due to disuse, inadequate nutrient intake, and excessive loss of minerals from the body.
	Multiple myeloma	Bone pain either localized or general. Caused by invasive destruction of bone by malignant plasma cells of the bone marrow. X-rays show characteristic punched-out areas in the bone.
Bony swelling	Malignant tumor	May be accompanied by bone pain. Frequently associated with a pathological fracture. Location of swelling usually diagnostic of type of tumor. Tumor may be primary in origin or metastatic from breast, prostate gland, thyroid gland, kidney, stomach, or bronchus.

Muscles are examined for their shape, size, tone, consistency, and strength against resistance. The contour of each muscle group is inspected bilaterally. The shape follows the normal anatomical configuration for each group and is normally symmetrical.

The size of the muscle mass is determined by measuring the circumference of each extremity at various points with a tape measure (Figure 17-6). The muscles of the upper extremities are measured first. Both upper extremities are in the same relaxed position and measurements are taken at the same places. The same method of measurement is done on the lower extremities. When all measurements are made, a diagram is drawn showing the location and circumference of each measurement. These data then serve as a baseline for future assessments.

Muscles are palpated with the client in a relaxed position to determine their tone and consistency. Relaxed muscle is normally soft, pliable, and nontender. Contracted muscle feels firm (Table 17-8).

There are several maneuvers useful for general screening of muscle strength. The client squeezes the examiner's hand, does a deep knee bend, rises to a standing position, walks on the heels, and walks on the toes. Normal muscle strength permits the client to perform these exercises easily. Specific tests for muscle strength against resistance are usually carried out in a systematic manner while testing passive range of motion. These tests are described in more detail in the next section of this chapter.

Testing for muscle sensation and deep tendon reflexes are considered an integral part of assessing both the musculoskeletal and neurological systems. These tests are completely outlined in Chapter 18.

Joints are examined for color, shape, size, range of motion, and force against resistance. During assessment of the joints, the muscles, tendons, and bones responsible for their movement are also inspected and palpated.

First, the examiner systematically inspects each joint for color, shape, and size. The color of the skin over the joint reflects the individual's normal skin pigmentation. The shape and size of the joint depends on its location and function. Each joint is palpated for temperature, shape, size, and pain. Normal joints reflect the skin temperature of other body parts. Their shape and size depends on their specific location and function. The examiner locates the joint capsule based on knowledge of the anatomy of the individual joint and attempts to palpate the synovial membrane. Normally, the synovial membrane is not palpable.

Next each joint is put through active and passive range of motion to determine the degree of movement. The range of joint motion gives the examiner information about muscle function, ligament support, and the general condition of the articular surfaces.

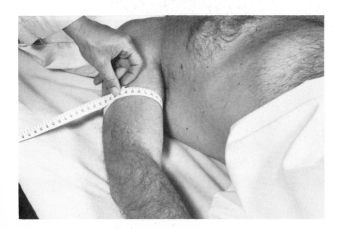

Figure 17-6. *Measurement of the muscle mass.*

Table 17-8 Selected Muscle Abnormalities

Finding	Condition	Description
Atrophy	Cerebral vascular accident Diabetic neuropathy Multiple sclerosis Muscular dystrophy Polyneuritis	Loss of muscle mass. Usually apparent on inspection. Slow to develop. Results from damage to muscle tissue or motor nerves which leads to disuse. Frequently associated with paralysis.
Tremors 　Fine, rapid 　Slow at rest 　Action or 　intention	 Thyrotoxicosis Chronic alcoholism Anxiety states Parkinson's syndrome Cerebellar disease Multiple sclerosis	Ranges from a slight twitching of a single muscle to extensive convulsive movements of the entire body. Occurs during or after voluntary movement. Tremors do not occur during sleep. The examiner notes when they occur in relation to body movement, the skeletal muscles involved, and the amplitude.
Fasciculations	Denervation of muscle fibers	Slight twitching in a resting muscle. Readily observable by the examiner. Frequently accompanied by muscle atrophy and weakness.
Pain/tenderness 　Trauma 　Infections	 Muscle strain Hematoma of the muscle Influenza Rubella Polymyalgia	Differentiated from bone and joint pain by squeezing muscles between thumb and index finger. Pain is usually accompanied by muscle tenderness. Trauma produces localized pain that may radiate. Systemic infections produce a nonspecific, systemic muscle pain.
Paralysis	Cerebral vascular accident Multiple sclerosis Myasthenia gravis Polyneuritis Trauma to nerves	Decreased or absent motor power of muscles caused by damage to motor nerves or muscle fibers. If chronic, associated with muscle atrophy.

Range of motion is either active or passive. Active range of motion is the voluntary movement of the joint. Passive range of motion is tested when the examiner moves the joint through all of its motions. The examiner always tests active range of motion first. Passive range of motion is tested if there is limitation of movement during active range of motion. Normally, active and passive range of motion are equal. When they are not equal, passive range of motion is usually a more reliable test than the actual range of motion present in a joint (Table 17-9).

Goniometry is the procedure used for measuring range of motion of the joints. A goniometer is a simple protractor with arms and a scale that indicates degrees. It is placed against the joint and the range of motion of the joint is then measured (Figure 17-7).

Finally, each major joint is tested against resistance to measure the power of movement present (Table 17-10). These movements are carried out for each of the major joints of the body, including neck, lumbar spine, shoulders, elbows, wrists, fingers, hips, knees, ankles, and toes.

The Cervical Spine. Inspection of the cervical spine initially involves evaluating the movements and position of the head. Usually, the head is perpendicular to the shoulders, is held erect, and moves in tandem with the rest of the body. The regions of the neck are also inspected for color and pulsations.

Table 17-9. Selected Joint Abnormalities

Finding	Condition	Description
Joint pain	Arthritis Gout	Joint is usually swollen and tender to palpation. The skin over the joint is reddened and warm. Motion is limited and crepitus may occur on movement. Synovial membrane feels boggy. The examiner notes the location, duration, and severity of the pain.
Stiffness	Osteoarthritis	Stiffness occurs after rest; disappears with movement of the joint. Signs of inflammation are minimal. May be grating noise with movement. Due to degeneration of articular cartilage. Epiphyses wear down. Weight-bearing joints most affected. Starts during middle years.

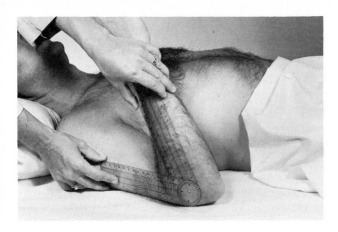

Figure 17-7. Goniometry.

To palpate the neck, the client is placed in a supine position. The examiner stands to one side of the client, supports the back of the neck with one hand, and palpates with the other.

The anterior region of the neck is palpated, with the examiner first moving from the hyoid bone to the thyroid cartilage to the cricoid cartilage and the adjacent thyroid rings. These structures are normally found in the midline of the anterior neck and are flexible and nontender. The posterior region of the neck is palpated while the examiner stands behind the client and supports the neck with the hands. The occiput, occipital protuberance (inion), mastoid process, and seven cervical vertebrae are palpated (Figure 17-8). These structures normally feel smooth and firm and are nontender.

Next the soft tissues of the neck are palpated, starting with the anterior neck and moving around to the posterior neck region. In the anterior neck region, the

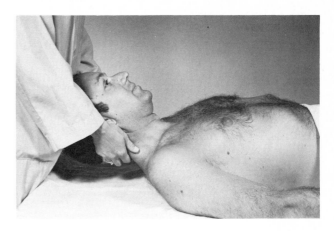

Figure 17-8. Palpation of the cervical spine.

sternocleidomastoid muscle and the supraclavicular fossa are palpated. With the client seated, the trapezius muscle in the posterior neck region is palpated. With the client in a relaxed position, the neck muscles normally feel smooth and soft (Table 17-11).

Range of motion in the cervical spine includes the movements of flexion, extension, lateral bending, and rotation (Tables 17-14, 17-15).

The Lumbar Spine. Initially the examiner inspects posture and movements of the lumbar spine as the client removes clothing. The client normally bends and twists spine naturally without evidence of stiffness or pain.

Palpation of the lumbar spine requires that the client remain standing. The examiner sits behind the client with the thumbs on the vertebral line at the interspace between L4 and L5. The fingers rest on top of the iliac crests, (Figure 17-9).

The posterior aspect of the lumbar spine is palpated first. The examiner palpates the lumbar vertebrae superior and inferior to the L4-L5 interspace, and the posterior coccyx. Normally the examiner feels the bony prominences of each spinous process. There are five lumbar vertebrae and a fused mass of five sacral and four coccygeal vertebrae, which are normally nontender.

After palpating the posterior bony lumbar spine, the soft tissues in the area are palpated. This includes the spinous ligaments, the iliac crest, the sciatic nerve, the anterior abdominal muscles, and the inguinal area. The soft tissues of this area are usually soft and smooth without bulges or spasms (Table 17-11).

Normal range of motion of the lumbar spine involves flexion, extension, lateral bending, and rota-

Table 17-10. Grading of Muscle Strength against Resistance

Grade 0	0%	Zero (0)	No evidence of contractility
Grade 1	10%	Trace (T)	Slight contractility but no joint motion
Grade 2	25%	Poor (P)	Complete motion with gravity eliminated
Grade 3	50%	Fair (F)	Barely complete motion against gravity
Grade 4	75%	Good (G)	Complete motion against gravity and some resistance
Grade 5	100%	Normal (N)	Complete motion against gravity and full resistance

Source: E. L. DeGowin and R. L. DeGowin. *Bedside Diagnostic Examination*, 3rd edition. New York: The MacMillan Company, 1976.

Table 17-11.   Selected Cervical and Lumbar Spine Abnormalities

Finding	Description	Possible Conditions
Neck pain	Dull pain begins in the occipital area and moves over the head to the eye region. Usually described as behind the eye. Pain can be reproduced by palpation of posterior cervical muscles.	Nuchal headache
	Due to degeneration of the cervical vertebra. Pain frequently extends to occipital area, shoulder and arm. Accompanied by parasthesias of the hand and crepitus on movement. Biceps reflex is diminished or absent. Occurs after 50 years of age.	Cervical spondylosis
Low back pain	Pain may be gradual or sudden in onset. Pain in the buttock radiating down the lateral aspect of the leg to the toes may be present (sciatica). Pain increases with coughing or sneezing. Tenderness, limited motion, muscle spasm, and lateral deviation toward the affected side are all present.	Prolapsed intervertebral disc

tion. It is important to remember that flexion of the spine is slight when compared to flexion of the extremities. It is limited by the size of the vertebral bodies and the force exerted by the adjacent ligaments (Tables 17-14 and 17-15).

The Shoulder. The examiner begins inspection of the shoulder on ambulatory clients as the client walks into the room. Symmetry and rhythm of the shoulder motion are evaluated. Normal movement is smooth and efficient; during walking, the movement of each shoulder is coordinated with the movement of the opposite lower extremity.

Next, the shoulder is more closely inspected for anatomical structure by comparing it with the opposite shoulder. The examiner looks for symmetry in the clavicle, scapula, and deltoid regions. The shoulders are normally symmetrical.

The examiner prepares to palpate the shoulder by standing behind the seated client. The examiner gently cups the hands and places them on the deltoid using firm but gentle pressure to palpate. The suprasternal notch is located, and then the sternoclavicular joint is palpated. The examiner palpates laterally across the clavicle to the shoulder articulations. The shoulder joint and the vertebral and lateral borders of the scapula are palpated posteriorly (Figure 17-10).

Next the examiner palpates the muscles and bursa in the shoulder area. The size, shape, and consistency of the muscle tissue are noted, and the muscle tone is evaluated. Usually the size and shape of the muscles are consistent with the normal anatomical structure; the muscle tissue is soft and nontender. If the client complains of tenderness, its exact location is determined (Table 17-12).

Six movements are evaluated in range of motion of the shoulder joint. These include abduction and adduction, external and internal rotation, and flexion and extension. As the client performs these movements, the examiner assesses the motion for symmetry, rhythm, and limitation of motion (Tables 17-14, 17-15).

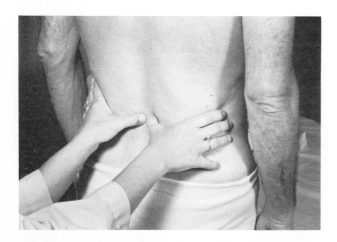

Figure 17-9. *Palpation of the lumbar spine.*

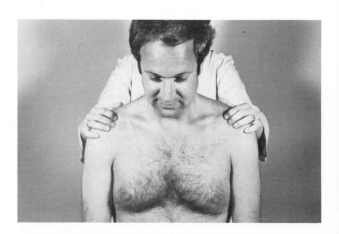

Figure 17-10. *Palpation of the shoulder.*

The Elbow. The elbow is inspected for shape, size, color, and carrying angle. The examiner assesses the entire area for shape and size of the joint. The elbow joints are normally symmetrical and conform to the normal anatomical structure. The examiner also evaluates the carrying angle of the elbow joint. This is the angle formed by the longitudinal axis of the upper arm and the longitudinal axis of the forearm. In men this angle is approximately 5 degrees; in women it measures 10 to 15 degrees. Normally, the elbow fits comfortably at the client's waist just above the iliac crest.

To palpate the elbow, the examiner stands at the client's side and abducts and extends the arm with the elbow flexed at 90 degrees. The joint and the soft tissues around the elbow are palpated with the elbow flexed at 90 degrees and the shoulder slightly abducted and extended. The ulnar nerve, triceps muscle, brachioradialis, cubital fossa, and biceps tendon are all palpated. Normally the elbow joint has three bony prominences that are palpable. The soft tissues feel smooth and soft (Table 17-12, Figure 17-11).

Four movements of the elbow joint are evaluated in range of motion: flexion and extension of the joint and supination and pronation of the forearm. The test for pronation is a continuous movement following supination. During these tests the examiner observes the client from either the front or the side. The client sits or stands and performs active range of motion with both elbows at the same time (Tables 17-14 and 17-15).

The Wrist and Hand. The examiner notes the position and motion of the hands as the client enters the room. Normally they swing naturally at the sides in a smooth and synchronous movement. After initially observing the gross movement of the hands, their anatomic structure is more closely inspected. The ex-

aminer notes the position of the hand at rest. Normally the fingers are slightly flexed.

Next the palmar surface of the wrist and hand is inspected. The palmar creases are closely examined. The normal shape of the palm is concave. The palmar surfaces of both hands are compared for shape, size, scars, lesions, and callouses. Normally the hands are approximately symmetrical. Usually the dominant hand is larger, with deeper creases and more callouses.

Finally, the dorsal side of both hands and wrists is inspected. The creases appear symmetrical. The fingers normally vary in length, but no one finger is excessively longer or shorter than the others. The examiner asks the client to make a fist and inspects the knuckles, comparing both hands. Normally the most prominent knuckle is at the middle finger.

Palpation of the wrist and hand involves palpating both the skin and the underlying bony prominences. The examiner's thumb is placed proximal to the client's thumb, and the examiner's fingers are proximal to the client's fifth finger on the two bony processes of the wrist. Palpation proceeds toward the distal part of the hand with special attention given to the skin as well as to bony prominences (Figure 17-12).

The metacarpals, the metacarpophalangeal joints, the phalanges, and the interphalangeal joints are palpated. These structures are symmetrical in both size and shape. The soft tissues in and around the wrist and hand are also palpated. Normally these tissues feel soft and smooth (Table 17-12).

In assessing range of motion of the wrist, six movements are evaluated: flexion and extension of the wrist, ulnar and radial deviation of the wrist, and supination and pronation of the forearm. While test-

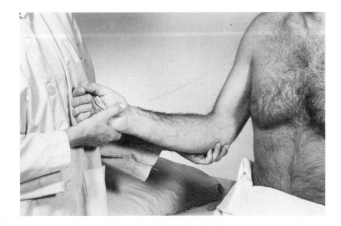

Figure 17-11. Palpation of the elbow.

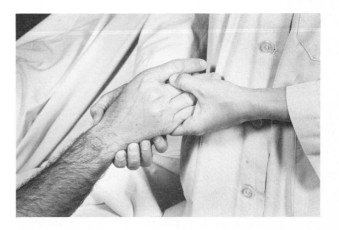

Figure 17-12. Palpation of the wrist and hand.

Table 17-12.   Selected Abnormalities of the Upper Extremities

Location	Finding	Description	Possible Conditions
Shoulder	Pain	Dull pain in shoulder without history of trauma. Elevation of arm between 60 and 120° produces severe pain. Localized tenderness at the acromion tip. Movement may product crepitus. May be acute or chronic in nature.	Supraspinatus tendinitis
Elbow	Swelling	Characterized by an accumulation of fluid in the olecranon bursa due to inflammation or trauma. Swelling is localized and fluctuant. May be accompanied by pain and limited movement.	Olecranon bursitis
Wrist	Decreased motor and sensory function	Due to narrowing of the carpal tunnel, resulting in compression on the medial nerve of the hand. Inability to flex fingers and tingling of the fingers are common findings.	Carpal tunnel syndrome
Finger	Swelling	Characterized by an enlarged joint, which is sensitive to palpation. Stiffness may be present with limited range of motion.	Arthritis
		Characterized by unilateral swelling and tenderness of the distal interphalangeal joint. Bony nodules (Heberden's nodes) may be palpated on dorsal and lateral surfaces of joint.	Osteoarthritis
	Pain	Characterized by pressure in the distal end of finger due to pus. Very painful; if localized known as felon. May spread to hand and tendon sheaths with swelling, red streaks, and tenderness along tendon sheaths. Axillary lymph nodes may be enlarged and tender to palpation.	Infection of finger tufts
		Hangnail infection, which starts in soft tissue around nail. Swelling, tenderness, and pus may be present around nail base.	Paronychia

ing range of motion, the client sits or stands with the examiner directly in front (Tables 17-14 and 17-15).

Range of motion of the hand involves the following movements: finger flexion and extension, finger abduction and adduction, thumb flexion and extension, palmar abduction and adduction of the thumb, and opposition (Tables 17-14 and 17-15).

The Hip. Inspection of the hip begins while observing the client's gait. Efficiency and symmetry of movement are noted. The client's stance is also observed. From the side there is normally a slight anterior curvature of the lumbar spine (lordosis). In front, the anterior iliac crests are in alignment. In the back, the gluteal folds are inspected; they become deeper with hip extension and tend to flatten with flexion of the hip (Figure 17-13).

While the anterior hip is palpated, the client may stand or lie down (Figure 17-14). The examiner stands in front of the client to palpate the iliac crest and tubercle and the greater trochanter. To palpate the posterior hip, the client is repositioned on the side with the superior hip flexed. The posterior iliac spines, the greater trochanter, the ischial tuberosity, and the sacroiliac joints are palpated. Normally all of these structures are palpable. The head of the femur can be felt and is usually movable.

Soft tissue palpation includes palpation of the muscles of the hip region, the bursa near the trochanter, and the sciatic nerve. All of these structures are normally palpable and the femoral vessels pulsate (Table 17-13).

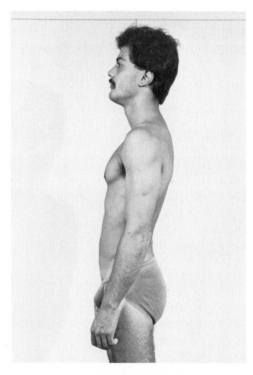

Figure 17-13. Normal curvature of the spine.

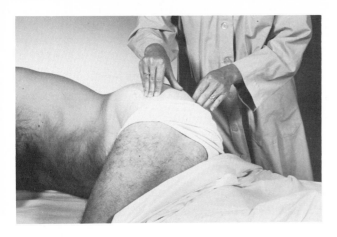

Figure 17-14. Palpation of the hip.

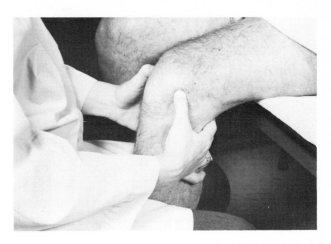

Figure 17-15. Palpation of the knee.

The hip joint is the most stable and the most mobile of all joints. Range of motion of the hip includes flexion, extension, abduction, adduction, external rotation, and internal rotation (Tables 17-14 and 17-15).

The Knee. The knee is initially inspected during the observation of the client's gait. The gait is natural and smooth with the knee flexed during swing phase, extended during heel strike, and then flexed for the remainder of the stance phase. Any unusual movements of the knee are noted.

The knee is more closely inspected with the client standing and knees fully extended. The examiner inspects the contour of the knee joint and the muscles directly above it. Normally, the knees are symmetrical, at the same level, with a slight lateral angle. The knees are then observed from the side. Normally there is no flexion, and both knees are completely extended.

In order to palpate the knee, the examiner sits facing the client while the client sits on the edge of the examination table with legs dangling. The client's leg is held between the examiner's legs for palpation (Figure 17-15). The knee is easiest to palpate in the flexed position, as the bony landmarks are more prominent and the muscles and tendons are more relaxed.

The anterior and lateral aspects of the knee joint are palpated with the examiner's thumbs while the fingers are anchored in the popliteal space. After palpating the bony landmarks and grooves, the soft tissues in the area of the knee are palpated. The quadriceps, bursa, medial and lateral meniscus, and the gastrocnemius muscle are palpated. The bony landmarks are normally smooth and easily defined. The soft tissues are soft, pliable, and nontender (Table 17-13). Range of motion in the knee involves the

movements of flexion and extension and internal and external rotation (Tables 17-14 and 17-15).

The Ankle and Foot. Inspection of the ankle and foot begins with evaluating the client's shoes since many foot problems distort the normal shape of the shoe. Normally shoes wear symmetrically without excessive wear on one part of the sole, scuffed toes, or broken-down insteps. Creases are normally present across the tops of both shoes. The client's shoes are removed, and the examiner inspects them for hard protrusions, wrinkled linings, or rough edges.

Normally the toes on both feet are in proportion to one another. The toes are flat and straight with thick pads on the bottoms. The examiner observes for callouses or any abnormally hard areas.

The color of the foot is observed. In the nonweightbearing position it is lighter than the rest of the body. In the weightbearing position it darkens slightly. The shape of the foot is also evaluated. Normally the dorsal aspect is dome-shaped as a result of the longitudinal arch.

To begin palpation of the ankle and foot, the client sits on the edge of the examining table, facing the examiner. The examiner anchors the foot by firmly holding the heel with one hand and palpates the medial and lateral aspect of the foot with the other hand (Figure 17-16). The ankle joint and plantar surface area are then palpated. Bony structures of the foot are normally palpable. The skin is normally smooth, soft, and pliable (Table 17-13).

There are two movements of the ankle joint: dorsiflexion and plantar flexion. Movements of the foot include inversion and eversion, adduction and abduction, and flexion and extension.

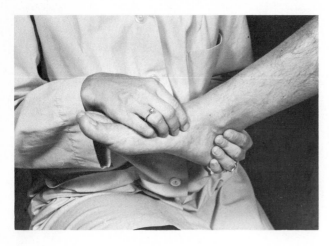

Figure 17-16. Palpation of the ankle and foot.

Life Cycle Variations

Childhood

There are several important characteristic features of the infant skeleton:

The head is approximately one-fourth of the infant's total body height.

The skull is eight times the size of the face.

The thorax has a round shape.

The legs are proportionately shorter than the trunk.

The vertebral column has only a cervical curvature.

The epiphyses of long bones are made of cartilage.

The arm and leg movements of the infant are vague. The upper body moves awkwardly due to the

Table 17-13.   Selected Abnormalities of the Lower Extremities

Location	Finding	Description	Possible Conditions
Hip	Pain	Boring pain in the hip extending to knees and back. Client walks with a limp. Crepitus is present on motion. Joint stiffness present after rest, relieved by exercise. Joint capsular swelling is palpable.	Osteoarthritis
Knee	Swelling	Localized swelling that occurs in the subcutaneous tissues over the patella in the area of the prepatellar or infrapatellar bursa. Swelling is fluctuant. Due to chronic trauma to the knee.	Bursitis
		Swelling around the patella obliterates natural hollows of the knee and is usually diffuse. Frequently assumes a horseshoe shape. Swelling may be due to excess synovial fluid, blood or pus.	Fluid in the knee
Ankle and foot	Swelling	Unilateral swelling from residual edema due to trauma. Usually localized around the malleoli.	Sprain
		Unilateral swelling from residual edema due to trauma. Usually generalized, involving the entire foot. May extend up the tibial shaft.	Fracture
		Bilateral swelling of ankles and feet most commonly due to cardiac insufficiency. May also be due to lymphatic or pelvic obstruction to venous return.	Decreased venous return
Toe	Flexion	Characterized by flexion of proximal and distal interphalangeal joints accompanied by hyperextension of the metatarsophalangeal joints. Usually all toes are involved. Callouses frequently develop on dorsal and plantar surfaces of toes.	Claw toes
		Characterized by flexion of proximal interphalangeal joint accompanied by hyperextension of the metarsophalangeal and distal interphalangeal joints. Usually involves only the second toe. Callous frequently develops on the proximal interphalangeal joint.	Hammer toes
	Swelling	Characterized by soft, swollen tissue due to moisture between toes. Most frequently found between fourth and fifth toes. Palpation produces tenderness.	Soft-tissue corns
		Characterized by swelling on the interphalangeal joints. Develops most often in areas of excessive pressure, particularly the fifth toe. Palpation may produce tenderness.	Hard-tissue corns
	Tenderness	Characterized by tenderness of the great toe. Medial and lateral corners of the toenail grow into surrounding skin. Swelling of the adjacent soft tissue occurs. Tissue is tender, warm, boggy to palpation.	Ingrown toenail

Table 17-14   Tests for Active Range of Motion

Joint	Motion	Test
Cervical spine	Flexion	The client is instructed to bend the head forward and touch the chin to the chest.
	Extension	The client is instructed to bend the head backward and look at the ceiling.
	Lateral bending	The client is instructed to tilt the head and try to touch the left ear to the left shoulder and the right ear to the right shoulder.
	Rotation	The client is instructed to turn the head and try to touch the chin to the right shoulder and then to the left shoulder.
Lumbar spine	Flexion	The client is instructed to bend forward and try to touch the toes.
	Extension	The client is instructed to bend backward as far as possible with the examiner's hand supporting the lower spine.
	Lateral bending	The client is instructed to bend as far to the right and as far to the left as possible.
	Rotation	The client is instructed to twist the shoulders to the right and then to the left.
Shoulder	Abduction and external rotation	The client is instructed to reach behind and touch the superior, medial (upper, inner) angle of the opposite scapula with fingers.
	Internal rotation and abduction	The client is instructed to reach across chest and touch the opposite shoulder joint. Then client is asked to reach behind and touch the inferior, medial (lower, inner) angle of the opposite scapula with fingers.
Elbow	Flexion	The client is instructed to bend the elbows and touch the hands to the front of the shoulders.
	Extension	The client is instructed to straighten out elbows as much as possible.
	Supination	The client is instructed to bend the elbows to 90° and hold them tightly against the waist. The client is asked to hold a pencil in each fist, palms facing downward, and then turn the fists until the palms are facing upward.
	Pronation	The client is instructed to bend the elbows to 90° and hold them tightly against the waist. The client is asked to hold a pencil in each fist, palms facing upward, and then turn the fists until the palms are facing downward.
Wrist	Flexion	The client is instructed to bend the wrist, moving the palmar surface of the hand down.
	Extension	The client is instructed to bend the wrist, moving the dorsal surface of the hand upward.
	Ulnar deviation	The client is instructed to bend the wrist toward the little finger side of the hand.
	Radial deviation	The client is instructed to bend the wrist toward the thumb side of the hand.
	Supination	See Table 17-2.
	Pronation	See Table 17-2.
Hand	Finger flexion	The client is instructed to make a tight fist.
	Finger extension	The client is instructed to open the hand and extend the fingers.
	Finger abduction	The client is instructed to spread the fingers apart as far as possible.
	Finger adduction	The client is instructed to close the fingers together tightly.
	Thumb flexion	The client is instructed to move the thumb over to the base of the little finger.
	Thumb extension	The client is instructed to bend the thumb away from the rest of the fingers.
	Palmar abduction	The client is instructed to move the thumb upward, away from the palm of the hand.
	Palmar adduction	The client is instructed to move the thumb back to touch the palm of the hand.
	Opposition	The client is instructed to touch the tips of each of his four fingers with the thumb.

Table 17-14 Tests for Active Range of Motion (continued)

Joint	Motion	Test
Hip	Flexion	The client is instructed to bring the knees as far as possible toward the chest without bending the back.
	Extension	While the client is sitting, client is instructed to fold the arms across the chest, keep the back straight, and get up from the chair.
	Abduction	While the client is standing, the client is instructed to spread the legs as far apart as possible.
	Adduction	With the legs spread apart, the client is instructed to bring them back together and then cross the right leg over the left and the left leg over the right.
	External rotation	The client is instructed to place the lateral side of the foot on the opposite knee. Repeat this for both sides.
	Internal rotation	There are no adequate active tests.
Knee	Flexion	The client is instructed to do a deep knee bend.
	Extension	The client is instructed to stand up from a deep knee bend or to sit on the edge of the examining table and extend the leg out straight.
	External rotation	The client is instructed to rotate the foot outward (laterally).
	Internal rotation	The client is instructed to rotate the foot inward (medially).
Ankle	Dorsiflexion	The client is instructed to walk on the heels.
	Plantar flexion	The client is instructed to walk on the toes.
Foot	Inversion	The client is instructed to walk on the outer (lateral) borders of the feet.
	Eversion	The client is instructed to walk on the inner (medial) aspects of the feet.
	Adduction	The client is instructed to move the foot inward without twisting it.
	Abduction	The client is instructed to move the foot outward without twisting it.
	Toe flexion	The client is instructed to walk on the toes.
	Toe extension	The client is instructed to extend the toes.

porportionately oversized head. There is a wide range of motion in all body joints. The legs appear bowed and the feet appear flat. The feet may also assume an abnormal position due to fetal positioning. This normally corrects itself by the second year.

As the child grows, the extremities lengthen and the head becomes proportionately smaller. The vertebral column develops a lumbar curve by one year of age. At the age of two the child's legs are knock-kneed and the feet are slightly pronated. The child has a wide-based stance and the gait appears somewhat unbalanced. The lower extremities straighten in the older child and the gait gradually becomes more balanced.

Control of body movement occurs in stages from infancy to childhood. The infant first learns to hold the head in space, then crawls and later learns to move around while sitting. Eventually, when the body weight can be supported by the lower extremities, the child learns to stand and then to walk.

The development of motor function of the musculoskeletal system is summarized in Appendix 10 and 11.

Adolescence

During adolescence the bones and muscles continue to grow and develop. This growth is much more pronounced in males than in females. In addition, the efficiency of the muscle cells continues to develop. Rapid growth of muscles and bones during this period may cause less coordinated body movements.

Pregnancy

Due to the increase in abdominal size during the latter months of pregnancy, the active range of motion of the lumbar spine may be more difficult for the client and slightly decreased from normal. Otherwise, musculoskeletal structure and function are within normal limits for the pregnant woman.

Late Adulthood

From early adulthood until the mid-30s, the processes of bone formation and bone destruction balance each other. During these years the focus of bone formation is bone growth and the maintenance and repair of bone tissue. Sometime during the third decade, however, bone destruction begins to exceed bone formation, which causes changes in individual bones and in the skeletal framework.

The size of bones changes with increasing age. Bones become proportionately smaller. This change in size is due to specific physiological alterations that occur in the individual bones.

Table 17-15. Passive Range of Motion and Resistance Tests

Joint Movement	Passive Test	Resistance Test	Illustration
Flexion and extension of the <u>cervical spine</u>	With the client's head in the neutral position, the examiner's hands are on either side of the client's head, which is bent forward; extension of the cervical spine is accomplished by the examiner tilting the client's head backward. Approximate normal range of motion: cervical spine flexion 45° cervical spine extension 55°	Flexion. The examiner's hands are placed on the client's forehead and xyphoid process, and pressure is applied. The client is asked to bend the head forward and touch the chin to the chest. Extension. The examiner's hand is placed on the occipital bone, and pressure is applied. The client is asked to bend the head backward as far as possible.	
Lateral bending of the cervical spine	With the client's head in a neutral position, lateral bending or flexion of the cervical spine is accomplished by the examiner tilting the client's head to the right and then to the left so that the right and then the left ear approximates the corresponding shoulder. Approximate normal range of motion: right cervical spine lateral bending 40° left cervical spine lateral bending 40°	The examiner's hands are placed on the left and right temporal bones and pressure is applied. The client is asked to bend the head to the left and then to the right without moving the shoulders.	
Rotation of the <u>cervical spine</u>	With the head in the neutral position, rotation of the cervical spine is accomplished by the examiner moving the client's head to the right and then to the left so that the chin approximates the right and then the left shoulder (a "no" motion). Approximate normal range of motion: right cervical spine rotation 70° left cervical spine rotation 70°	The examiner's hands are placed on the client's temples and pressure is applied. The client is asked to move the head to the right so the chin is close to the right shoulder and to the left so the chin is close to the left shoulder.	
Flexion and extension of the <u>lumbar spine</u>	With the spine in the neutral position, flexion of the lumbar spine is accomplished by the examiner bending the client forward at the waist with the client's fingertips directed toward the floor; extension of the lumbar spine is accomplished by the examiner bending the client backward at the waist. Approximate normal range of motion: lumbar spine flexion 75-90° lumbar spine extension 30°	Flexion. The examiner holds the client's legs. The client is asked to touch toes. Extension. The examiner's hands are placed on the scapulae, and pressure is applied. The client is asked to bend the head and shoulders backward without using the hands.	
Lateral bending of the lumbar spine	With the spine in the neutral position, lateral bending or flexion of the lumbar spine consists of the examiner bending the client's trunk to the left and to the right laterally at the waist. Approximate normal range of motion: right lumbar spine lateral bending 35° left lumbar spine lateral bending 35°	Usually not tested.	
Rotation of the <u>lumbar spine</u>	With the spine in the neutral position, rotation of the thoracolumbar spine is accomplished by the examiner twisting the client's shoulders first to the left and then to the right. Approximate normal range of motion: right thoracolumbar spine rotation 30° left thoracolumbar spine rotation 30°	The examiner's hands are placed on the anterior aspects of the right and left shoulders. With the client seated, the examiner asks the client to touch the right shoulder to the left knee and the left shoulder to the right knee.	

Table 17-15 Passive Range of Motion and Resistance Tests (*continued*)

Joint Movement	Passive Test	Resistance Test	Illustration
Abduction and adduction of the shoulder joint	With the arm in the neutral position of the body, abduction of the shoulder joint is accomplished by the examiner moving the client's arm outward and upward. Adduction of the shoulder joint is accomplished by returning the arm toward the midline of the body and continuing this motion in an upward direction beyond the midline of the body. Approximate normal range of motion: abduction of the shoulder joint 180° adduction of the shoulder joint 45°	Usually not tested.	
External and internal rotation of the shoulder joint	With the elbow held at a 90° angle, external rotation of the shoulder joint is accomplished by the examiner rotating the client's arm upward around the shoulder joint. Internal rotation of the shoulder joint is accomplished by holding the elbow at a 90° angle and rotating the arm in the opposite direction. Approximate normal range of motion: external rotation of the shoulder joint 40-45° internal rotation of the shoulder joint 55°	External rotation. The examiner's hands are placed on the dorsal aspect of the wrist. The client is asked to swing the arm forward as if pitching a ball overhead. Internal rotation. The examiner's hand is placed on the volar aspect of the wrist. The client is asked to swing the arm backward and point toward the ceiling.	
Flexion and extension of the shoulder joint	With the arm in the neutral position, flexion of the shoulder joint is accomplished by the examiner bending the client's arm forward at the shoulder. Extension is accomplished by holding the client's arm above the elbow and extending the arm from the shoulder. Approximate normal range of motion: flexion of the shoulder joint 90° extension of the shoulder joint 45°	Flexion. The examiner's hands are placed on the upper arm and pressure is applied. The client is asked to bring the arm up and forward. Extension. The examiner's hands are placed on the posterior upper arm proximal to the elbow and apply pressure. The client is asked to bring the arm down and backwards.	
Flexion and extension of the elbow joint	With the arm in the neutral position, flexion of the elbow joint is accomplished by the examiner holding the client's elbow against the waist and drawing the forearm upward. The elbow joint is extended when the arm is moved to the neutral position. Approximate normal range of motion: flexion of the elbow joint 135-150° extension of the elbow joint 0-5°	Flexion. The examiner's hands are placed on the client's lower arm and apply pressure. The client is asked to bring the right hand to the right shoulder and the left hand to the left shoulder. Extension. The examiner's hands are placed on the dorsal aspect of the client's lower arm and apply pressure. The client is asked to straighten the arm from the elbow.	
Pronation and supination of the forearm	With the forearm in the neutral position, pronation of the forearm is accomplished by the examiner holding the client's elbow flexed at 90° at his waist and turning the forearm so that palm of the hand is facing downward. With the forearm in the neutral position, supination of the forearm is accomplished by turning the forearm so the palm of the hand is facing upward. Approximate normal range of motion: supination of the forearm 90° pronation of the forearm 90°	Pronation. The examiner's hand is placed around the client's wrist. The client is asked to turn the hand inward so the palm faces down. Supination. The examiner's hand is placed around the client's wrist. The client is asked to turn the hand outward so the palm faces up.	

Table 17-15   Passive Range of Motion and Resistance Tests (*continued*)

Joint Movement	Passive Test	Resistance Test	Illustration
Flexion and extension of the wrist joint	With the hand in the neutral position, flexion of the wrist is accomplished by the examiner bending the palmar surface of the client's hand downward. This is also known as palmar flexion. With the hand in the neutral position, extension of the wrist is accomplished by the examiner bending the dorsal surface of the client's hand upward. This is also known as dorsiflexion. Approximate normal range of motion: flexion of the wrist joint — 80° extension of the wrist joint — 70°	Flexion. The examiner's hand is placed on the palmar surface of the client's hand and applies pressure. The client is asked to bend the hand down against the examiner's hand. Extension. The examiner's hand is placed on the dorsal surface of the client's hand and applies pressure. The client is asked to bend the hand back against the examiner's hand.	
Ulnar and radial deviation of the wrist joint	With the hand in the neutral position, ulnar deviation is accomplished by the examiner moving the client's hand laterally toward the ulnar or little finger side of the hand. With the hand in the neutral position, radial deviation is accomplished by the examiner moving the client's hand laterally toward the radial or thumb side of the hand. Approximate normal range of motion: ulnar deviation of the wrist joint — 30° radial deviation of the wrist joint — 20°	Not normally done.	
Flexion and extension of the finger joints	With the finger in a neutral position, flexion of the finger is accomplished by the examiner bending each joint of the client's finger down toward the palmar surface of the hand. The finger joints are extended when the finger is in a neutral position. Approximate normal range of motion: flexion of the finger joints: metacarpophalangeal joint — 90° proximal phalangeal joint — 100° distal phalangeal joint — 90° extension of the finger joints metacarpophalangeal joint — 30-45° proximal phalangeal joint — 0° distal phalangeal joint — 20°	Flexion. The examiner's fingers are placed on the palmar surface of the client's finger between the joints and apply pressure. The client is asked to bend the finger down at all three joints. Extension. The examiner's fingers are placed on the dorsal surface of the client's finger between the joints and apply pressure. The client is asked to straighten the fingers.	
Abduction and adduction of the finger joints	With the finger in a neutral position and the joints isolated, abduction of the finger is accomplished by the examiner moving the client's finger laterally away from the other fingers; adduction of the finger is accomplished by the examiner moving the client's finger laterally toward the other fingers. Approximate normal range of motion: abduction of the finger joint — 20° adduction of the finger joint — 0°	Abduction. The examiner attempts to push the client's fingers together as the client is asked to spread the fingers apart. Adduction. The examiner attempts to pull the client's fingers apart as the client is asked to press the fingers together.	

Table 17-15 Passive Range of Motion and Resistance Tests (*continued*)

Joint Movement	Passive Test	Resistance Test	Illustration
Flexion and extension of the <u>thumb</u> joints	With the thumb in a neutral position, flexion of the thumb is accomplished by the examiner bending each joint of the client's thumb down toward the palmar surface of the hand. The thumb joints are extended when the thumb is in a neutral position. Approximate normal range of motion: Flexion of the thumb joint 　metacarpophalangeal joint　50° 　interphalangeal joint　90° Extension of the thumb joint 　metacarpophalangeal joint　0° 　interphalangeal joint　20°	Flexion. The examiner's finger is placed on the palmar surface of the distal thumb and applies pressure. The client is asked to bend the thumb down to the palm. Extension. The examiner's finger is placed on the dorsal surface of the distal thumb and applies pressure. The client is asked to straighten the thumb.	
Abduction and adduction of the <u>thumb</u> joint	With the thumb in a neutral position, abduction of the thumb is accomplished by the examiner moving the client's thumb away from the palm of the hand; adduction of the thumb is accomplished by the examiner moving the client's thumb back toward the palm of the hand. Approximate normal range of motion: 　abduction of the thumb joint　70° 　adduction of the thumb joint　0°	Abduction. The examiner's finger is placed on the dorsal side of the thumb and applies pressure. The client is asked to move the thumb away from the fingers. Adduction. The examiner's finger is placed on the distal end of the thumb and applies pressure. The client is asked to move the thumb toward the index finger.	
Opposition of the <u>thumb</u> and fingers	With the thumb held in the neutral position, opposition of the thumb and fingers is accomplished by the examiner moving the client's thumb to touch each fingertip. Approximate normal range of motion: 　Normally the thumb can touch the tip of each finger.	The examiner's thumbs are placed on the palmar surface of the fingers and thumbs. The client is asked to touch the tip and base of each finger with the thumb.	
Flexion and extension of the <u>hip</u> joint	With the hip held in a neutral position, while the client is lying supine, flexion of the hip is accomplished by the examiner bending the client's thigh up onto the chest. With the hip held in a neutral position while the client is lying prone, extension of the hip is accomplished with the examiner's hand under the client's thigh and lifting the entire leg up. Approximate normal range of motion: 　flexion of the hip joint　120° 　extension of the hip joint　30°	Flexion. The examiner's hands are placed on the anterior surface of the client's thigh and pressure is applied. The client is asked to bring the knee up to the trunk. Extension. The examiner's hands are placed on the dorsal surface of the client's thigh and apply pressure. The client is asked to raise the leg upward.	
Abduction and adduction of the <u>hip</u> joint	With the hip in the neutral position, while the client is lying supine, abduction of the hip is accomplished by the examiner pulling the client's leg laterally outward; adduction of the hip is accomplished by the examiner moving the client's leg over the midline of body and across the other leg. Approximate normal range of motion: 　abduction of the hip joint　45-50° 　adduction of the hip joint　20-30°	Abduction. The examiner's hands are placed on the lateral surface of the client's thigh and apply pressure. The client is asked to move the leg laterally outward. Adduction. The examiner's hands are placed on the medial surface of the client's thigh and pressure is applied. The client is asked to bring the legs together.	

Table 17-15 Passive Range of Motion and Resistance Tests (*continued*)

Joint Movement	Passive Test	Resistance Test	Illustration
External and internal rotation of the hip joint	With the hip in the neutral position while the client is lying supine, external rotation of the hip is accomplished by the examiner holding the client's foot and twisting the leg outward; internal rotation of the hip is accomplished by twisting the leg inward. Approximate normal range of motion: external rotation of the hip joint 45° internal rotation of the hip joint 35°	External rotation. The examiner's hand is placed on the medial surface of the ankle and pressure is applied. The client is asked to pivot the hip outward so the foot twists inward. Internal rotation. The examiner's hand is placed on the lateral surface of the ankle and pressure is applied. The client is asked to pivot the hip inward so the foot twists outward.	
Flexion and extension of the knee joint	With the knee held in a neutral position, flexion of the knee is accomplished by the examiner bending the client's lower leg back toward the buttocks. The knee is extended when it is held in a neutral position. Approximate normal range of motion: flexion of the knee joint 135° extension of the knee joint 0°	Flexion. The examiner's hand is placed on the posterior surface of the ankle and pressure is applied. The client is asked to bend the lower leg back toward the buttocks. Extension. The examiner's hand is placed on the anterior surface of the ankle and pressure is applied. The client is asked to straighten the lower leg.	
External and internal rotation of the knee joint	With the knee held in the neutral position, external rotation of the knee is accomplished by the examiner turning the client's tibia toward the outside of the leg; internal rotation of the knee is accomplished by the examiner turning the client's tibia to the inside. Approximate normal range of motion: external rotation of the knee joint 10° internal rotation of the knee joint 10°	Not normally done.	
Dorsiflexion and plantar flexion of the ankle joint	With the ankle in the neutral position, dorsiflexion of the ankle is accomplished by the examiner holding the client's heel and pulling up on the foot; plantar flexion is accomplished by pushing down on the foot. Approximate normal range of motion: dorsiflexion of the ankle joint 20° plantar flexion of the ankle joint 50°	Dorsiflexion. The examiner's hand is placed on the dorsal surface of the foot and pressure is applied. The client is asked to bend the foot up. Plantar flexion. The examiner's hand is placed on the plantar surface of the foot and pressure is applied. The client is asked to bend the foot down.	
Inversion and eversion of the foot joints	With the foot held in the neutral position, inversion of the foot is accomplished by the examiner holding the client's heel and twisting it laterally; eversion of the foot is accomplished by twisting the heel medially. Approximate normal range of motion: inversion of the foot joints 5° eversion of the foot joints 5°	Inversion. The examiner's hand is placed on the medial surface of the first metatarsal bone and pressure is applied. The client is asked to move the toes inward. Eversion. The examiner's hand is placed on the lateral surface of the fifth metatarsal bone and pressure is applied. The client is asked to move the toes outward.	
Adduction and abduction of the foot joints	With the foot held in the neutral position, adduction of the foot is accomplished by the examiner holding the client's heel and moving the foot inward laterally without twisting it; abduction of the foot is accomplished by moving the foot outward laterally. Approximate normal range of motion: adduction of the foot joint 20° abduction of the foot joint 10°	Not normally done.	

Table 17-15 Passive Range of Motion and Resistance Tests *(continued)*

Joint Movement	Passive Test	Resistance Test	Illustration
Flexion and extension of the toe joints	With the toe in the neutral position, flexion of the toe is accomplished by the examiner bending the client's toe downward toward the plantar surface of the foot; extension of the toe is accomplished by bringing the toe straight up. Approximate normal range of motion: flexion of the toe joint 45° extension of the toe joint 70-90°	Flexion. The examiner's finger is placed on the plantar surface of the toes and pressure is applied. The client is asked to bend the toe down. Extension. The examiner's finger is placed on the dorsal surface of the toe and pressure is applied. The client is asked to point the toe upward.	

The calcification, texture, and shape of bone change with age. Bone is lost from the inside (endosteal surfaces) and is gained on the outside (periosteal surfaces). Compact bone in the diaphyses of long bones decreases. The size of the medullary cavities increases. This causes the bone to become rigid, brittle, and hollow. As a result it is not as capable of withstanding the stresses of compression. The density and strength of bone decreases and the older adult is at high risk for fractures.

Because there is an increase of bone on the periosteal surfaces, bone projections and margins increase in size. This causes spurs and ridges and makes bony processes more prominent.

Bone tissue at the articulation surfaces also increases, enlarging and deforming the joints. The synovial fluid thickens and the hyaline cartilage degenerates. These changes cause decreased active and passive range of motion; the elderly client frequently complains of joint stiffness. Joint pain and compensatory changes in gait, particularly during the stance phase, may also occur.

Skeletal muscle fibers also degenerate. Muscle is slowly replaced by collagen tissue, a process known as fibrosis. The connective tissue interferes with the oxygen and nutrient supply to muscle. Force of contraction decreases, and there is a decrease in muscle bulk accompanied by a generalized muscle weakness.

When assessing the musculoskeletal system of the aging client, the examiner focuses on the functional abilities of the client rather than on age or medical diagnoses. During inspection of posture and gait, the examiner notes any changes in general body posture and the use of special aids for ambulation. The older client usually presents a picture of generalized flexion. Changes in the vertebral bones and cartilaginous discs cause the vertebrae to collapse slightly. The vertebral column has a stooped (kyphotic) curvature. The hips and knees are flexed when standing and the client's gait may be shuffling. This may be due to decreased motor function or to decreased sensory stimulation on the foot pads of the bottoms of the feet.

Inspection and palpation of the upper and lower extremities usually reveal decreased muscle mass, tone, and strength. Atrophy of the peripheral muscles is usually symmetrical. The hands appear thin and bony and the arms and legs are thin and flabby due to muscle wasting.

Muscle cramps tend to occur with increasing frequency with aging. Cramps usually occur at night and are aggravated by excessive exercise. Usually only one muscle group is involved, such as the neck, calf, or thigh muscles. The cramping is due to involuntary, painful muscle contractions.

The joints are inspected for swelling and deformities. Previous deformities usually become more pronounced with age. The joints in the hands may enlarge or become disfigured. There may also be redness and localized or diffuse swelling. The range-of-motion tests are generally normal but frequently reveal impaired mobility. The joints in the fingers, hips, and knees are particularly susceptible to stiffening. The examiner notes the presence of any crepitation, joint tenderness, or pain.

Anatomy and Physiology

The nervous system consists of the brain, spinal nerve cord, and millions of nerve cells (neurons). Nerve cells are characterized by many processes; their specialized functions include irritability and conductivity. The overall function of the nervous system is to store, process, and transmit information. It is a communication system of the highest order.

Anatomically, the nervous system consists of two divisions: the central nervous system (brain and spinal cord) and the peripheral nervous system (cranial, spinal, and peripheral nerves). The autonomic nervous system includes neurons from both the central nervous system and the peripheral nervous system. These neurons specifically innervate smooth muscle, cardiac muscle, and glands.

A pertinent review of the anatomy and physiology of the nervous system focuses on the areas evaluated in the neurological assessment. These areas involve parts of both the central and peripheral nervous systems and include the cerebrum, cranial nerves, cerebellum, motor and sensory pathways, and reflexes.

The Cerebrum

The brain (cerebrum or encephalon) is the enlarged end of the central nervous system that is encased within and protected by the skull. The brain integrates sensory and motor functions and carries out higher-level functions that deal with behavior, learning, and language.

The brain itself is an integrated mass of nerve dendrites and axons that interconnect and form a communications network with endless possibilities for programming information. Nine-tenths of the body's ten billion neurons are found in the brain. The normal brain reaches its maximum weight around 20 years of age, and then its size slowly decreases with age.

The outer layer of the cerebrum, the cerebral cortex, is only a few millimeters thick and is composed of nerve cell bodies. These bodies give the cortex a grayish color. The surface of the cortex is very irregular with many fissures (sulci) that run between the numerous convolutions (gyri). Fissures are deep folds of cortex that separate the convolutions or raised areas of the cerebrum. This convoluted configuration of the cerebral cortex increases the surface area of the cortical tissue without increasing the total size of the brain.

The cerebral cortex is divided into the right and left main cerebral hemispheres by a deep fissure known

Chapter 18

Assessment of the Neurological System

Objectives

The examiner will be able to do the following

1. Test the function of cranial nerves
2. Test cerebellar function
3. Test the function of motor nerves
4. Test the function of sensory nerves
5. Test the reflex activity
6. Recognize abnormalities of the neurologic system
7. Record the information obtained

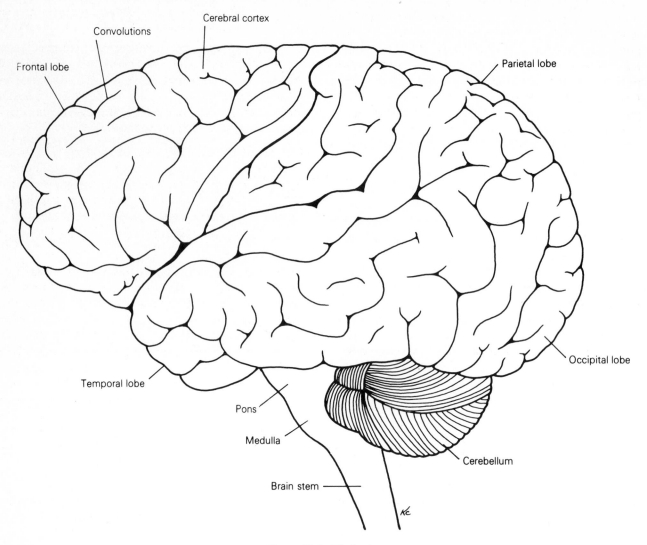

Figure 18-1. The brain.

as the medial longitudinal fissure. Each hemisphere is further divided into four functional lobes by lesser fissures: the frontal lobe, parietal lobe, temporal lobe, and occipital lobe (Figure 18-1).

In the frontal lobe is the motor cortex, which contains neurons responsible for the control of motor function. The motor cortex controls body movements, not specific muscles. In addition to controlling voluntary muscle movements, the frontal lobe also plays a role in intellectual functions, personality characteristics, and expression of speech. Motivation, vigilance, and emotional behavior are controlled through the limbic system. The limbic system is a group of neurons that interconnects parts of the frontal and temporal lobes with the thalamus and hypothalamus as well as many other parts of the central nervous system. Though the function of the limbic system is

not completely understood, stimulation of various limbic areas produces a wide variety of behavioral changes. The frontal lobes seem to function as overseer or executor of all other higher cerebral functions.

The parietal lobe contains the primary area for sensory perception and provides the ability to perceive, localize, and discriminate tactile stimuli and body part position. It is also involved in the recognition of the size, weight, and texture of objects and controls the ability to understand written words. The temporal lobe contains the centers for comprehensive speech and for interpretation of the sensations of taste and smell. The chief function of the occipital lobe is visual perception.

In addition to the specialized function of the lobes, each hemisphere is specialized. The left cerebral hemisphere is specialized for language, some skilled motor acts, certain analytical processes such as arithmetic, and certain aspects of memory. The right hemisphere may be more important in spatial relationships and nonverbal reasoning. Most people (85 percent) are right-handed, probably reflecting the dominance of language and other functions in the left hemisphere. Recent studies have shown that the right hemisphere may process emotional sounds such as crying and laughing and be involved in musical discrimination.

Cranial Nerves

Twelve pairs of nerves emerge from the base of the brain and send sensory and motor fibers mainly to the head and neck region. Most leave the cranium through small foramina in the skull. Some of the nerves have both sensory (afferent) and motor (efferent) fibers; others have only sensory fibers or only motor fibers. The cranial nerves are numbered from front to back in the order they arise from the brain. They also have specific names based on their anatomical distribution or their physiological function (Figure 18-2).

Cranial Nerve I. The olfactory nerves (15 to 20 in number) arise from the upper third of the nasal chamber. Composed of special sensory fibers, their receptors are located in the nasal mucosa. The fibers pass through the skull via the ethmoid bone to the olfactory bulb. From there the fibers run to the olfactory cortex, a portion of which is located in the temporal lobe. The olfactory nerves are responsible for olfaction or the sense of smell.

Cranial Nerve II. The optic nerve is a sensory nerve whose receptors are located in the retina of the eye. It passes through the optic foramen and meets the nerve from the opposite eye forming the optic chiasm. Approximately one-half of the fibers of each optic nerve cross via the optic chiasm through the optic tract to the opposite side of the brain and run through the thalamus and white matter to the occipital lobe. Thus, the optic nerve from each eye contains sensory fibers from only that eye, while the optic tracts contain fibers from both eyes. Besides vision, the optic nerve forms the afferent (sensory) half of the pupillary light reflex.

Cranial Nerve III. The oculomotor nerve is a motor nerve whose fibers originate in the midbrain and run to the muscles of the eye and pupil. Inferior fibers supply the superior rectus and levator palpebrae superioris (muscle of the upper eye lid). Inferior fibers innervate the inferior oblique, medial recti, and in-

ferior recti muscle. The inferior fibers also supply the ciliary muscle of the lens and the sphincter muscle of the iris, which constrict the pupil. The oculomotor nerve is thus responsible for extrinsic eye muscle movement, movement of the upper eyelid, pupillary constriction, and accommodation.

Cranial Nerve IV. The trochlear nerve is a motor nerve that travels a similar path as the oculomotor nerve. The motor fibers supply the superior oblique muscle of the eyes. The trochlear nerve is responsible for movement of the eye medially and inferiorly.

Cranial Nerve V. The trigeminal nerve has both sensory and motor fibers. It emerges from the pons. The trigeminal nerve supplies sensory fibers to the face and anterior scalp, and motor fibers to the four muscles of mastication. Its sensory fibers are divided into three main parts: the ophthalmic (V_1), the maxillary (V_2), and the mandibular (V_3). The ophthalmic division (V_1) has receptors located in the lacrimal glands, conjunctiva, skin of the upper eyelid, scalp, forehead, mucus membranes, and skin of the nose. The maxillary division (V_2) has receptors on the sides of the face, nose, upper lip, lower eyelids, and the upper teeth. The mandibular division (V_3) has receptors in the lower jaw and teeth. A separate motor division controls the muscles of mastication.

Cranial Nerve VI. The abducens nerve is a motor nerve that supplies the lateral rectus eye muscle. It originates in the pons and the floor of the fourth ventricle. It is responsible for abduction of the eye.

Cranial Nerve VII. The facial nerve has both sensory and motor fibers. The sensory receptors are located in the taste buds of the anterior two-thirds of the tongue. The fibers follow the path of the eighth cranial nerve and eventually terminate in the pons. The motor nerves originate in the pons and supply the facial muscles. The facial nerve is responsible for taste sensation on the anterior two-thirds of the tongue and for facial movements. It also supplies the ipsilateral lacrimal apparatus and certain salivary glands.

Cranial Nerve VIII. The acoustic (auditory) nerve is a sensory nerve with two divisions: the cochlear and the vestibular nerves. The receptors of the cochlear nerve are found in the organ of Corti in the cochlea of the inner ear. The cochlear nerve is responsible for hearing. The receptors for the vestibular nerve are found in the semicircular canal and utricle of the inner ear. Some of its fibers run to the cerebellum. The vestibular portion of the eighth cranial nerve is responsible for equilibrium.

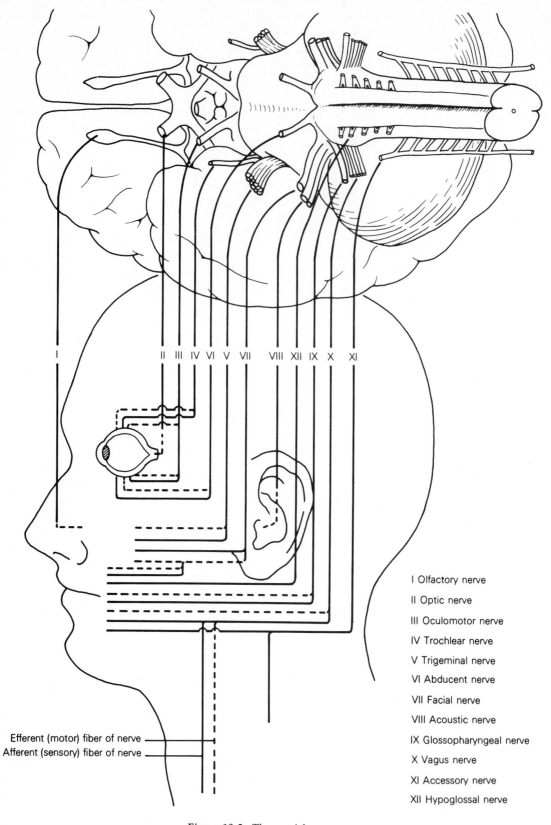

I Olfactory nerve

II Optic nerve

III Oculomotor nerve

IV Trochlear nerve

V Trigeminal nerve

VI Abducent nerve

VII Facial nerve

VIII Acoustic nerve

IX Glossopharyngeal nerve

X Vagus nerve

XI Accessory nerve

XII Hypoglossal nerve

Efferent (motor) fiber of nerve

Afferent (sensory) fiber of nerve

Figure 18-2. The cranial nerves.

Cranial Nerve IX. The glossopharyngeal nerve is composed of both sensory and motor fibers. The sensory fiber has receptors for taste on the posterior one-third of the tongue, epiglottis, soft palate, and tonsils. The motor fiber supplies the stylopharyngeus muscle of the pharynx. The glossopharyngeal is responsible for taste sensations on the posterior one-third of the tongue, sensation of the palate and the pharynx, and swallowing movements.

Cranial Nerve X. The vagus nerve contains both sensory and motor fibers, which are widely distributed over the body. Sensory vagal receptors are found in the pharynx, larynx, trachea, bronchi, lungs, carotid body, heart, esophagus, stomach, small intestine, and gallbladder. Motor fibers originate in the medulla and innervate muscles of the pharynx, larynx, and abdominal viscera. The vagus mediates sensation from the pharynx and larynx. It also mediates motor function for swallowing and for movements of the vocal cord, uvula, and soft palate.

Cranial Nerve XI. The accessory nerve is a motor nerve. Most of its fibers originate in the first six segments of the spinal cord and emerge through the spinal root to supply the sternocleidomastoid and trapezius muscles. The accessory nerve is responsible for the shrugging movements of the shoulders and the side-to-side turning movements of the head.

Cranial Nerve XII. The hypoglossal nerve is composed of motor fibers that originate in the medulla and supply the muscles of the tongue. It is responsible for tongue movements.

The Cerebellum

The cerebellum is located dorsal to the brain stem (Figure 18-1). It is attached to the brain stem by three pairs of peduncles. It is roughly divided into two hemispheres with a middle, connecting portion known as the vermis. The outer layer of the cerebellum is composed of cortical gray matter. Like the cerebrum, there are numerous fissures and gyri in the cerebellar cortex. However, unlike the cerebrum, these convolutions are much less prominent.

The internal portion of the cerebellum is composed of short and long nerve fiber tracts. The short nerve tracts conduct impulses between the outer cerebellar cortex and the inner cerebellum. The long tracts conduct impulses between the cerebellum and various parts of the brainstem and spinal cord. The nerve fibers of the longer tracts pass through the three pairs of peduncles providing the cerebellum with a direct connection to the medulla, spinal cord, pons, midbrain, thalamus, and motor cortex.

The major functions of the cerebellum include the maintenance of skeletal muscle coordination and equilibrium and the control of posture. There are many theories about the functions of the cerebellum, though most physiologists consider coordination to be its main function.

The coordination of muscle activity by the cerebellum is closely connected to the control of muscle movement by the motor cortex. Coordinated, smooth, steady, efficient muscle movements are the result of cerebral plus cerebellar neural activity. The motor cortex starts muscle movement; impulses from the cerebellum fine tune those movements once they have begun. The cerebellum also controls rapid muscle movements by integrating the time and force needed for the movement with data on the position and final location of the moving part.

Another portion of the cerebellum is apparently responsible for maintaining posture. It receives information from cortical and subcortical areas of the cerebrum as to what the posture should be and from afferent sensory pathways as to what the posture actually is. The cerebellum integrates all of this information unconsciously. If there is a discrepancy between the two pieces of information, it sends impulses to the motor cortex to correct the muscle action. Thus, posture is maintained.

The final function of the cerebellum involves the maintenance of equilibrium. The cerebellum receives afferent impulses from the vestibular apparatus in the middle ear indicating the orientation of the head in space. If disequilibrium is present, efferent impulses are then returned to the appropriate muscles to correct the condition.

Motor Pathways

Motor neurons conducting impulses from the central nervous system to skeletal muscles compose the motor pathways. Numerous motor fibers conduct impulses from various areas of the cerebral cortex down to all levels of the spinal cord and out to the skeletal muscles after synapse in the cord.

The motor pathways are divided into pyramidal and extrapyramidal tracts. The pyramidal tracts (corticospinal tracts) are composed of upper motor neurons that originate in the cerebral cortex and merge in the medulla, forming pyramids. Most of their fibers cross over in the medulla and travel down the corticospinal tract on the opposite side in the white matter of the spinal cord. The motor fibers that do not cross over (decussate) extend down the spinal cord tracts on the same side as the cerebral cortex from which they originated. The corticospinal tract fibers synapse with interneurons in the gray matter. The interneurons of the cord then synapse with lower motor neurons. The lower motor neurons emerge from the spinal cord at various levels via the anterior (ventral) nerve root. From there the lower motor neurons travel directly to the skeletal muscles (Figure 18-3).

The extrapyramidal tracts consist of motor pathways in the spinal cord other than the corticospinal tracts. These motor fibers originate in the cerebral cortex, thalamus, basal ganglia, cerebellum and brain stem. They extend down the cord, terminate in the gray matter, and synapse with an interneuron, which in turn synapses with the lower motor neuron fiber.

The most significant extrapyramidal tracts are the reticulospinal tracts. These tracts are responsible for large, automatic muscle movements such as those used in walking, running, or swimming. They also play a role in producing emotional expressions. Smiling and frowning are examples of expressions that are mediated by the extrapyramidal tracts.

Sensory Pathways

Sensory pathways consist of sensory neurons that run from the periphery of the body to the spinal cord or brain stem and then to the higher centers of the cerebral cortex. These pathways are composed of first order, second-order, and third-order neurons. Receptors of first-order neurons are found in the periphery (skin and muscles); their axons terminate in the gray matter of the spinal cord and the brain stem. Second-order neurons conduct sensory impulses from the spinal cord or brain stem to the thalamus. Third-order sensory neurons run from the thalamus to the post-

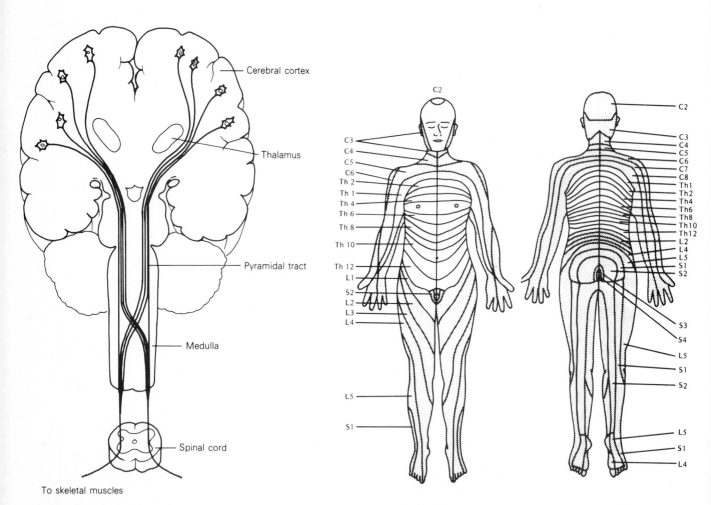

Figure 18-3. *Pyramidal (corticospinal) tracts.*

Figure 18-4. *Dermatome map.*

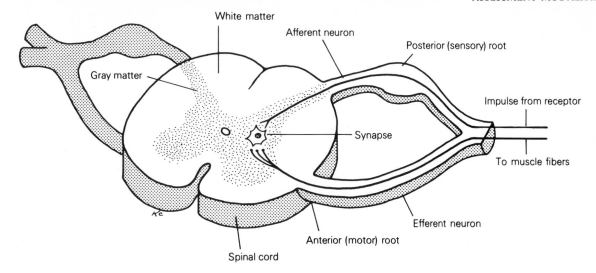

Figure 18-5. Reflex arc.

central gyrus in the parietal lobe, which is the higher center for sensory recognition in the cerebral cortex.

The first-order sensory neurons enter the spinal cord at different levels. The peripheral area innervated by a specific spinal cord segment is known as a dermatome (Figure 18-4).

The first-order sensory neuron enters the spinal cord via the posterior (dorsal) nerve root. Different courses are followed by sensory fibers subserving different functions. Pain and temperature synapse in spinal cord gray matter within a few levels of root entry and cross to the opposite side of the spinal cord, ascending via the second-order neuron in the lateral spinothalamic tract to synapse in the thalamus. Position and vibration sense, on the other hand, ascend without synapse via the posterior columns of the cord and synapse in the lower brain stem before crossing to the contralateral side via the medial leminiscus. A third sensation, light touch, also synapses in the cord and passes upward both curved and uncrossed to the thalamus via the anterior spinothalamic tract. When these impulses reach the ventral posterior lateral nucleus of the thalamus, they are relayed via the third-order neuron to the post-central gyrus of the cerebral cortex.

Reflexes

A simple reflex arc consists of a sensory (afferent) neuron with a receptor, a central nervous system synapse (intermediary), and a motor (efferent) neuron with an effector. A reflex is the muscle action that results from a stimulus applied to a receptor site, causing a nerve impulse to travel over a reflex arc.

Spinal nerves are arranged segmentally and emerge from the spinal cord by way of an anterior (efferent or motor) and a posterior (afferent or sensory) root. A sensory stimulus is received by the sensory receptor and the impulse is carried by the afferent neuron via the posterior (sensory) root to the spinal cord. In the gray matter of the spinal cord, the afferent neuron synapses with the efferent neuron, which exits the spinal column via the anterior (motor) root. The efferent neuron carries the impulse to the selected muscle fibers (effectors) to cause a muscle action. This is the simplest pathway of a reflex arc (Figure 18-5).

Spinal reflexes are under indirect control of the cerebral cortex, which may facilitate or inhibit the reflex. The term *reflex* usually refers to only involuntary responses mediated at the cord level. The normal reflex response to a specific stimulus is always the same; it happens quickly, and it is not generally under conscious control, although it may be increased symmetrically by anxiety states.

Assessment Modalities

Preparation

The purpose of a neurologic assessment is threefold: (1) to determine the absence or presence of nervous system dysfunction, (2) to determine the location and extent of nervous system dysfunction, and (3) to determine the degree to which the healthy portion of the client's nervous system compensates for the dysfunction.

Cerebral Function

The neurological system is examined by using the techniques of inspection, palpation, and percussion. The instruments necessary include a tuning fork, reflex hammer, ophthalmoscope, test tubes, calipers, safety pin, Snellen eye chart, tape measure, cotton ball, tongue depressor, test tubes, and newspaper.

Evaluation of the nervous system proceeds in steps from higher levels of integration to lower levels of function. The nervous system itself is not directly accessible to examination; therefore, assessment of its function is dependent on peripheral indicators of nervous system activity. These indicators include general cerebral function, cranial nerve integrity, cerebellar function (coordination and balance), motor function, sensory function, and reflex activity.

The extent of the neurologic assessment depends on the client's chief complaint or findings from the history and physical examination. Portions of the assessment, such as evaluation of cerebral and motor function, are often integrated throughout the history and physical examination. Most health assessements on well clients require only a screening neurologic assessment.

Assessment of cerebral function includes general and specific functions. Testing of general function is called the *mental status examination* (Chapter 3). Assessment of specific cerebral functions includes cortical sensory interpretation, cortical motor integration and language (Tables 18-1 and 18-2).

The temporal, parietal, and occipital lobes of the cerebrum are essential to cortical sensory interpretation of the environment through hearing, feeling, and seeing. Auditory sensations are mediated through the temporal lobe; tactile sensations, through the parietal lobe; and visual sensations, through the occipital lobe.

Cortical motor integration involves understanding what the desired action is, remembering how to do it, and having the motor strength to complete the action. The client is instructed to protrude tongue, snap fingers, and repeat sentences after the examiner. Normally the client performs these actions without difficulty or hesitation.

The client normally communicates with verbal and written language as well as with gestures. Speech is the motor aspect of communication. A general evalu-

Table 18-1.   Specific Cerebral Functions

Cerebral Function	Description of Test	Normal Response
Auditory recognition	The examiner instructs the client to identify familiar sounds with the eyes closed.	The client identifies familiar sounds accurately.
Auditory-verbal comprehension	The examiner asks the client to answer specific questions and carry out instructions such as "Please walk across the room."	The client responds to a series of questions and instructions with relevancy that shows understanding of what the examiner has said.
Visual recognition	The examiner asks the client to identify familiar objects such as a paper clip, pencil, or wristwatch.	The client identifies familiar objects accurately.
Visual-verbal comprehension	The examiner asks the client to read a paragraph from a newspaper and explain its meaning.	The client reads the paragraph accurately and explains its meaning, which shows understanding of what has been read.
Skilled motor act performance	The examiner instructs the client to close a safety pin, drink from a cup, and write with a pen.	The client performs a series of skilled motor acts smoothly and with ease.
Motor speech	The examiner instructs the client to imitate different sounds such as "do, ra, me, fa, so, la, te."	The client imitates different sounds distinctly and clearly.
Automatic speech	The examiner instructs the client to repeat a series learned in the past such as the days of the week or the months of the year.	The client repeats a learned series accurately.
Writing	The examiner instructs the client to write name and address, the name of a familiar object, a simple sentence, and then one word with his eyes closed and open.	The client correctly writes name and address, the name of a familiar object, a simple sentence, and one word with eyes closed and then with eyes open.

Table 18-2. Selected Sensory Recognition Abnormalities

Finding	Condition	Lobe Involvement
Inability to recognize sounds	Auditory agnosia	Temporal
Inability to recognize objects through feeling	Tactile agnosia	Parietal
Inability to recognize objects through sight	Visual agnosia	Occipital

ation of normal speech reveals a smooth stream of talk. Words are spoken clearly in distinct syllables and are consistently understandable by the examiner. Gestures reflect the spoken word and are used appropriately. The client consistently gives relevant answers to questions.

Cranial Nerves

In addition to information about the integrity of the central nervous system, evaluation of the cranial nerves gives the examiner information about the effectiveness of twelve of the most important receptors and effectors in the body. The cranial nerves are tested alone or in groups, depending on their specific functions. Both motor and sensory functions are evaluated. Several of the cranial nerve checks may be incorporated into other parts of the physical examination and do not have to be repeated unless there is some question about the client's responses (Tables 18-3 and 18-4).

Table 18-3. Cranial Nerve Function

Cranial Nerve	Description of Test	Normal Response
I. Olfactory Nerve Motor function. None. Sensory function. Mediates the sensation of olfaction (smell) high in the nasal chamber.	Motor function tests. None. Sensory function tests. Before testing the olfactory nerve, the examiner assesses the patency of both nasal passageways. The client is instructed to close one nostril with the finger and close the eyes. A familiar odor such as coffee, tea, or tobacco is placed under the open nostril. Pungent odors are not used. The client is asked to identify the odor. Each nostril is tested separately several times. (Figure 18-6)	Client accurately identifies 2 of 3 odors.
II. Optic Nerve Motor Function. None. Sensory function. Mediates the sensation of vision in the retinal layer of the eyeball.	Motor function tests. None. Sensory function tests. Visual acuity. The examiner tests visual acuity with a Snellen chart and newspaper print. If the client wears corrective lenses, the examiner tests for visual acuity with and without the lenses. Visual fields. See Chapter 7. Optic discs, vessels, retinal periphery. A neurological evaluation of the optic nerve is not complete without a thorough ophthalmoscopic examination (Chapter 7).	Chapter 7 Chapter 7 Chapter 7
III. Oculomotor Nerve Motor function. Supplies the ocular muscles that control upward, downward and medial eye movement, and elevation of the eyelid.	Motor function tests. Cranial nerves III, IV and VI are tested as one unit because they all supply muscles that control eye movements. Extraocular movements are evaluated by asking the client to follow the examiner's finger as it moves in the horizontal, vertical, and oblique directions of gaze. (Figure 18-7)	Chapter 7

Table 18-3.   Cranial Nerve Function (*continued*)

Cranial Nerve	Description of Test	Normal Response
Sensory function. Mediates the response to accommodation and light in the pupil.	Sensory function tests. The examiner darkens the room prior to examining the pupils. First, the size, shape, and equality of both pupils are assessed. The pupillary accommodation reflex is tested by asking the client to focus on a distant object and then a close object as the examiner observes for pupillary constriction. The pupillary light reflex is tested by bringing a light from the side and shining it into the eye. Each eye is tested separately. The examiner observes for both direct and consensual pupillary reflexes.	Chapter 7
IV. Trochlear Nerve		
Motor function. Supplies the ocular muscles that control downward and medial eye movement.	Motor function tests. See motor function tests for oculomotor nerve.	Chapter 7
Sensory function. None.	Sensory function tests. None.	
VI. Abducens Nerve		
Motor function. Supplies the ocular muscles that control lateral eye movement.	Motor function tests. See motor function tests for oculomotor nerve.	Chapter 7
Sensory function. None.	Sensory function tests. None.	
V. Trigeminal Nerve		
Motor function. Supplies the masseter, temporal, and diagastric muscles that control jaw movement and mastication.	Motor function tests. The examiner observes the symmetry of the client's jaw while the mouth is open. The examiner instructs the client to clamp the jaws tightly together and then palpates the masseter and temporal muscles. (Figure 18-8)	The jaw is symmetrical without deviation to one side. The masseter and temporal muscles are the same size and shape on both sides and feel firm and smooth.
Sensory function. Mediates the sensations of light pressure, pain, temperature, and vibration in the anterior half of the scalp, face, and buccal mucosa.	Sensory function tests. The examiner instructs the client to close the eyes and tests for the presence of light pressure by lightly touching a wisp of cotton to both sides of the forehead, cheeks, and jaw and asking if the client feels the sensation and if both sides are equally sensitive. The presence of pain is tested using a pinprick; temperature, using hot and cold objects; and vibration, using a vibrating tuning fork, following the same procedure. (Figure 18-9)	The client feels light pressure, a pinprick, hot and cold objects, and vibration on all areas of the forehead, cheeks, and jaw. Both sides of the face are equally sensitive.
Also mediates the corneal reflex in the cornea.	The corneal reflex is tested by touching the cornea lightly with a wisp of cotton. (The cornea, not the sclera, must be stimulated.) (Figure 18-10)	The client blinks. The response may be diminished in a client who wears contact lenses.
	The maxillary reflex (jaw jerk) is also tested. The examiner instructs the client to open the mouth slightly and then taps the center of the chin with a reflex hammer. (Figure 18-11)	Sudden, slight closing movements of the jaw.
VII. Facial Nerve		
Motor function. Supplies the muscles of the face that control facial expressions.	Motor function tests. To evaluate facial expressions the examiner instructs the client to imitate as the examiner wrinkles the forehead, smiles, frowns, raises eyebrows, looks at the ceiling, and whistles. (Figure 18-12a-d)	The client performs all facial expressions. Facial movements are symmetrical.
	Then the eyelid muscles are tested by instructing the client to close the eyes while the examiner tries to open them. (Figure 18-12e)	The client opens eyes against resistance.

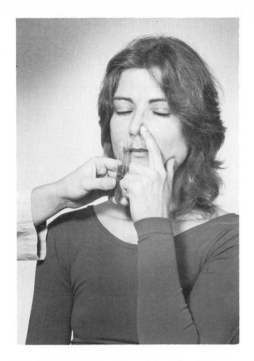

Figure 18-6. Olfactory nerve sensory function test.

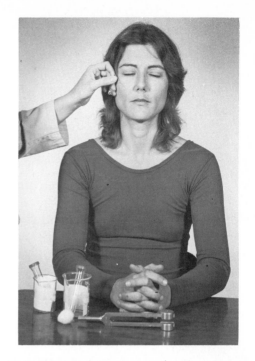

Figure 18-9. Trigeminal nerve sensory function tests.

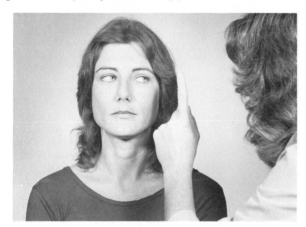

Figure 18-7. Oculomotor nerve motor function test.

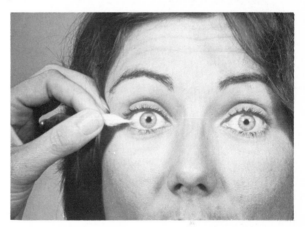

Figure 18-10. The corneal reflex.

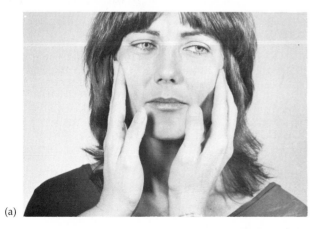

(a)

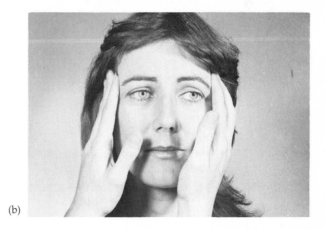

(b)

Figure 18-8. Trigeminal nerve motor function tests: (a) palpation of the masseter muscles; (b) palpation of the temporal muscles.

303

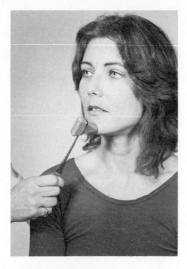

Figure 18-11. *Testing the maxillary reflex.*

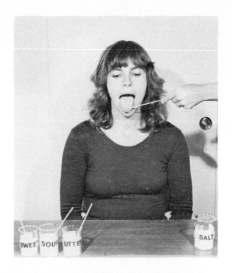

Figure 18-13. *Facial nerve sensory function tests.*

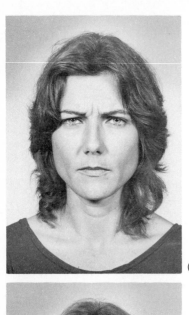

(a)

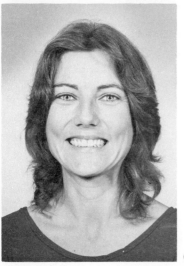

(b)

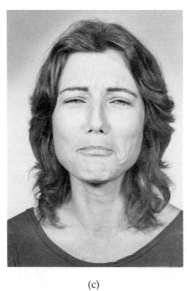

(c)

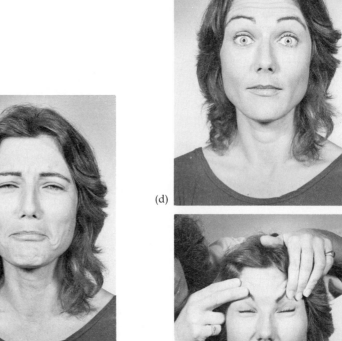

(d)

(e)

Figure 18-12. *Facial nerve motor function tests: (a) facial expression—wrinkles forehead; (b) facial expressioin—smiles; (c) facial expression—frowns; (d) facial expression—raises eyebrows; (e) eyelid muscle test.*

Table 18-3. Cranial Nerve Function (*continued*)

Cranial Nerve	Description of Test	Normal Response
Sensory function. Mediates the sensation of taste in the anterior two-thirds of the tongue.	Sensory function tests. Taste is tested by applying solutions of salt, sweet, sour, and bitter to both sides of the anterior tongue. The client is instructed to leave the tongue protruded until able to identify the taste and then take a sip of water after each application. The bitter taste is tested last since the taste remains in the mouth. (Figure 18-13)	The client accurately identifies the taste sensations of salt, sweet, sour, and bitter on both sides of the anterior tongue.
VIII. Acoustic Nerve		
Motor function. None.	Motor function tests. None.	
Sensory function. Mediates the vestibular function (equilibrium) of the vestibular apparatus in the inner ear and the auditory function (hearing) of the cochlea in the inner ear.	Sensory function tests. First, the examiner observes the auditory canal to assess the canal and drum. Tests for vestibular function are not routinely done during a physical examination. Tests for cochlear function include hearing, lateralization, and bone and air conduction (Chapter 8).	Chapter 8
IX. Glossopharyngeal Nerve	Motor function tests. Cranial nerves IX and X are tested as one unit because they are anatomically and physiologically similar.	
Motor Function.		
Supplies the pharyngeal muscles that control swallowing and the gag reflex.	The examiner inspects the soft palate for symmetry. The client is instructed to say "ah" and the examiner notes the movement of the palate. The examiner strokes one side of the soft palate with an applicator to test the palatal relfex.	Chapter 9
	The gag reflex is tested by touching each wall of the pharynx with a tongue depressor or applicator.	The palate rises and the pharyngeal muscles contract producing the gag reflex.
	The examiner tests swallowing by instructing the client to drink water and observing the swallow.	The client swallows water easily without choking or passage of water through the nose.
Sensory function. Mediates the sensation of taste on the posterior one-third of the tongue.	Sensory function tests. The presence of taste is tested following the same procedure used to test the anterior tongue. See sensory function of the facial nerve.	The client accurately identifies the taste sensations of salt, sweet, sour, and bitter on both sides of the posterior tongue.
X. Vagus Nerve		
Motor Function. Supplies muscles of the palate, pharynx, and larynx that control movement of the palate, swallowing, gag reflex, and phonation. It also supplies muscles of the thoracic and abdominal organs, and mediates heart rate, bronchial constriction, gastric secretion, and peristalsis.	Motor function tests. See motor function tests for glossopharyngeal nerve. The examiner evaluates the client's speech for clarity. The autonomic functions of the vagus are usually assessed system by system during the physical examination (Chapters 10, 11, and 13).	The client speaks clearly without hoarseness.
Sensory function. Mediates sensation in the walls of the heart, lungs, and gastrointestinal viscera.	Sensory function tests. Not done in a routine physical examination.	

Table 18-3. (*continued*)

Cranial Nerve	Description of Test	Normal Response
XI. **Accessory Nerve** Motor function. Supplies the trapezius and sternocleidomastoid muscles that control head, neck, shoulder movements and the pharyngeal muscles that control swallowing.	Motor function tests. The sternocleidomastoid and trapezius muscles are examined for symmetry, size, and shape. To test the sternocleidomastoid muscle, the client is instructed to push the head to one side against the examiner's hand. The sternocleidomastoid muscle on the opposite side is then inspected and palpated. To test the trapezius muscle, the client is instructed to shrug the shoulders against the downward resistance of the examiner's hands. The examiner then evaluates the symmetry, size, and strength of the trapezius muscle as it contracts. (Figure 18-14)	The sternocleidomastoid and the trapezius muscles on both sides are symmetrical, equal in size, and firm to palpation. The client pushes and shrugs against the examiner's hands with equal strength.
Sensory function. None.	Sensory function tests. None.	
XII. **Hypoglossal Nerve** Motor function. Supplies muscles of the tongue that control swallowing and articulation of speech sounds.	Motor function tests. The examiner evaluates the tongue for size, shape, and symmetry. The client is instructed to protrude the tongue as far as possible. The examiner observes if the tongue protrudes straight, how far it protrudes, and if it is without tremors. The client is then instructed to protrude the tongue and push it from side to side against a tongue depressor. The examiner notes the strength of the tongue movements (Figure 18-15).	Chapter 9
	Articulation is tested by instructing the client to repeat a phrase containing many words with the letters d, l, n, and t.	Speech sounds are clear and crisp. Words are recognized.
Sensory function. None.	Sensory function tests. None.	

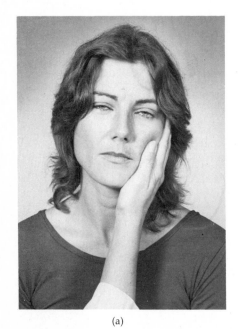
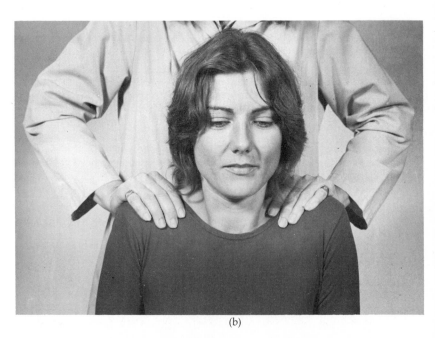

(a)

(b)

Figure 18-14. *Accessory nerve motor function tests: (a) sternocleidomastoid muscle test; (b) trapezius muscle test.*

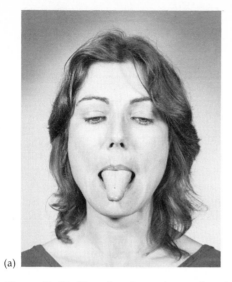 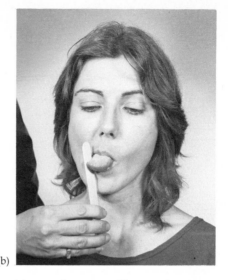

(a)   (b)

Figure 18-15. *Hypoglossal nerve motor function test: (a) protrudes tongue; (b) protrudes tongue and pushes it against a tongue depressor.*

Table 18-4.   Selected Cranial Nerve Abnormalities

Finding	Condition	Description
Loss of sense of smell	Anosmia (Cranial Nerve I)	Cannot distinguish odors; frequently not aware of condition. May be due to inflammation of nasal mucosa or lesion of olfactory bulb or tract. Distortions of smell are usually caused by lesions of the sinuses.
Weakness, atrophy of muscles of mastication	Myasthenia gravis Amyotrophic lateral sclerosis (ALS) (Cranial Nerve V)	Difficulty in chewing; unable to close mouth. In myasthenia gravis, this is due to progressive fatiguability of muscles. In ALS this is due to degeneration of the motor component of the trigeminal nerve.
Rigidity of muscles of mastication	Tetanus (Cranial Nerve V)	Rigid, sustained, tonic spasm of the jaw muscles known as "lockjaw." Frequently induced by bright lights or loud noises. Due to toxic action of Clostridium tetanii on myoneural junctions.
Severe facial pain along a branch of the trigeminal nerve	Trigeminal neuralgia (Tic Douloureux) (Cranial Nerve V)	Excruciating, paroxysmal pain; frequently involves chin and lips. Induced by cold air, shaving, chewing. Accompanied by muscle spasms, tearing, and excessive salivation. Cause felt to be arterial loops physically irritating Cranial Nerve V.
Flaccid paralysis of the face	Bell's palsy (lower motor neuron) (Cranial Nerve VII)	Cannot elevate eyebrow or wrinkle forehead. Only one eye closes when closing both eyes. Usually sudden onset. Cause unknown.
	Hemiparesis (upper motor neuron)	Can elevate eyebrow and wrinkle forehead. Eyelids close normally. Cannot show teeth or puff out cheeks.
Loss of sense of taste	Ageusia (Cranial Nerve VII)	Inability to distinguish sweet, sour, salty, and bitter tastes. May be unilateral (lesions of the tractus solitarius) or bilateral (lesions of the midpons.)
Lateral deviation of the uvula and soft palate	Vagal nerve lesion (Cranial Nerve X)	Unilateral weakness; palate and uvula deviate to the strong side because the muscles on the weak side are unopposed.
Pain in the neck and limitation of motion	Neck trauma (Cranial Nerve XI)	Fixed posture of the neck with localized swelling or tenderness upon palpation; pain on movement. May be due to injury or rupture of cervical vertebrae or soft tissues.
Lateral deviation of the head	Torticollis (Cranial Nerve XI)	Head flexed to one side; one sternocleidomastoid more prominent than the other. If chronic, face and skull may be asymmetrical. Usually congenital.
Lateral deviation of the tongue	Paralysis of the tongue (Cranial Nerve XII)	Tongue deviates toward the weak side; atrophy and fasciculations may be present. Due to unilateral nerve damage or upper motor neuron lesion.

Cerebellar and Proprioceptive Function

Testing cerebellar function involves evaluation of posture, coordination, and balance (proprioception). For the client to perform coordination and balance tests accurately, the cerebellum and its afferent and efferent pathways must be intact. In addition, the vestibular apparatus and proprioceptive mechanisms must be functioning properly. The examiner evaluates the client's ability to perform all the tests smoothly and accurately. Inability to perform any one test is not necessarily indicative of cerebellar dysfunction. (Tables 18-5 and 18-6).

Table 18-5. Cerebellar and Proprioceptive Function

Function	Description of test	Normal Response
Coordination	The examiner instructs the client to touch the finger to the nose, first with one hand and then with the other hand, with eyes open and then with eyes closed. Next the client touches the finger to the nose and then touches the examiner's finger, which is held approximately 18 inches from the client. The examiner then changes the position of the fingerwith increasing speed as the clientrepeats the movement several times with both hands.	The client touches the finger to the nose and to the examiner's finger smoothly, without tremor, and in rapid succession, accurately gauging distance. (Figure 18-16a and b)
	The client is instructed to pat the knees with the palms and backs of the hands in rapid alternating movements. The client is asked to touch each finger to the thumb of the same hand as rapidly as possible.	The client supinates and pronates the hands smoothly and at regularly timed intervals without clumsiness. The client touches each finger to the thumb smoothly and at regularly timed intervals without clumsiness. (Figure 18-16c, d, and e)
	The client is instructed to sit down and run each heel down the opposite shin, then draw a "figure eight" in the air with each foot, and finally point to the examiner's hand with each big toe.	The client runs the opposite heel down each shin, draws a "figure eight" and points to the examiner's hand with each foot in an accurate and smooth manner. (Figure 18-16f, g, and h)
Balance	The client is instructed to stand erect, feet together with eyes open and then with eyes closed. The examiner stands nearby and observes the amount of swaying, (Romberg test) (Figure 18-17a).	Some swaying is normal. A significant amount of swaying is abnormal and, if noted, the client is asked to hop on one foot and then the other. Romberg is either present or absent; present if swaying or falling increases with eyes closed.
	The client is asked to walk normally with eyes open and with eyes closed. The client is then instructed to walk in tandem fashion, placing each foot heel to toe (Figure 18-17b).	The client's gait is smooth and natural. Arm movements are coordinated with leg movements. Posture is erect. Client walks a straight line in tandem fashion balancing self. Posture is erect. Turns are smooth.
	The client is instructed to stand on one foot and then the other foot with eyes closed. (Figure 18-17c).	Client stands on each foot for approximately 5 seconds without losing balance. Posture is erect.

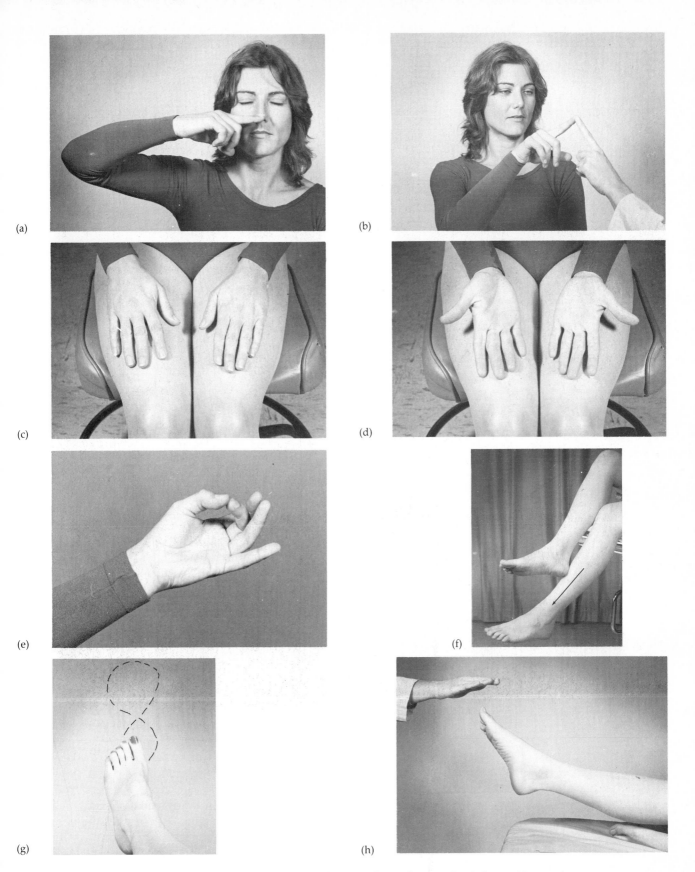

Figure 18-16. *Coordination testing: (a) touches nose; (b) touches examiner's finger; (c) pronation of hands; (d) supination of hands; (e) touches each finger to the thumb; (f) runs heel down shin; (g) draws a figure 8; (h) points to examiner's hand with the foot.*

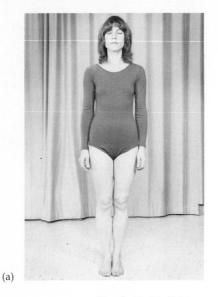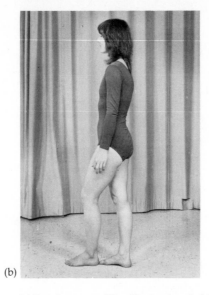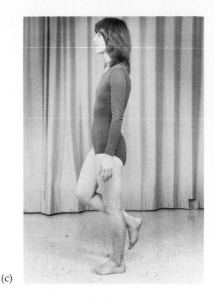

Figure 18-17. *Balance testing: (a) Romberg test; (b) walks tandem fashion; (c) stands on one foot with eyes closed.*

Table 18-6. Selected Cerebellar and Proprioceptive Abnormalities

Finding	Condition	Description
Wide-based, uncoordinated, rigid gait	Ataxia (cerebellar gait)	History of falling frequently; tends to stagger and lurch when walking; not alleviated by visual orientation. Cerebellar disorder due to impairment of position sense.
Illusion of environment whirling	Vertigo (vestibular dysfunction)	Usually accompanied by nausea and vomiting. No motion felt with eyes closed. May have nystagmus. Due to vestibular disease.
Unsteady, weak, vague feeling of turning	Dizziness (proprioceptive dysfunction)	Sense of disturbed relation to space, frequently difficult to describe. No sense of environment whirling. Has many causes other than proprioceptive disorders.

Motor System

Tests for motor system function include inspection of muscle size, tone, strength, symmetry, contour, and involuntary muscle movements. Muscles are palpated for consistency and percussed for irritability or myotonia. Muscles and joints are put through active and passive range of motion with and without resistance. (Chapter 17).

Sensory System

Testing the sensory system involves assessing the sensory function of the peripheral nerves. The primary forms of sensation include light touch, superficial pain, temperature, vibration, deep pressure pain, motion and position. Only light touch, pain, position, and vibration are done routinely. The discriminatory sensations include two-point discrimination, point localization, texture discrimination, stereognostic function, graphesthesia, and extinction phenomenon.

The client keeps the eyes closed for all the tests. The forehead, cheeks, hands, forearms, upper arms, trunk, feet, lower legs, thighs, and perineal and perianal areas are tested. In testing the extremities the examiner usually begins distally and proceeds proximally (Table 18-7). Throughout the assessment, the examiner uses uniform intensity while applying stimuli to corresponding sites, and compares the ability to perceive sensation on both sides of the body and extremities. The stimuli are applied systematically to various sites at different times to prevent the client from learning a pattern of responses. It is important for the examiner to keep in mind that a decrease in sensation (hypoesthesia) occurs more often than an absence of sensation (anesthesia).

It is difficult to evaluate sensory testing because of the subjective nature of the sensations and the preconceived, culturally influenced responses by the client. If sensory changes are present, the examiner notes and maps their location. Distribution may be unilateral, bilateral, dermatomal, or peripheral (Table 18-8).

Table 18-7.   Sensory System

Sensation	Description of Test	Normal Response
Primary Forms of Sensation		
Light touch	The examiner lightly touches a wisp of cotton to the skin and instructs the client to say "yes" when the sensation is perceived. The examiner compares the sensitivity of both sides of the body and of the distal parts of the extremities with the proximal parts. (Figure 18-18)	The client says "yes" each time sensation is perceived.
Superficial pain	The examiner lightly touches the point of a pin to the skin and follows the method described above.	The client says "yes" with each pinprick. Intensity of the prick is the same in all areas.
Temperature	Test tubes containing hot and cold water are touched to the skin. The client is instructed to indicate whether the sensation is "hot" or "cold." The rest of the procedure is the same as the preceding. It is not necessary to test temperature sensation if superficial pain sensation is present.	The client says "hot" and "cold" accurately with each sensation.
Vibration	The examiner touches a vibrating tuning fork to bony prominences at the wrist, shoulder, ankle, shin, knee, and hip. The client is instructed to say "yes" when the vibration is first perceived and "now" when the vibration stops. Sensitivity is compared on both sides of the body and on distal and proximal areas of the extremities.	The client accurately indicates the beginning and end of the vibratory sensation at each bony prominence tested. The intensity of the vibration is the same for all areas of the body.
Deep pressure pain	The examiner applies pressure to the superolateral aspect of the eye orbit and squeezes the Achilles tendon, calf, and forearm muscles. The client indicates the presence of sensitivity as preceding. (Figure 18-19)	The client says "yes" each time pressure is applied.
Motion and position	The examiner passively moves the fingers and toes in different directions. The client is asked to identify the direction of movement of the fingers and toes including the final position. (Figure 18-20)	The client accurately indicates the direction of movement and final position of the fingers and toes.
Cortical and Discriminatory Forms of Sensation		
Two-point discrimination	The examiner touches various parts of the body with two sharp points (calipers) simultaneously. The client is asked to indicate whether one or two points are felt. The examiner can vary the distance between the two points.	The client indicates that two points are felt at all areas touched.
Point localization	The examiner asks the client to locate the spot touched. The examiner touches the arms, legs, abdomen, and trunk.	The client accurately locates all areas touched.
Texture discrimination	The examiner places familiar materials, such as cotton, wool, and corduroy, in the client's hands for identification. (Figure 18-21)	The client identifies the materials correctly by feel.
Stereognostic function	The examiner places familiar objects, such as a key, paper clip, and button, in the client's hands for identification.	The client identifies the objects correctly by feel.
Graphesthesia	The examiner draws letters and numbers with a blunt object on the palms of the client's hands, on the back, and on other parts of the body. The client is asked to identify the letters and numbers. Both sides are compared. (Figure 18-22)	The client accurately identifies the letters and numbers on both sides of the body.
Extinction phenomenon	The examiner touches two points simultaneously on corresponding sides of the body. The client is asked to indicate that the sensation is on one or both sides.	The client indicates sensation on both sides.

Table 18-8. Selected Sensory System Abnormalities

Findings	Condition	Description
Bilateral sensory loss of the lower extremities	Peripheral neuropathy	May be accompanied by paresthesias, weakness, lower extremity pain. Usually diminished deep tendon reflexes and vibratory sensation. Frequently due to diabetes mellitus.
	Spinal cord abnormality	Similar to peripheral neuropathy with paresthesias, weakness, pain; reflexes usually increased; bladder function often involved.
Loss of discriminatory sensation	Lesion of the cortex	May be accompanied by loss of motion and position sense and loss of stereognosis. Lesions of the cortex are due to vascular impairment, tumors, or trauma.

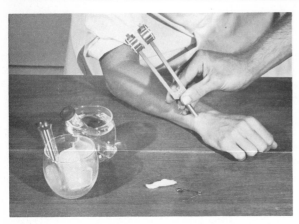

Figure 18-18. Sensation testing for light touch, superficial pain, temperature, and vibration.

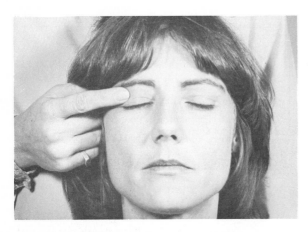

Figure 18-19. Sensation testing for deep pressure pain.

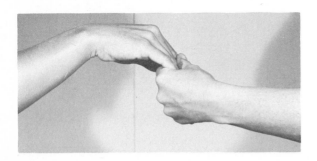

Figure 18-20. Sensation testing for motion and position.

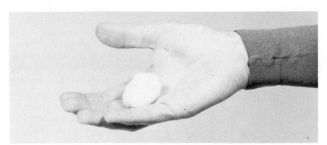

Figure 18-21. Sensation testing for texture discrimination.

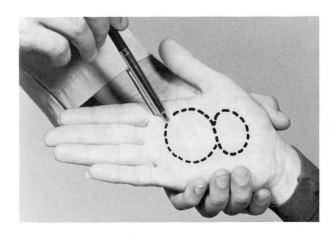

Figure 18-22. Graphesthesia.

Reflexes

Reflexes are important from the standpoint that a reflex response deviating from normal frequently indicates neurological pathology. Thus, the evaluation of reflex activity is a valuable tool in the assessment of nervous system function.

During this part of the neurological assessment, the examiner tests both deep tendon and superficial reflexes. Deep tendon reflexes are lower motor neuron reflexes. Testing deep tendon reflexes provides the examiner with information about the integrity and function of the reflex arcs and spinal cord centers without the influence of higher centers in the brain. Superficial reflexes, on the other hand, reflect upper motor neuron function, from which they receive facilitation. Testing superficial reflexes gives the examiner information about the integrity of the upper motor neurons, from the cortex through the spinal cord.

To test the deep tendon reflexes (DTRs), the client is first instructed to relax the part of the body being tested. The limb is then positioned so that the involved muscle is slightly stretched. The examiner supports the limb loosely and then taps briskly but firmly on the tendon or bony prominence with a rubber reflex hammer. This stimulus normally causes the muscle suddenly to stretch further; the normal response is a slight contraction of the muscle. The stimulus is always applied with equal intensity to corresponding symmetrically positioned parts of the body (Tables 18-9 and 18-12).

Table 18-9.   Deep Tendon Reflexes

Reflex	CNS level	Description of Test	Normal Response
Biceps	Cervical 5,6 (Primarily C5)	The examiner places the client's arm over the opposite forearm and holds client's elbow. The client is instructed to relax the arm completely. The examiner places the thumb at the insertion of the biceps tendon superior to the antecubital fossa and taps the thumbnail with the narrow rubber end of the reflex hammer. (Figure 18-23)	Contraction of the biceps muscle resulting in slight flexion of the forearm at the elbow joint. Normally the examiner sees or feels a slight jerk of the biceps muscle.
Brachioradialis	Cervical 5, 6 (Primarily C6)	The examiner supports the client's arm in the same manner used to test the biceps reflex. The styloid process of the radius is located proximal to the wrist. The examiner taps the process with the flat rubber end of the reflex hammer. (Figure 18-24)	Slight flexion of the elbow joint and pronation of the forearm. Slight flexion of the fingers and hand may also occur.
Triceps	Cervical 6,7, 8 (Primarily C7)	The examiner supports the client's arm in the same manner used to test the biceps reflex. The examiner taps at the insertion of the triceps tendon superior to the olecranon with the narrow rubber end of the reflex hammer. (Figure 18-25)	Contraction of the triceps muscle, resulting in extension of the arm at the elbow joint.
Patellar	Lumbar 2,3,4 (Primarily L4)	The examiner instructs the client to sit on the edge of the examining table with the legs dangling free, palpates the soft tissue depression on both sides of the patellar tendon, taps the tendon with the flat rubber end of the reflex hammer. (Figure 18-26)	Contraction of the quadriceps muscle, resulting in extension of the leg at the knee joint.
Achilles	Sacral 1, 2 (primarily S1)	With the client sitting on the edge of the table with the legs dangling, the examiner dorsiflexes the foot slightly. The insertion of the Achilles tendon is located by palpating the soft tissue depressions on both sides of it. The tendon is then tapped with the flat rubber end of the reflex hammer. (Figure 18-27)	Contraction of the triceps surrae muscle, resulting in plantar flexion of the foot.

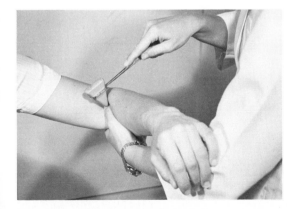

Figure 18-23. Biceps reflex testing.

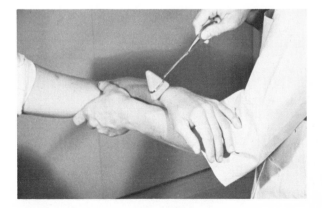

Figure 18-24. Brachioradialis reflex testing.

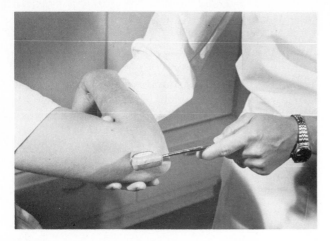

Figure 18-25. *Triceps reflex testing.*

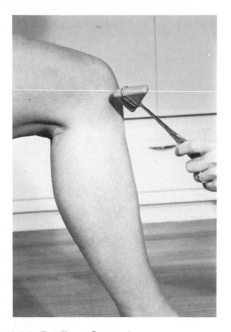

Figure 18-26. *Patellar reflex testing.*

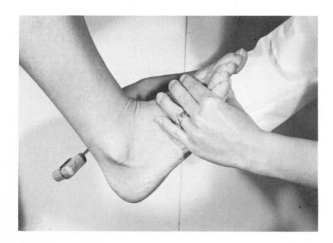

Figure 18-27. *Achilles reflex testing.*

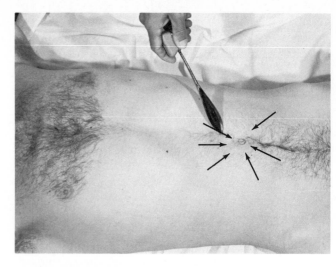

Figure 18-28. *Abdominal reflex testing.*

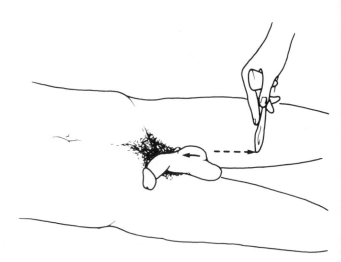

Figure 18-29. *Cremasteric reflex testing.*

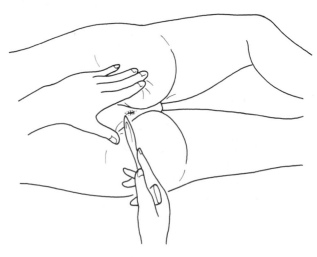

Figure 18-30. *Glutal reflex testing.*

314

Table 18-10. Superficial Reflexes

Reflex	CNS Level	Description of Test	Normal Response
Upper abdominal	Thoracic 7, 8, 9	The client lies supine. With the handle end of the reflex hammer, the examiner strokes the skin from the upper abdominal quadrants toward the umbilicus observing the movement of the umbilicus (Figure 18-28).	Umbilicus moves up and toward area being stroked. Slight abdominal muscle contraction observable.
Lower abdominal	Thoracic 11, 12	The client lies supine. With the handle end of the reflex hammer, the examiner strokes the skin from the lower abdominal quadrants toward the umbilicus observing the movement of the umbilicus (Figure 18-28).	Umbilicus moves down and toward area being stroked. Slight abdominal muscle contraction observable.
Cremasteric (males)	Thoracic 12 Lumbar 1,2	With the client supine, the examiner strokes the medial side of the upper thigh using the handle end of the reflex hammer (Figure 18-29).	Contraction of the cremaster muscle, which pulls the scrotal sac upward on the side stroked.
Gluteal	Sacral 3, 4, 5	With the client lying prone, the examiner separates the buttocks and strokes the perianal skin with the handle end of the reflex hammer (Figure 18-30).	Contraction of the external and anal sphincter muscles.
Plantar	Sacral 1, 2	The examiner runs the handle end of the reflex hammer from the heel of the foot up the lateral border of the sole, turning medially and going across the ball of the foot underneath the great toe (Figures 18-31 and 32).	Flexion of the toes. Prior to the age a child walks, the normal response is extension and fanning of the toes.

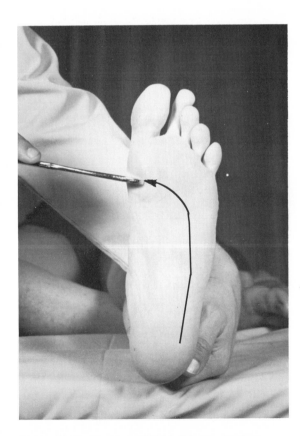

Figure 18-31. Plantar and Babinski reflex testing.

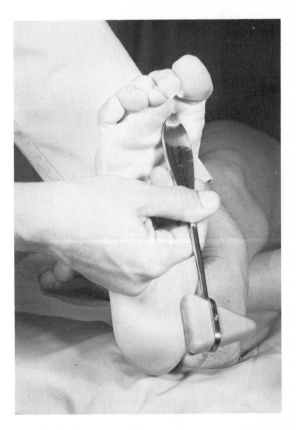

Figure 18-32. Positive plantar reflex.

315

Deep tendon reflexes are assessed for presence or absence, strength and rapidity. They are graded on a scale of 0 to 4+:

0—absent; no response is elicited; may be indicative of disease.

1+—slightly diminished; below normal response is elicited.

2+—normal; average response is elicited.

3+—stronger or brisker than normal response is elicited; not necessarily indicative of disease.

4+—very brisk; hyperactive response is elicited; associated with clonus; frequently indicative of disease.

When reflexes are absent or slightly diminished, a method known as reinforcement is used to increase reflex activity. The client is instructed to contract isometrically those muscles of the body not being tested. For example, the client is asked to clench the teeth, clench the fists, or hook the fingers together of both hands and pull. The reflex is then tested in the usual manner.

The superficial reflexes require stimulation of the skin. The client is instructed to relax, and the examiner strokes the skin with the handle of the reflex hammer. Enough moderately sharp pressure is exerted on the handle to depress the skin. Superficial reflexes are also assessed for presence or absence, strength, and rapidity (Table 18-10).

Several reflexes, if elicited, are often considered to be indicative of pathology. These include the Babinski reflex, Gordon's reflex, the grasp reflex, and the finger flexor reflex (Table 18-11).

Table 18-11. Pathological Reflexes

Reflex	Description of Test	Abnormal Response
Babinski	The examiner stimulates the sole of the client's foot with the method described for eliciting the plantar reflex.	Extension (dorsiflexion) of the great toe with fanning of the other toes. This may be a normal response prior to 18 months of age. The Babinski sign is present or absent. (Figure 18-33)
Gordon's	The examiner firmly squeezes the client's calf muscles on both legs.	Extension (dorsiflexion) of the great toe with fanning of the other toes. (Figure 18-34)
Grasp	The examiner places the index and middle fingers on the palm of the client's hand between the thumb and index finger and draws the fingers across the client's palm.	The client grasps the examiner's fingers with the fingers. (Figure 18-35 a and b)
Finger flexor	The examiner depresses and then releases the client's distal phalanx.	Flexion of the thumb and other finger. (Figure 18-36)

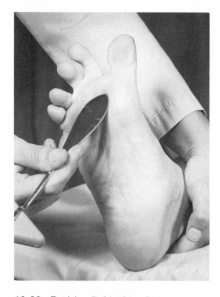

Figure 18-33. *Positive Babinski reflex.*

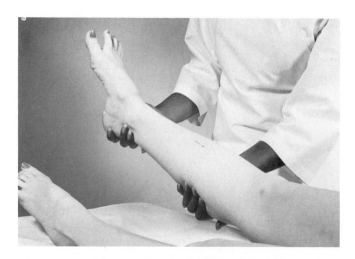

Figure 18-34. *Positive Gordon's reflex.*

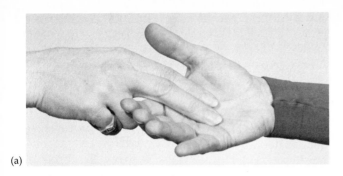

(a)

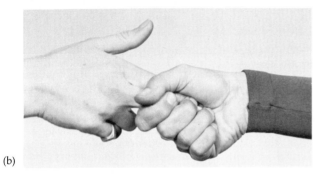

(b)

Figure 18-35. *Grasp reflex: (a) testing for grasp reflex; (b) positive grasp reflex.*

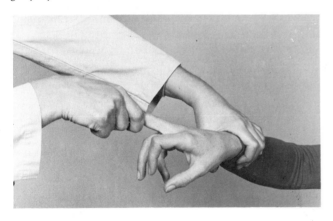

Figure 18-36 *Positive finger flexor reflex.*

Life Cycle Variations

Childhood

At birth the spinal nerves are fully myelinated, mature, and functioning. The cerebral cortex, brain stem, and spinal cord, however, are not fully myelinated. As the child grows, myelinization of the nervous system progresses in a cephalocaudal, proximodistal direction.

All nervous system tissues grow rapidly during early childhood. By the end of the first year the child has all the brain cells. These cells continue to grow in size and complexity; by the age of two the child's brain has reached 90 percent of its mature size. Throughout the rest of childhood there is a slow, steady increase in neural tissue growth until the child reaches maturity.

The special senses—taste, smell, touch, hearing, and vision—are well-developed at birth. The integration of these senses with higher cerebral cortex centers is still immature, however, and develops gradually over a period of years. The senses of taste and smell are, perhaps, most discriminating at birth. The sense of touch is first developed during infancy and is followed by the development of hearing and vision.

The development of vision during childhood is an excellent example of neural growth. During infancy, the child perceives simple shapes. The ability to perceive differences in complex shapes develops over a period of years. Accommodation begins at approximately nine months of age; changes in refraction continue to occur over the life span. The tendency toward hyperopia increases until the age of eight, when the

Table 18-12. Selected Reflex Abnormalities

Findings	Condition	Description
Diminished or absent deep tendon reflexes	Lower motor neuron lesion	
	Peripheral neuropathy myopathy	Usually accompanied by muscle weakness and atrophy.
	Tabes dorsalis	Absent deep tendon reflexes with loss of sensation on the same side. Reduction of reflex may result from lesion of sensory (afferent) or motor (efferent) arc or reflex.
Hyperactive deep tendon reflexes, diminished superficial reflexes, and present Babinski sign.	Upper motor neuron lesion Pyramidal tract lesion Stroke, tumor of brain or spinal cord	
	Amyotrophic lateral sclerosis Trauma to brain or spinal cord	Usually accompanied by hemiparesis and expressive or receptive aphasia.

eyeball has reached its adult size. At that time emmetropia occurs. By the end of the first year, eye muscle movements are fully developed.

Deep tendon and superficial reflexes are normally present in the infant, though they may be variable. Several infant reflexes are present and normal at birth and disappear within a few months to a couple of years. Normal infant reflexes are discussed in detail in Table 18-13.

Intellectual, emotional, social, and motor development proceed in an orderly fashion during the first five years of childhood as the nervous system myelinizes and matures. Neural development during the first five years is summarized in Table 18-13 and Appendix 10 and 11.

Table 18-13.   Infant Reflexes

Reflex	Testing Procedure	Normal Response
Rooting	With the infant supine, the examiner holds the head in the midline and the hands against the chest. With the other hand, the examiner strokes the perioral skin at the corners of the mouth.	Infant turns head toward the stimulus and opens mouth. Present from birth to approximately 4 months while awake and 7 months while asleep. (Figure 18-37a)
Sucking	With the infant supine, the examiner places a nipple or a finger 3 to 4 centimeters into the mouth.	Infant immediately begins vigorous, rhythmical sucking. Present from birth to approximately 4 months while awake and 7 months while asleep. (Figure 18-37b)
Tonic neck	With the infant supine, the examiner slowly turns the infant's head to one side and holds it for a few seconds. After response is illicited, the procedure is repeated for the other side.	Infant assumes the "fencing" position: arm and leg on side to which head is turned extend, while opposite arm and leg flex. Present from birth to approximately 6 months. (Figure 18-37c)
Moro	With the infant supine, the examiner elevates the head a few centimeters off the examining surface. After the infant's head relaxes, the examiner suddenly releases the head and allows it to fall back onto the examiner's hand. Can also be illicited by producing a sudden loud noise or by jarring the examining surface.	Infant extends arms and fingers and flexes hips and knees slightly. Present from birth to approximately 4 months. (Figure 18-37d)
Palmar grasp	With the infant supine, the examiner places a finger into the infant's hand and presses the palmar surface.	Infant flexes all of the fingers around the examiner's finger. Present from birth to approximately 4 months. (Figure 18-37e)
Placing	Examiner holds the infant upright with the dorsum of one foot lightly touching the under edge of the examining table.	Infant simultaneously flexes hips and knees while the foot is placed on top of the table. Present from birth to approximately 6 weeks. (Figure 18-37f)
Stepping	Examiner holds the infant upright with the soles of the feet lightly touching a flat surface.	Infant "walks" forward. Present from birth to approximately 6 weeks. (Figure 18-37g)
Spontaneous crawling (Bauer's response)	With the infant prone, the examiner presses lightly on the soles of the feet.	Infant makes crawling movements which are increased with pressure on the feet. Present from birth. (Figure 18-37h)
Plantar grasp	With the infant supine, the examiner places thumbs against the balls of the infant's feet near the toes.	Infant flexes all toes. Present from birth to approximately 12 months. (Figure 18-37i)
Babinski	With the infant supine and legs semiflexed, the examiner scratches the sole of the foot along the lateral aspect, beginning at the heel and scratching toward the toes.	Infant fans the toes. Present from birth until myelinization is completed. (Figure 18-37j)

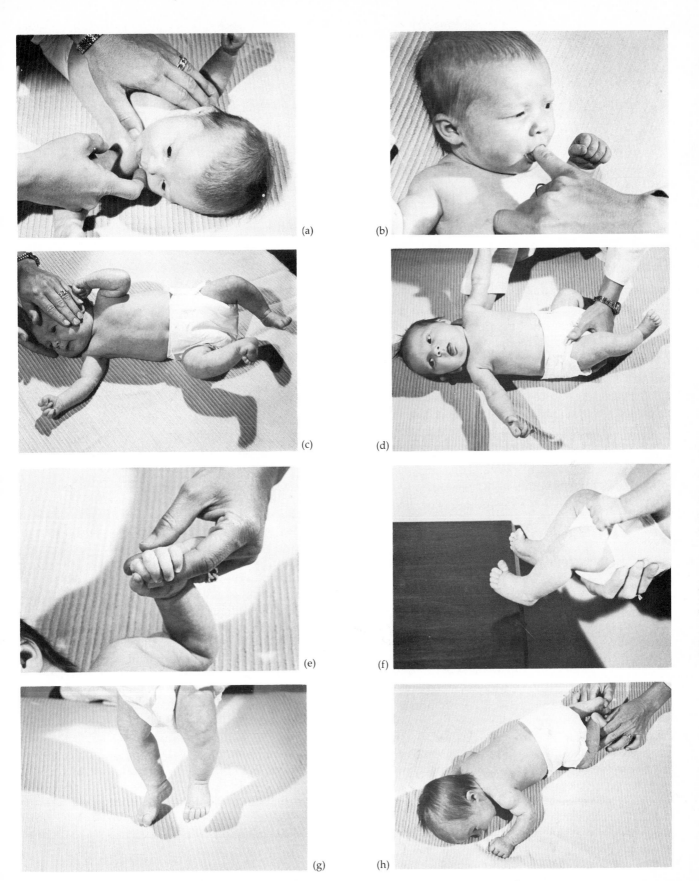

Figure 18-37. *Infant reflexes: (a) rooting reflex; (b) sucking reflex; (c) tonic neck reflex; (d) Moro reflex; (e) palmar grasp reflex; (f) placing reflex; (g) stepping reflex; (h) spontaneous crawling reflex.*

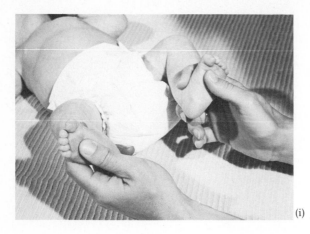
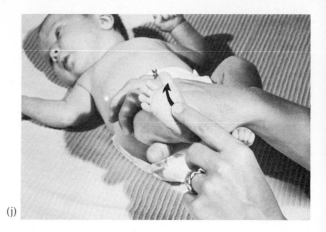

(i)   (j)

Figure 18-37 (continued): (i) plantar grasp reflex; (j) Babinski reflex.

Late Adulthood

The changes in the structure and function of the nervous system as the adult matures are many and varied. Significant facts about aging and the nervous system are as follows:

1. The weight of the brain decreases due to a decrease in the number and size of viable neurons.

2. The functions of the brain are maintained with use.

3. Demyelinization of nerve axons increases and the speed of nerve impulses decreases.

4. Muscle action and reaction time slow down.

5. Sensory nerves degenerate faster than motor nerves.

6. Taste, hearing, and vision become less discriminatory.

With aging, the cognitive processes of the cerebral cortex show a slight decline. There is little decrease in basic intelligence and learning ability. Changes in learning performance are usually due to faulty perception, shortened attention span, decreased motivation, and declining physical health. The more irrelevant information the older adult has to sort, the more the learning performance declines. To test the capacity to learn, the older adult must be given information in a concise, clear, and meaningful manner.

Changes in memory also occur in the older adult. Short-term memory declines slightly, and there is usually a significant decrease in long-term memory. However, the ability to recall past events is usually unimpaired.

Degenerative changes in the sensory system are significant and frequently lead to misperceptions of the environment. Illusions and hallucinations are frequently faulty perceptions of surrounding stimuli and not signs of mental illness or organic brain changes.

Hearing loss is a major sensory deficit of aging. The number of receptor cells in the cochlea decrease with age; the ability to hear high-pitched sounds is gradually lost. This change seems to occur more frequently in men than in women.

Visual acuity declines significantly after 50 years of age. The function of the rods decreases; the older person has more difficulty adapting to the dark and distinguishing light intensities. In addition, the pupil is smaller, and less light hits the retina. Finally, with advancing age the lens starts to yellow and causes the retina to be less sensitive to blue light.

The number of taste buds decreases, particularly those responsible for sweet sensations. Atrophy of the olfactory nerve fibers frequently causes a decrease in the sense of smell.

The sense of touch is diminished, and frequently the elderly need more intense and varied stimulation to feel objects. The sensation of pain may also be diminished in some individuals, although this is difficult to evaluate. Many older adults live with chronic pain and accept it as part of "growing old." Others deny the existence of pain because of the fear of what it may mean. Because of the subjective component of pain, changes in pain sensitivity in later adulthood are not clear.

Reflex activity in the healthy adult is normal; all deep tendon and superficial reflexes are present. Some elderly individuals may have slightly diminished deep tendon reflexes, which is still considered within the normal range. Absent ankle jerks in patients over 70 are not considered pathological unless associated with other signs and symptoms.

The hematologic system includes the bone marrow, circulating blood, lymph nodes, spleen (Chapter 13), and fixed tissue macrophages. This system has diverse functions such as oxygen transport (red blood cells), blood coagulation (platelets), inflammation (white blood cells), and immune response (lymphocytes and plasma cells).

Chapter 19

Assessment of the Blood and Lymph Nodes

Bone Marrow and Circulating Blood Cells

The bone marrow, one of the largest organs in the body, is the principal site for blood cell formation. The cells produced by the bone marrow include the red blood cells (erythrocytes), platelets, and white blood cells (leukocytes). In the adult, active bone marrow is found in the vertebral bodies, ribs, skull, sternum, pelvis, and proximal humerus and femur. The bone marrow is also a major organ involved in antibody synthesis and in the recognition and removal of aging and abnormal red blood cells. Under certain pathologic conditions, blood cell formation can occur in the liver and spleen; this is termed extramedullary hematopoiesis.

The functions of the erythrocyte are to transport oxygen from the lungs to the tissues, and carbon dioxide from the tissues to the lungs. The red blood cell is a non-nucleated biconcave disc. It is filled with hemoglobin, a complex protein to which oxygen and carbon dioxide are bound. The erythrocyte also contains complex enzyme systems, which provide energy and maintain hemoglobin in a functional state. Hemoglobin concentration varies with age (Table 19-1). Oxygen diffuses from the alveolar gas into the erythrocyte, binds to hemoglobin, and is carried to the peripheral capillaries. There it diffuses into the interstitial fluid and thus into the tissues. Carbon dioxide diffuses from the tissues, binds directly with hemoglobin for transport to the lungs, diffuses into the alveoli, and is exhaled.

Platelets are formed in the bone marrow and circulate in the peripheral blood. They have two major functions in blood coagulation: the formation of an initial plug in a hole in a vessel wall and provision of the phospholipid necessary for blood coagulation.

There are three types of white blood cells (leukocytes): granulocytes, monocytes, and lymphocytes. The total number of leukocytes and the percentage of each specific type present (differential count) vary with age (Table 19-1). Granulocytes are subdivided into neutrophils, basophils, and eosinophils. The

Objectives

The examiner will be able to do the following:

1. Recognize abnormalities in the complete blood count and coagulation testing
2. Palpate regional lymph nodes
3. Record the information obtained

Table 19-1. Normal Leukocyte Count, Differential Count, and Hemoglobin Concentration at Various Ages

PERCENTAGE OF TOTAL

TOTAL LEUKOCYTES (X10³/mm₃)			NEUTROPHILS		
AGE	MEAN	RANGE	TOTAL	BAND	SEGMENTED
Birth	18.1	9-30	61	9	52
Week 1	12.2	5-21	45	7	39
Month 12	11.4	6-18	31	3	28
Year 4	9.1	6-16	42	3	39
Year 6	8.5	5-15	51	3	48
Year 10	8.1	5-14	54	3	51
Year 14	7.9	5-13	56	3	53
Year 18	7.7	5-13	57	3	54
Year 21	7.4	5-11	59	3	56

AGE	EOSINOPHILS	BASOPHILS	LYMPHOCYTES	MONOCYTES	HEMOGLOBIN (g/100 ml. blood) MEAN	RANGE	
Birth	2	0.6	31	6	19.3	17-21	
Week 1	4	0.4	41	9	17.9	15-20	
Month 12	3	0.4	61	5	11.6	9-15	
Year 4	3	0.6	50	5	12.6	10-16	
Year 6	2	0.6	42	5	12.7	10-16	
Year 10	3	0.5	38	4	13.0	11-16	
Year 14	2	0.5	37	5			
Year 18	3	0.5	35	5			
Year 21	3	0.5	34	4	15.8	14-18	(Male)
					13.9	12-16	(Female)

neutrophils protect against most bacterial infections by migrating to the invading organism, ingesting it, and destroying it. The basophil is believed to play a part in immediate hypersensitivity reactions and allergic disorders. The exact function of the eosinophil is not known, although it shares most of the responses of the neutrophil to bacteria; in addition, it is strongly associated with immune complexes, allergic disorders, and parasite infestations.

The monocyte originates in the bone marrow, spends a short period in the peripheral blood, and enters the tissue, where it fulfills its major function as a macrophage. These tissue macrophages are phagocytic cells and serve in protective reactions against certain microorganisms, remove damaged or dying cells and cellular debris, and interact with lymphoid cells in certain stages of immunologic reactions.

There are two major classes of lymphocytes, which are functionally different but morphologically similar. The first are the B-lymphocytes and B-memory cells, which are involved in immediate hypersensitivity reactions. Upon activation they proliferate rapidly, and differentiate into specific antibody-producing cells and plasma cells. The B-memory cells have a long life span, recirculate in the peripheral blood, and are essential in the anamnestic response to antigen stimulation. The anamnestic response is a shortening of the time required for antibody formation and is the basis of immunization in booster shots. This can occur because several of the antigen-processing steps are eliminated when the B-memory cells are activated. The second group are the T-lymphocytes; they function primarily in delayed hypersensitivity reactions in the defense against certain microorganisms (such as tuberculosis), viruses, and protozoa, and in transplantation and tumor immunity.

Lymph Nodes

Lymph nodes are complex structures that have evolved as sites of interaction between antigens and fixed cells within the lymph nodes (Figure 19-1). Antigens are substances that the body recognizes as foreign; they are carried by draining lymph and circulating blood cells. The lymph enters the lymph node by numerous afferent lymphatic vessels, which pierce

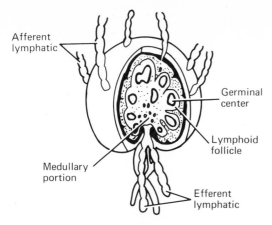

Figure 19-1. Structure of a lymph node.

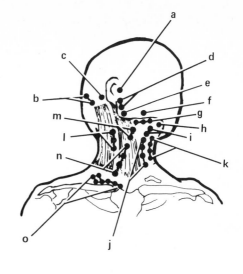

the convex side of the capsule, and courses through the node. It exits via a single efferent vessel at the hilum of the node. The center of the lymphoid follicles contains large lymphocytes, macrophages, and plasma cells and is termed the *germinal center*. Lymphocytes enter the node via hilar blood vessels, pass through the blood vessel lining, transverse the node, and exit via the efferent lymphatics. Upon antigenic stimulation, the cellular elements of the lymph node proliferate, which causes it to become enlarged and sometimes tender. This is referred to as reactive hyperplasia.

The major lymph node bearing areas of the body are depicted in Figure 19-2. Lymph from portions of the body distal to the lymph node drains through the lymph nodes before it returns to the blood via the thoracic duct and superior vena cava. When foreign organisms or substances are present in lymphatic drainage, the lymphoid system recognizes them and initiates an immunologic response.

Blood Coagulation

Blood coagulation is the process by which damaged blood vessel walls are repaired and the integrity of the vascular system is restored. It can be thought of as a cascade sequence (Figure 19-3). Plasma coagulation

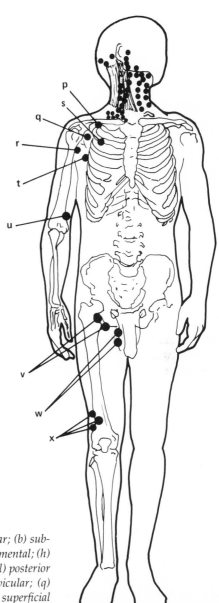

Figure 19-2. Distribution of the major lymph-node-bearing areas: (a) preauricular; (b) suboccipital; (c) postauricular; (d) parotid; (e) retropharyngeal; (f) suprahyoid; (g) submental; (h) submandibular; (i) thyrolinguofacial; (j) internal jugular; (k) deep cervical chain; (l) posterior cervical; (m) tonsillar; (n) superficial cervical; (o) supraclavicular; (p) infraclavicular; (q) intermediate; (r) brachial; (s) mammary; (t) scapular; (u) epitrochlear; (v) superior superficial inguinal; (w) inferior superficial inguinal; (x) posterior popliteal.

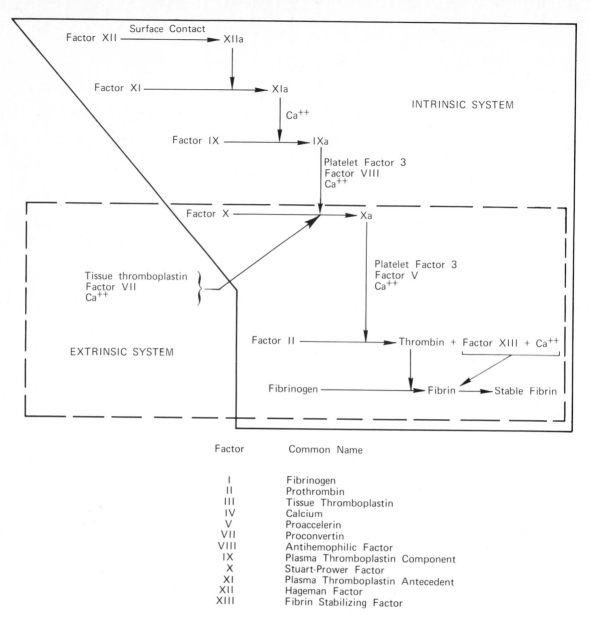

Factor	Common Name
I	Fibrinogen
II	Prothrombin
III	Tissue Thromboplastin
IV	Calcium
V	Proaccelerin
VII	Proconvertin
VIII	Antihemophilic Factor
IX	Plasma Thromboplastin Component
X	Stuart-Prower Factor
XI	Plasma Thromboplastin Antecedent
XII	Hageman Factor
XIII	Fibrin Stabilizing Factor

Figure 19-3. Cascade sequence of blood coagulation.

factors circulate as inactive proteins, which are sequentially converted into active proteins during clotting. This process causes the formation of a fibrin clot. This fibrin clot is the primary mechanism by which the body repairs defects in blood vessel walls. The coagulation of blood can occur via either of two pathways. The intrinsic system describes coagulation resulting from the activation of the plasma coagulation factors by surface contact. This primarily occurs upon exposure of tissue in blood vessel walls when they are damaged. The extrinsic system describes clotting in which the initial step involves release of tissue thromboplastin. Since thromboplastin is a substance present in the tissues, it is extrinsic to the circulation.

Tissue thromboplastin is released with tissue injury of almost any kind.

Assessment Modalities

Preparation

The major modalities for evaluating the hematologic system are laboratory testing and palpation of the spleen (Chapter 13) and regional lymph nodes. In addition, inspection of the skin, mouth, and eyes contributes to the assessment (Table 19-2). The client is

Table 19-2. Selected Abnormalities of Skin, Mouth, and Eye Appearance

Finding	Condition	Explanation for Finding
Pallor	Anemia (decreased hemoglobin level)	Decreased blood flow through skin and conjunctival capillaries.
Cyanosis	Excess unsaturated hemoglobin (chronic lung disease, right-to-left cardiac shunts)	Unsaturated hemoglobin is bluer than oxygenated hemoglobin.
Jaundice	Hemolytic anemia (abnormal breakdown of red blood cells)	The breakdown of red blood cells releases hemoglobin, which is converted into bilirubin, and this stains the skin and sclera a yellowish color.
Petechiae and ecchymoses	Thrombocytopenia	Hemorrhage into the skin due to decreased platelets.
Excoriation	Hodgkin's disease	Intense itching, but cause is not known.
Leg ulcers	Sickle cell anemia	Probably due to thrombosis of skin capillaries.
Plethora	Polycythemia	Increased blood flow through the skin.

disrobed and draped, and the examiner explains the need for venipuncture for laboratory testing.

Laboratory Testing

The two most valuable laboratory testing devices are the complete blood count (CBC) and coagulation studies.

Complete Blood Count. The complete blood count usually includes the following tests: (1) white blood cell count (WBC)—total number of leukocytes/milliliter; (2) hemoglobin (Hgb)—weight of hemoglobin/milliliter; (3) red blood cell count (RBC)—total number of red blood cells/milliliter; (4) hematocrit (Hct)—percentage of blood comprised of red blood cells; (5) mean corpuscular volume (MCV)—average size of each red blood cell; (6) mean hemoglobin concentration (MCH)—average amount of hemoglobin/red blood cell; and (7) mean corpuscular hemoglobin concentration (MCHC)—average percentage of each red blood cell that is hemoglobin. The platelet count is also often included; it enumerates the number of platelets/milliliter. The differential white count enumerates the percentages of leukocytes that are segmented neutrophils, band neutrophils, lymphocytes, monocytes, eosinophils, and basophils. These are the only cells normally found in the peripheral blood, although under pathologic conditions many other types of cells may appear (Appendix 9).

Leukocytosis is the absolute increase in the peripheral blood leukocyte concentration, without regard to cell immaturity, type, or percentage. In the adult this is usually greater than 12,000 cells/cubic milliliter. The term *left shift* refers to an increased percentage of immature neutrophils in the peripheral blood. Granulocytosis commonly means an increase in the number of neutrophilic granulocytes, although technically it applies to all granulocytes. Similarly, granulocytopenia means an absolute decrease in the number of neutrophilic granulocytes. Lymphocytosis and lymphopenia relate to an absolute increase and decrease in lymphocytes, respectively. Eosinophilia, basophilia, and monocytosis refer to an absolute increase in eosinophils, basophils, and monocytes. *Thrombocytopenia* and *thrombocytosis* are terms used to express a decrease and increase in platelets respectively (Table 19-3).

Abnormalities of the red blood cells are usually expressed as anemia or polycythemia. Anemia is defined as a decreased amount of hemoglobin in the peripheral blood. In the male this is less than 14 grams/milliliter; in females, less than 12 grams/milliliter. The MCV, MCH, and MCHC are referred to as the red blood's indices and are calculated from the hemoglobin, hematocrit, and red blood cell count (Appendix 9). The MCV is used in a morphologic classification of anemias with the MCH and MCHC sometimes useful in subclassfications. The morphologic classification subdivides anemias as follows: (1) macrocytic anemia—elevated MCV; (2) normocytic anemia—normal MCV; and (3) microcytic-hypochromic anemia—decreased MCV and MCH (Table 19-4). A pathophysiologic classification of anemia subdivides into the following categories: (1) anemia due to decreased red blood cell production, (2) anemia due to increased red blood cell destruction, and (3) anemia due to acute blood loss.

Table 19-3. Selected Abnormalities of Leukocytes and Platelets

Finding	Condition	Causative Factors of Finding
Leukocyte Count:		
Neutrophils		
More than 8,000 cells/mm^3.	Neutrophilia (granulocytosis)	Exercise, physical and emotional stress, bacterial, mycotic, viral and parasitic infections, neoplasia, drugs, leukemia
Fewer than 1,500 cells/mm^3.	Neutropenia (Granulocytopenia)	Drug-induced, viral, and rickettsial infections, specific bacterial infections, severe bacterial sepsis, leukemia, bone marrow replacement
Lymphocytes		
More than 4,000 cells/mm^3.	Lymphocytosis	Acute infectious lymphocytosis, whooping cough (pertussis), toxoplasmosis, cytomegalic virus infection, infectious mononucleosus, leukemia
Fewer than 1,500 cells/mm^3.	Lymphopenia	Immunoglobulin disorders, lymphocyte destruction as in radiation therapy or chemotherapy, Hodgkin's disease, sarcoidosis, renal failure
Eosinophils		
More than 450 cells/mm^3.	Eosinophilia	Parasitic infections, allergic disorders, dermatoses, neoplasia
Basophils		
More than 50 cells/mm^3.	Basophilia	Hypersensitivity reactions, chronic granulocytic leukemia, tuberculosis, ulcerative colitis
Monocytes		
More than 500 cells/mm^3.	Monocytosis	Collagen vascular disease, neoplasia, tuberculosis, subacute bacterial endocarditis, syphilis, leukemia
Platelet count:		
More than 400,000 platelets/mm^3.	Thrombocytosis	Chronic inflammatory diseases, neoplasia, exercise, hematologic malignances
Fewer than 100,000 platelets/mm^3.	Thrombocytopenia	Aplastic anemia, bone marrow replacement, drugs, radiation therapy, severe iron deficiency, infections, disseminated intravascular coagulation, idiopathic thrombocytopenic purpura, thrombotic thrombocytopenic purpura, platelet antibodies, hypersplenism

Table 19-4. Morphologic Classification of Anemia

Finding	Condition	Causative Factors of Finding
Hemoglobin less than 12 grams% in females, less than 14 grams% in males	Macrocytic-MCV greater than 100μ^3	Pernicious anemia Vitamin B-12 deficiency Folic acid deficiency Alcoholic liver disease
	Normocytic-MCV 80-100μ^3	Acute blood loss Hemolytic disorders Poisons and drugs Malignancy Anemia of chronic disease Hypersplenism Bone marrow failure
	Microcytic-hypochromic-MCV less than 80μ^3	Iron deficiency
	MCHC less than 31 grams/100 ml RBC	Chronic lead poisoning Thallasemia syndrome Chronic blood loss

Absolute polycythemia is an increased total body red blood cell mass and is either primary or secondary. Primary polycythemia (polycythemia rubra vera) is a premalignant proliferation of erythroid precursors and usually involves all the elements of the bone marrow. Secondary polycythemia is a red blood cell hyperplasia usually due to decreased oxygen saturation of the blood (Table 19-5).

Coagulation Testing. When blood is collected for coagulation testing, it is mixed with an anticoagulant, which binds the plasma calcium to prevent activation of the coagulation cascade. The prothrombin time (PT) measures the coagulant activity of the extrinsic system (Figure 19-3). It is used to screen for deficiencies in factors I, II, V, VII, and X, and is particularly useful in following clients on coumadin therapy because this anticoagulant depresses factor VII levels. The activated partial thromboplastin time (PTT) measures the coagulation activity of the intrinsic system and thus is a screen for all of the coagulation factors except VII and XIII (Figure 19-3). It is also very useful in monitoring heparin therapy, which acts as an antithrombin and thus prolongs the PTT. The bleeding time test is a measure of the duration of bleeding from a standardized skin wound and thus evaluates the interaction between platelets and capillaries (Appendix 9 and Table 19-6).

Regional Lymph Node Palpation

The lymph nodes are palpated with the tips of the middle fingers. The examiner palpates in a slow, gentle, rotary motion, moving systematically from one region to the next, and comparing contralateral sides. Normal lymph nodes are not palpable. Palpable nodes exist due to acute inflammation, prior inflammation, or neoplasia. Lymph nodes are palpated to determine the following characteristics: location, size, tenderness, degree of fixation (movable, matted or fixed), and texture (hard, firm, or soft). Cervical lymph nodes up to 1.0 centimeter in diameter are often felt in preadolescence and are believed to result from the frequency of upper respiratory tract infections in this age group. "Shotty" lymph

Table 19-5. Common Causes of Absolute Polycythemia

Finding	Condition	Causative Factors of Finding
Hemoglobin greater than 18 grams%	Secondary polycythemia	Chronic lung disease and right-to-left shunts in cardiovascular disease
	Primary polycythemia	Premalignant hyperplasia of the red blood cell elements of the bone marrow

Table 19-6. Causes of Prolonged Coagulation

Finding	Condition	Causative Factors of Finding
Prothrombin time—2 sec. longer than control	Factor deficiency	Liver disease
	Anticoagulant therapy	Presence of coumadin
	Fibrinogen deficiency	Afibrinogenemia, liver disease, and disseminated intravascular coagulation
	Fibrin-fibrinogen split products present	Disseminated intravascular coagulation
Partial thromboplastin time—5 sec. longer than control	Factor deficiency	Hemophilia or von Willebrand's disease
	Fibrinogen deficiency	Afibrinogenemia, liver disease, disseminated intravascular coagulation
	Fibrin-fibrinogen split products present	Disseminated intravascular coagulation
	Anticoagulant therapy	Presence of heparin
Bleeding time prolonged greater than controls	Hemorrhagic tendency	Thrombocytopenia von Willebrand's disease Functional platelet defects as in aspirin ingestion

nodes—firm, freely movable, and nontender—are common in the occipital, axillary, and inguinal regions. These are due to common infections of the scalp, hands, feet, and genitalia and the resulting antigenic stimulation and reactive hyperplasia of the regional lymph nodes.

The lymph nodes of the head and neck are examined from either an anterior or posterior approach with the client sitting. When the anterior approach is used the head is controlled with the hand not used for palpation (Figure 19-4). In the posterior approach, the neck is flexed to relax the musculature, which enables simultaneous bilateral palpation (Figure 19-5). This approach is preferred since asymmetry can be detected immediately. The examiner begins in the occipital region and proceeds as follows: occipital and posterior auricular, submaxillary and submental, upper and deep cervical, superficial cervical, lower deep cervical, and supraclavicular nodes. When the axillae are palpated the client may be sitting or supine. The examiner supports and slightly abducts the ipsilateral arm with one arm and uses the other hand to palpate. The pads of the fingertips reach high into the axillae and press lightly against the chest wall; the examiner moves the fingers inferiorly. The examiner proceeds along the edge of the pectoral muscle, in the central axillae, and along the edge of the latissimus dorsi

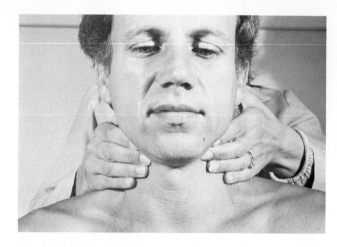

Figure 19-5. Posterior approach to palpation of the head and neck lymph nodes.

muscle (Figure 19-6). To examine the epitrochlear nodes, the examiner supports the arm as if shaking the client's hand, and uses the other hand to palpate the medial aspect of the arm just above the medial epicondyle of the humerus (Figure 19-7). The inguinal nodes are palpated with the client supine (Figure 19-8). The posterior popliteal nodes are found in the middle of the upper half of the popliteal fossae and are examined with the knees flexed (Figure 19-9 and Table 19-7).

Life Cycle Variations

Childhood and Adolescence

In children, anemia is usually due to blood loss, blood destruction, decreased production, or replacement of the bone marrow by either leukemia or cancer. These

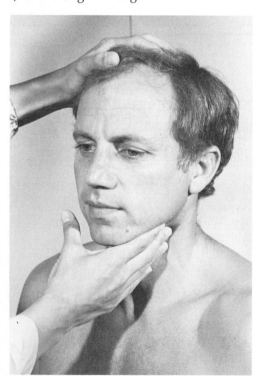

Figure 19-4. Anterior approach to palpation of the head and neck lymph nodes.

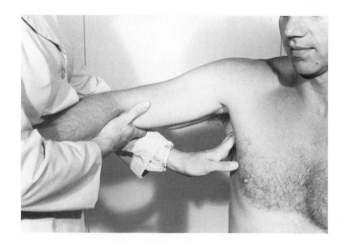

Figure 19-6. Palpation of the axillary lymph nodes.

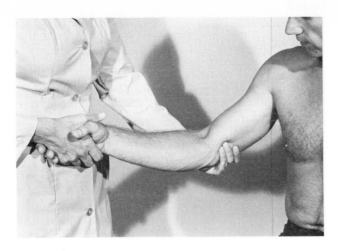

Figure 19-7. *Palpation of the epitrochlear lymph nodes.*

processes are usually age specific. In the newborn, common causes are blood loss due to placenta previa or shunting during a twin delivery and hemolytic disease of the newborn. In the first year of life, destructive processes such as sickle cell anemia and thalassemia manifest themselves. From 12 to 30 months the major cause is iron deficiency due to poor eating habits. Among one- to six-year olds, anemia due to bone marrow replacement by leukemia is a frequent cause of anemia. Leukemia is the most common neoplasm in children. Acute leukemia is the most frequent form and occurs with sudden onset of elevated white blood count with large numbers of immature cells.

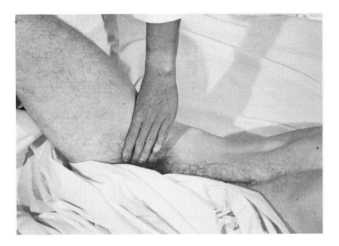

Figure 19-8. *Palpation of the inguinal lymph nodes.*

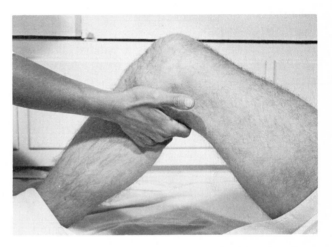

Figure 19-9. *Palpation of the posterior popliteal lymph nodes.*

Table 19-7.   Common Causes of Lymph Node Enlargement (Lymphadenopathy)

Finding	Condition	Explanation for Findings
Localized lymphadenopathy	Acute lymphadenitis	Bacteria and toxins cause acute inflammation.
	Cat-scratch fever	Acute inflammation.
	Tuberculosis	Granulomatous inflammation.
	Lymphoma	Replacement by primary neoplasia.
	Metastatic carcinoma	Replacement by metastasizing malignant cells.
Generalized lymphadenopathy	Hodgkin's disease	Replacement by primary neoplasia of lymphoid system.
	Lymphoma	
	Chronic lymphocytic leukemia	
	Drug therapy	Phenylbutazine, dilantin, isoniazide, and many antithyroid and antileprosy drugs cause a nonspecific enlargement.
	Infectious mononucleosis	Nonspecific reactive changes particularly of cervical lymph nodes.
	Rubella	Nonspecific reactive changes particularly of occipital lymph nodes.
	Rheumatoid arthritis	Generalized reactive changes, but greatest in drainage areas of involved joints.
	Sarcoidosis	Infiltration by noncaseating epitheloid granulomas.
	Toxoplasmosis	Reactive adenitis due to toxoplasma organism.

It is characteristic of infancy, childhood, and early adolescence for the lymph nodes to respond to stimuli with pronounced swelling and hyperplasia. This enlargement may persist for a long period of time and is most noticeable in the head and neck, particularly with upper respiratory tract infections. Often the hyperplastic lymphoid tissue causes secondary effects such as the middle ear disorders associated with enlarged tonsils and adenoids. Lymphomas are relatively rare in children. Hemorrhagic diseases often manifest themselves in childhood and adolescence, and usually need specialized coagulation studies to establish their etiology. (Table 19-8).

Pregnancy

In pregnancy the only common hematologic problem is anemia. Because there is an expanded blood volume during pregnancy, the pregnant woman may appear mildly anemic even though red blood cell mass is unchanged. With a tremendous demand for iron and folate, the developing fetus preferentially takes these nutrients from the mother and causes her to become deficient. Iron deficiency is most common in mothers who have closely spaced pregnancies and breast feed. Folate deficiency is common in mothers on poor diets. Mixed iron and folate deficiencies are frequent in the lower socioeconomic groups, with women who often do not take supplemental prenatal vitamins, have closely spaced pregnancies, and have poor dietary habits.

Late Adulthood

In the elderly, there is little change in the complete blood count. Iron deficiency anemia is less frequent in the aged and when present is often due to chronic blood loss from neoplasms of the gastrointestinal or genitourinary tract. Chronic liver disease and chronic renal failure are also often associated with anemia. Dietary deficiency of folate is not uncommon in the elderly on restricted diets and leads to a macrocytic anemia.

Chronic lymphocytic leukemia and chronic granulocytic leukemia are seen in the elderly. The incidence of lymphomas increases with age. Hemorrhagic tendencies in the elderly are usually due to thrombocytopenia caused by bone marrow replacement by leukemia or cancer or due to antineoplastic drugs.

Table 19-8.   Common Hemorrhagic Diseases in Childhood

Finding	Condition	Causative Factors of Finding
Bleeding tendency	Thrombocytopenia	Platelet destruction as in idiopathic thrombocytopenic purpura Bone marrow replacement in leukemia and cancer
	Abnormalities in prothrombin time and partial thromboplastin time	Congenital coagulation deficiencies as in the hemophilias
	Prolonged bleeding time	Thrombocytopenia Intrinsic platelet abnormality in von Willebrand's disease

Physiology

Fluid and Electrolyte Distribution

The body fluids are composed of water (solvent) and dissolved substances (solute). These fluids function mainly as a medium for chemical reactions and as a transportation system for nutrients and waste products.

The adult male body is composed of approximately 60 percent water. Since women have more body fat than men, and fat contains less cytoplasm than other tissues, the adult female body is composed of approximately 50 percent water. The body fluids are in two main compartments: intracellular and extracellular. The extracellular compartment further divides into two groups: the intravascular and the interstitial spaces (Figure 20-1). The body water is divided among the three compartments as follows:

Fluid Compartment	% of Body Weight
Intracellular	40%
Extracellular	20%
Interstitial	15%
Intravascular	5%
TOTAL	60%

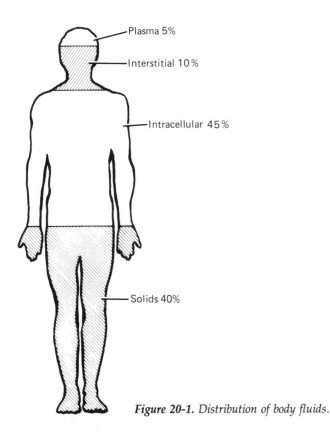

Figure 20-1. Distribution of body fluids.

Chapter 20

Assessment of Fluid and Electrolyte Balance

Objectives

The examiner will be able to do the following:

1. Recognize signs and symptoms of fluid volume deficit and fluid volume excess
2. Recognize signs and symptoms of electrolyte imbalance
3. Recognize abnormalities in serum electrolyte levels
4. Obtain accurate intake and output measurements
5. Record the information obtained

There is fluid in other parts of the body, such as the secretions of the stomach, liver, and pancreas; compared to total body fluid, their percentages are low. The various compartments are separated by a selectively permeable membrane which permits free passage of water and some of the dissolved substances between the vascular, interstitial, and intracellular fluid compartments.

Water is added to the body by three routes: oral liquids, water in food, and water of oxidation. The water of oxidation is a product of cellular metabolism. The metabolism of 100 calories produces 10 milliliters of water; therefore, a 2,000-calorie diet produces 200 milliliters of water. The major organs for water excretion are the kidneys, skin, lungs, and gastrointestinal tract (Table 20-1).

There is an obligatory amount of water excreted daily, regardless of fluid intake or hydration status. The skin excretes a daily minimum of 250 milliliters of water to help maintain body temperature. The kidneys excrete a minimum of 400 milliliters of urine (15 to 20 milliliters per hour), in order to excrete the end products of metabolism; the lungs excrete 350 milliliters of wa-

Table 20-1. Water Ingestion and Excretion in 24 Hours (measured in ml.)

Ingestion		Excretion	
Oral liquids	1,500	Kidneys	1,500
Food	700	Skin	350
Water of oxidation	200	Lungs	350
		GI tract	200
Total	2,400	Total	2,400

ter. Generally the water loss from the gastrointestinal tract equals the water gained from oxidation.

Adequate hydration is necessary for life. Inadequate hydration is called *volume deficit* and causes cell shrinkage from osmosis. If the shrinkage is severe, the cells may have irreversible damage and eventually die. A loss of 10 percent of the body fluids is serious; a loss of 20 percent of the body fluids is life-threatening (Table 20-2).

Excessive water in the body affects health by diluting dissolved substances. The amount of water an individual can safely ingest is directly related to the ability of the heart to pump the added volume and the kidneys to excrete it (Table 20-3).

Table 20-2. Volume Deficit

Findings	*Possible Causative Factors*	*Explanation for Findings*
Acute weight loss Thirst Little saliva, tears, or perspiration Dry mucous membranes Longitudinal wrinkling of tongue (furrows) Oliguria Hypotension	Vomiting Diarrhea Fistulous drainage	Loss of large volumes of fluid and electrolytes with no replacement causes concentrated body fluids and signs and symptoms of volume deficit, stimulation of the secretion of aldosterone, ADH, and the thirst mechanism.
	Decreased water intake	Concentration of body fluids causes signs and symptoms of volume deficit and stimulates the secretion of ADH and the thirst mechanism.
	Systemic infection with fever	For each 1° C. increase in body temperature, the need for water increases 15%. If adequate intake is not maintained, concentration of body fluids occurs.
	Diabetes insipidus	With the lack of ADH secretion, the kidneys are unable to reabsorb water or concentrate the urine. In this situation the serum values are the same as the other conditions, but the urine osmolality or specific gravity is greatly decreased and the urine volume is increased.
	Acute renal disease	During the diuretic phase of acute renal disease, the tubules are unable to concentrate the urine from the disease process.
	Burns	Excessive loss of salt and water through the skin causes the signs and symptoms of volume deficit.
	Hyperventilation	Excessive loss of water through the lungs causes the signs and symptoms of volume deficit.

The dissolved substances in the body fluids are electrolytes, sugars, proteins, and nitrogenous waste products. Electrolytes are substances that dissociate in solution into electrically charged ions and conduct an electrical current. Table salt, or sodium chloride (NaCl), is an example of a salt that dissociates into two electrolytes—sodium (Na^+) and chloride (Cl^-)—when in a solution and conducts an electrical current. If the water is removed, the electrolytes crystallize and form NaCl. NaCl is a salt, and does not conduct an electrical current.

There are two types of electrolytes: cations and anions. Cations are positively charged electrolytes, and anions are negatively charged electrolytes. In the body, solutions containing electrolytes have an equal number of cations and anions and are electrically neutral.

Electrolytes are counted, or measured, in milliequivalents per liter, mEq/L. A *milliequivalent* is a term that measures an electrolyte in terms of its chemical combining power. In considering the chemical activity of the solution, weight is not the significant factor: combining power is.

The normal function of cells depends upon the availability of water and electrolytes in the needed amount and correct location. The major constituents of the vascular fluid are Na^+ and Cl^-, while the major constituents of the intracellular fluid are K^+ and HPO_4^-. The interstitial fluid is almost identical to the vascular fluid in electrolyte composition, but the plasma contains larger amounts of proteinate to maintain the fluid volume within the blood vessels (Figure 20-2).

Serum Electrolytes

Serum electrolytes generally include sodium, potassium, chloride, and bicarbonate (measured as CO_2). Magnesium and phosphate are measured when an imbalance is suspected from the clinical findings (Table 20-4).

Table 20-4. Normal Serum Electrolyte Values (Measured in mEq/L)

Sodium (Na^+)	135-145
Potassium (K^+)	3.5-5
Calcium (Ca^{++})	4.5-5.5
Magnesium (Mg^{++})	1.5-2.5
Chloride (Cl^-)	95-105
Bicarbonate (CO_2 HCO_3^-)	23-28
Phosphate (PO_4^-)	2-4

Sodium. Sodium is the chief cation of the extracellular fluid; its primary function is the maintenance of extracellular fluid volume through its effect on osmolality. Since sodium regulates the volume of extracellular fluid, any change in sodium concentration causes a change in fluid volume. An increase in sodium increases extracellular fluid volume; a decrease in sodium decreases extracellular fluid volume.

The average American diet includes approximately 135 to 170 mEq. of sodium (8 to 10 grams) daily. This amount is far in excess of the 50 to 85 mEq. (3 to 5 grams) of sodium that the body daily needs to avoid a negative balance. Sodium is generally ingested as a salt—sodium chloride—which is present in foods and drinking water and added as a seasoning. Also, prepared foods have a large amount of sodium in the form of preservatives.

Sodium is primarily excreted in the urine, with the daily urine sodium output approximately equal to the daily sodium intake. Therefore, the sodium ingested in excess of the daily amount needed is excreted by the kidneys. Generally, only negligible amounts of sodium are lost through the skin, but during excessive sweating, large amounts are lost (Table 20-5).

Table 20-3. Volume Excess

Findings	Possible Causative Factors	Explanation for Findings
Weight gain Bounding pulse	Excessive fluid intake	The kidneys are unable to keep pace with the excessive intake.
Signs and symptoms of underlying disease process	Fluid retention Congestive heart failure Cirrhosis of the liver Nephrotic syndrome	The disease process stimulates aldosterone secretion, which causes sodium and water retention by the kidneys.
	Increased secretion of adrenocortical hormones	The kidneys retain sodium and water in response to the action of the hormones.

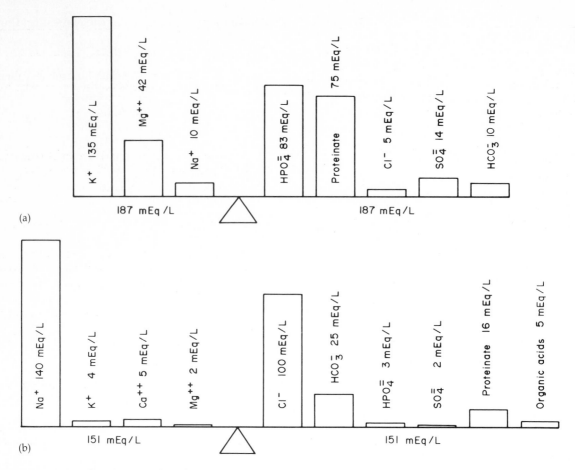

Figure 20-2. *Electrolyte distribution: (a) cellular electrolytes; (b) vascular electrolytes.*

Potassium. Potassium is the chief cation of the intracellular fluid and therefore maintains intracellular fluid volume, or cellular osmolality. Potassium is also necessary for the transmission of nervous impulses in the heart and striated muscles; is critical in the electrical functioning of the cells; and is necessary for the cellular transformation of carbohydrates into energy. Small quantities of potassium are found in the extracellular fluid. Therefore, it has little effect on serum osmolality.

The average daily intake of potassium is 80 to 200 mEq. Potassium is found in dairy products, meats, fruits, vegetables, and salt substitutes. There are 50 mEq. of potassium in three average bananas, six average oranges, three and one-half cups of tomato juice, or two cups of dried peaches.

Generally the amount of potassium ingested equals the amount of potassium excreted. Most of the potassium ingested (90 percent) is excreted in the urine (30-90 mEq/L); some (10 percent), in the feces (5-10 mEq/L). Only negligible amounts of potassium are

lost in perspiration, except in extreme conditions. The body is unable to conserve potassium as well as it conserves sodium. As a result, the kidneys continue to excrete potassium in the presence of a low-potassium intake. Since potassium is virtually in all foods, the excretion exceeds the intake only when a person is ingesting nothing by mouth or is taking diuretics (Table 20-6).

Calcium. Most of the body calcium (99 percent) is in the skeletal system and teeth, with only one percent present in the body fluids. Half of the calcium is nondiffusible since it is bound to proteins or other substances; half of it is diffusible because it is ionized. Only the diffusible calcium is effective in physiological mechanisms. Calcium is necessary for the formation and structure of bones and teeth. It is a constituent in mucoproteins, and mucopolysaccharides and is a coenzyme in blood coagulation. It is also important for smooth muscle contraction and neural transmission and function.

Table 20-5.   Sodium Imbalances

Findings	Possible Causative Factors	Explanation for Findings
Hyponatremia Na⁺ < 135 mEq/L Fatigue Confusion Apathy Anorexia Weakness Headache Hypothermia Tachycardia Hypotension Loss of skin turgor	Gastrointestinal losses Vomiting Nasogastric suction Ileostomy Fistulas Diarrhea	The body loses fluids with a high concentration of sodium.
	Nasogastric irrigation with water Repeated tap water enemas	The body loses fluids with a high concentration of sodium, plus a dilution of body fluids occurs from the absorbed water.
	Renal losses Inappropriate ADH secretion	The body fluids become diluted from the retention of water.
	Adrenal insufficiency (Addison's)	Increased sodium excretion in the urine as a result of the decrease in cortisone and mineralocorticoids and other corticosteroids.
	Salt-losing kidney	In chronic renal disease the kidneys are unable to conserve sodium.
	Diabetic acidosis	Diuresis of large quantities of glucose is associated with increased sodium excretion.
	Diuretics	Interference with sodium reabsorption increases sodium and water excretion.
	Skin losses Excessive perspiration	Moderate amounts of sodium are lost during extensive sweating. If large amounts of water are ingested, the severity of hyponatremia increases.
	Burns	Occurs when edema accumulates under the skin during the first few days after a burn. Edematous fluid includes sodium, chloride, water, and protein.
Hypernatremia Na⁺ > 145 mEq/L Signs and symptoms of volume deficit if associated with extracellular fluid loss	Inadequate water intake (volume deficit) Inability to drink fluids (comatose) Depression of thirst mechanism	Concentration of body fluids occurs from inadequate replacement of obligatory water losses.
	Excessive water loss (volume deficit) Diabetes insipidus	Urinary loss of water exceeds water intake.
	Salt poisoning Tube feedings with inadequate amount of water Overuse of salt tablets	Body fluids are overloaded with salt with an inadequate amount of ingested water to maintain the osmolality of body fluids.
Signs and symptoms of edema associated with volume excess	Sodium retention Congestive heart failure	Decreased cardiac output causes a decreased renal perfusion; therefore, sodium and water are retained and not excreted in the urine. Also aldosterone is secreted in response to the lowered renal perfusion.
	Cirrhosis of the liver Nephrotic syndrome	Due to decreased circulating blood volume from edema, aldosterone is secreted and the kidneys retain sodium and water.
	Cushing's Hyperaldosteronism Steroid therapy	Sodium and water are retained by the kidneys.

Table 20-6.   Potassium Imbalances

Findings	Possible Causative Factors	Explanation for Findings

Hypokalemia
  K⁺ < 3.5 mEq/L
Anorexia
Nausea
Vomiting
Decreased bowel sounds
Paralytic ileus
Muscular weakness
Decreased respiratory rate
Depression or absent deep tendon reflexes
Irregular pulse
Hypotension
	Inadequate intake
	  NPO with K⁺-free IVs
	  Alcoholism
	  Malnutrition
	  Starvation
		Kidneys are unable to adequately conserve potassium; although potassium intake is not meeting daily requirements, the urine contains 30-90 mEq/l of potassium.

	GI losses
	  Vomiting
	  Nasogastric suction
	  Fistulas
	  Ileostomy
	  Diarrhea
		The body loses fluids with a high concentration of potassium.

	Renal losses	
ECG	Renal tubular acidosis	Associated with an increased renal excretion of potassium.

Flat P
  Widened QRS
  Low and broadened T
  U-wave
	Diuretics (thiazides, mercurials, ethacrynic acid, furosemide)	The drug stimulates urinary excretion of potassium.

	Cushing's Hyperaldosteronism Steroid therapy	Potassium in the urine is increased from the hormonal action on the nephron.
	Extracellular to intracellular potassium shift Alkalosis	In alkalosis the cells release hydrogen and absorb potassium. There is no body loss of potassium. Hypokalemia can also cause alkalosis since Na⁺ and H⁺ move into the cells to replace the lost potassium. With more hydrogen in the cell, less is in the extracellular fluid and the pH rises.
	Recovery phase of diabetic acidosis	With the administration of insulin glucose is metabolized and potassium is also absorbed by the liver and muscle cells to aid in the conversion of glucose to glycogen.

Hyperkalemia
  K⁺ > 5 mEq/L
Flaccid paralysis
Decreased respiratory rate
Irregular heart beat progressing to cardiac arrest
Increased deep tendon reflexes
	Excessive intake
	  IV administration
	  Blood transfusion
		10-20 mEq/hr. is the maximum rate of administration for potassium. A faster rate can cause hyperkalemia and cardiac arrest.
		The older the blood, the more damaged cells there are. Each damaged cell releases K⁺ into the transfusion so that one unit of blood can have 10 mEq. of K⁺ or more. Blood administration through a needle smaller than 18 g. causes cell damage and the release of K⁺ into the transfusion.

	Oral intake exceeding renal tolerance	Since potassium is excreted by the kidneys, any decrease in urine output or inability of the kidneys to keep pace with K⁺ intake can cause hyperkalemia.

	Massive tissue trauma
	  Crushing injuries
	  Major surgery
	  Early stages of burns
	Acidosis
		Severe damage to the cells causes release of intracellular potassium into the body fluids.

	Adrenal insufficiency	In the presence of a low pH, H⁺ is absorbed by the cells and K⁺ is released. Serum K⁺ rises but there is no real gain in body K⁺ stores.
	Late-stage renal failure	Potassium is retained by the kidneys as a result of a decrease in the corticosteroids and mineralocorticosteroid (aldosterone). In advanced stages of renal disease the kidneys are unable to excrete the ingested potassium.

The major sources of calcium are dietary, in the form of milk and milk products. The average adult requires about .65 gram/day. The bones and teeth provide a ready reservoir for calcium. Since calcium is relatively insoluble, it is poorly absorbed by the intestines. Adequate supplies of vitamin D are needed for calcium absorption by the gastrointestinal mucosa.

Most of the calcium ingested is not absorbed but is excreted in the feces. Almost all that is absorbed is excreted by the kidneys in the urine. Therefore, virtually all calcium ingested is excreted.

Serum calcium is also affected by the levels of organic phosphate. Phosphate and calcium have an inverse relationship; when one is elevated, the other is decreased (Table 20-7).

Calcium is regulated by two hormones: calcitonin and parathyroid hormone. Calcitonin, a thyroid hormone, decreases serum calcium by inhibition of bone resorption. Bone resorption refers to the shift of calcium from the bones to the serum. Parathyroid hor-

Table 20-7. Calcium Imbalances

Findings	Possible Causative Factors	Explanation for Findings
Hypocalcemia $Ca^{++} < 4.5$ mEq/L (9 mg%) Confusion Circumoral tingling Tingling of palms of hands and feet Tetany Laryngeal stridor Carpopedal spasm Positive Trousseau Positive Chvostek Paresthesia Seizures	Decreased gastro-intestinal absorption Vitamin D deficiency	Lack of vitamin D decreases calcium absorption from the GI tract.
	Decreased parathyroid hormone	Lack of parathyroid hormone results in decreased calcium absorption from the gastrointestinal tract, decreased bone resorption of calcium, and increased renal excretion of calcium.
	Excessive phosphate	In renal insufficiency, phosphate is retained and causes the formation of a precipitate, calcium phosphate. This reduces the amount of ionized calcium.
	Magnesium deficiency	The release of calcium from the bones is inhibited.
	Citrated blood (massive transfusions)	The citrate binds calcium and therefore reduces the amount of ionized calcium in the body fluids.
	Correction of acidosis with bicarbonate	In the presence of a low pH (acidosis) the amount of ionized calcium increases. When the acidosis is reversed and the body fluids are more alkaline, the amount of ionized calcium decreases.
	Acute pancreatitis Massive infections of subcutaneous tissues Peritonitis	Precipitation of calcium in the diseased areas.
Hypercalcemia Ca^{++} 5.5 mEq/L (10.5 mg%) Confusion Lethargy Muscle weakness Constipation Renal colic Polyuria Increased deep tendon reflexes Gray or white opaque granular bands in cornea	Increased GI absorpiton Excessive vitamin D Milk-alkali syndrome	Vitamin D stimulates calcium absorption from GI tract. Increased ingestion of calcium from milk, milk products, and antacids exceeds renal output.
	Excessive parathyroid hormone	Increases calcium absorption from gastrointestinal tract, decreases renal excretion of calcium, and increases bone resorption of calcium.
	Bone destruction exceeding bone repair or regeneration. Prolonged immobilization	Bone production decreases from prolonged immobilization. Normal bone destruction continues, which causes an increased ionized calcium.
	Tuberculosis of bones	Excessive bone destruction causes increased ionized calcium.
	Cancer	Osteolytic metastases, calcium resorption from bone, immobilization, or production of parathormonelike hormone produces an increased amount of ionized calcium.

mone increases serum calcium by three mechanisms: increased gastrointestinal absorption, decreased renal excretion, and increased bone resorption.

Magnesium. Most body magnesium is in the bones and teeth, bound to protein, and in the skeletal and cardiac muscles. Only a small amount is ionized and in the serum.

Magnesium is essential to the enzyme systems and is vital for the formation of many organic compounds such as nucleoproteins and phospholipids. It is considered an integral part of all body cells and is necessary in carbohydrate and protein metabolism. In its ionized form in the extracellular fluid, magnesium causes the irritability of the central nervous system.

Magnesium is found in most foods; an adequate diet prevents any deficit. The best sources of magnesium are green vegetables, nuts, and whole grain cereals. The average magnesium intake is 20 to 40 mEq a day; two-thirds of the ingested magnesium is excreted in the feces. Vitamin D increases the absorption of magnesium in the gastrointestinal tract. The remaining one-third of the ingested magnesium that is absorbed is then excreted by the kidneys in the urine (Table 20-8).

Chloride. Chloride is the major anion of the extracellular fluid and generally changes proportionately with sodium; an increase in sodium causes an increase in chloride, and a decrease in sodium causes a decrease in chloride. Chloride ingestion and excretion are the same as sodium. Generally chloride is not the primary electrolyte in an imbalance but follows another electrolyte (sodium or hydrogen) to maintain electrical neutrality. Chloride is present in the extracellular fluid as ionized sodium chloride and in the stomach as ionized hyrochloric acid. Therefore, any loss of sodium in the extracellular fluid or hydrogen from the stomach causes a loss of chloride.

The findings and conditions of chloride disorders are the same as those for sodium. In addition, any loss of gastric secretions in large quantities, causes a loss of hydrochloric acid. Therefore, the body has less acid available and hence a hypochloremic metabolic alkalosis (Chapter 21).

Bicarbonate. Bicarbonate is not directly measured from the venous blood, but the total amount of carbon dioxide is. It is generally listed on the serum electrolytes as Tco_2 (total carbon dioxide), CO_2, CO_2 comb. (carbon dioxide combining power), or HCO_3^-. The total carbon dioxide equals the bicarbonate plus the dissolved carbon dioxide. Since the amount of carbon

Table 20-8.   Magnesium Imbalances

Findings	Possible Causative Factors	Explanation for Findings
Hypomagnesemia $Mg^{++} < 1.5$ mEq/L Mental depression Seizure Hyperactive deep tendon reflexes Muscle fasciculations Irregular rapid heart rate Hypertension	Inadequate intake Prolonged malnutrition Starvation Alcoholism Magnesium-free IVs for more than one week	The kidneys are unable to conserve adequate amounts of magnesium. A positive balance of magnesium is maintained by diet; if intake is reduced, a deficiency results.
	Impaired intestinal absorption Prolonged vomiting Nasogastric suction Diarrhea Ileostomies Fistulas	Associated with a loss of body fluids containing magnesium. The magnesium that is ingested is poorly absorbed in the gastrointestinal tract.
	Increased urinary losses (Diuretics)	Mercurial or thiazide diuretics promote magnesium excretion.
Hypermagnesemia $Mg^{++} > 2.5$ mEq/L CNS depression Hypotension Absent deep tendon reflexes Respiratory paralysis Complete heart block	Overuse of antacids containing magnesium, especially if renal failure is present	Intake of magnesium exceeds the ability of the kidneys to excrete magnesium.

dioxide dissolved is almost always less than 1 mEq/L, the terms Tco_2, CO_2, CO_2 comb., and HCO_3^- are used interchangeably.

Bicarbonate is a base and functions as a major component in acid-base balance. The amount of bicarbonate present in the body fluids is not as important as the ratio of bicarbonate to carbonic acid (20 parts of bicarbonate to 1 part of carbonic acid) (Chapter 21).

Phosphate. Phosphate is the major anion of the intracellular fluid; however, most of the body phosphate (90 percent) is in the bones and teeth. As with calcium, the bones and teeth provide a ready reservoir of phosphate if it is needed in the extracellular fluid. In the extracellular fluid, phosphate is in the ionized form, $PO_4^=$, and functions in the phosphate buffer system in the maintenance of acid-base balance. Phosphate is also necessary for cellular activity in carbohydrate metabolism and for the formation of nucleic acids, phosphoproteins, and phospholipids.

The major source of phosphate is in milk and milk products; in the presence of calcium, the insoluble salt calcium phosphate forms and is excreted in the feces. As with calcium, vitamin D increases intestinal absorption. Parathyroid hormone affects serum phosphate. Although parathyroid hormone increases intestinal absorption of phosphate, it stimulates renal secretion of phosphate. Therefore, the net result is that parathyroid hormone reduces serum phosphate.

Phosphate is excreted in the urine. When the serum level is low, less phosphate is excreted; when the serum level is high, more phosphate is excreted in the urine. Since calcium and phosphate have an inverse relationship in the serum, phosphate is increased when calcium is decreased (Table 20-9).

Homeostasis

The body maintains homeostasis of fluid and electrolytes by passive transport (osmosis, diffusion, and filtration) and active transport. Passive transport does not require expenditure of energy while active transport does.

Osmosis. Osmosis is the movement of water through a selectively permeable membrane from a dilute solution (hypotonic) to a concentrated solution (hypertonic). When two solutions are separated by a selectively permeable membrane, and one is concentrated and the other dilute, water moves from the dilute solution to the concentrated solution (Figure 20-3). The principle of osmosis is paramount in understanding fluid distribution.

Electrolytes and other dissolved substances do not move by osmosis, but they affect the speed of osmosis. The speed of osmosis is relative to the osmotic pressure of the two fluids. Osmotic pressure is the amount of pressure required to oppose osmosis, and is relative to the number of dissolved particles in solution. The greater the concentration of electrolytes in solution, the greater the osmotic pressure. Solutions with higher osmotic pressures pull water across selectively permeable membranes.

Table 20-9   Phosphate Imbalances

Findings	Possible Causative Factors	Explanation for Findings
Hypophosphatemia $HPO_4^= < 2$ mEq/L Anorexia Weakness Malaise	Inadequate intake Starvation Malnutrition Alcoholism	A positive balance of phosphate is generally maintained by diet, but if intake is greatly reduced for prolonged periods, a deficiency results.
	Inadequate gastrointestinal absorption Lack of vitamin D Malabsorption syndrome	Although intake is adequate, the gastrointestinal tract is unable to absorb adequate quantities to maintain a positive balance.
	Increased renal loss Hyperparathyroidism	Increased amounts of the parathyroid hormone cause the renal excretion of phosphate.
Hyperphosphatemia $HPO_4^= > 4$ mEq/L Signs and symptoms of tetany	Decreased renal excretion Renal insufficiency Hypoparathyroidism	Excretion of phosphate is reduced by the diseased kidney. Decreased amounts of parathyroid hormone cause a renal retention of phosphate.
	Excessive bone growth Infants Acromegaly	Associated with increased bone utilization of calcium, which reduces ionized calcium and increases ionized phosphate.

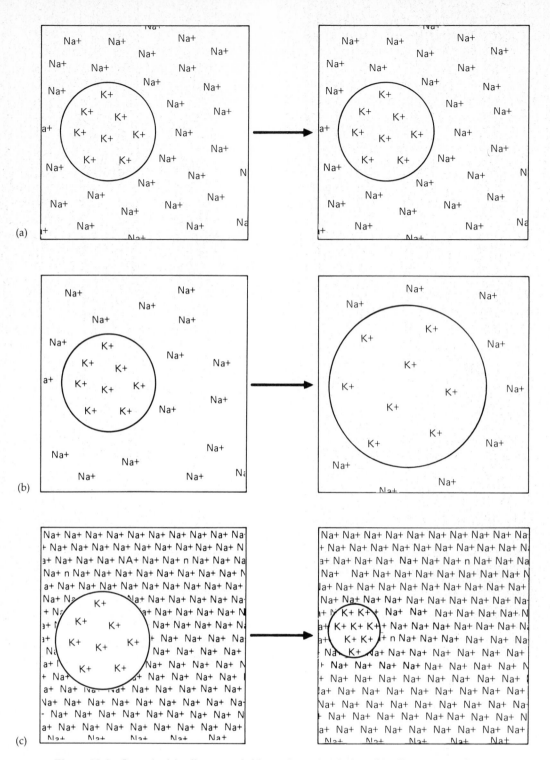

Figure 20-3. *Osmosis: (a) cell surrounded by an isotonic solution; (b) cell surrounded by a hypotonic solution; (c) cell surrounded by a hypertonic solution.*

Osmotic pressure is measured in milliosmoles per liter (mOsm/l). A millimole of a substance is the molecular weight of that substance in milligrams. A millimole is based on the weight of the substance. One millimole equals 1 milliosmole in substances that are dissociated. For instance, 1 millimole of sodium equals 1 milliosmole of sodium. But 1 mole of sodium chloride (NaCl) equals 2 milliosmoles since NaCl dissociates into Na^+ and Cl^-. One mole of calcium chloride ($CaCl_2$) equals 3 milliosmoles, since $CaCl_2$ dissociates into one Ca^+ and two Cl^-. Therefore, the osmotic pressure of a solution is simply the sum of all of the milliosmoles. This number is the osmolality of the solution.

The direction of osmosis is determined by knowing the osmotic pressure (osmolality). Serum osmolality is the sum of electrolytes in the blood and is measured in milliosmoles per liter. An approximation of serum osmolality is made by adding the number of milliequivalents of sodium and potassium, multiplied by two. For example, a person with a serum sodium of 147 mEq/L and a serum potassium of 4.5 mEq/L has an approximate serum osmolality of 303 mOsm/L. (147 + 4.5 = 151.5   151.5 × 2 = 303 mOsm/l).

Serum osmolality is increased if the serum is concentrated, either from water loss (volume deficit) or the addition of solute (hypernatremia). Serum osmolality is decreased if the serum is dilute, either from water gain (volume excess) or the loss of solute (hyponatremia).

The tonicity of a fluid describes the osmolality of the solution or its concentration. In the health field, all solutions are compared to the osmolality of the blood and extracellular fluid. An isotonic solution has the same osmolality as the blood, or approximately 300 mOsm/L. A hypotonic solution is a dilute solution with fewer dissolved particles than the blood and, therefore, has a lower osmolality than the blood. A hypertonic solution is a concentrated solution with more dissolved particles than the blood and, therefore, a higher osmolality.

In the body the greatest concern is the integrity of the cell, since any change in cellular function affects bodily function. If the cell is surrounded by an isotonic solution, the extracellular fluid, there is no net gain or loss of fluid (Figure 20-3). However, if the cell is surrounded by a hypotonic solution, it is surrounded by a dilute solution, water moves by osmosis into the cell, and the cell swells. If the cell is surrounded by a hypertonic solution, it is surrounded by a concentrated solution, water moves by osmosis from the cell, and the cell shrinks (Figure 20-3).

Any loss or gain of water or dissolved particles by the body affects the osmotic pressure of the extracellular fluid. Any change in the osmolality affects the amount of water in the cell. Some body processes are initiated or inhibited solely on the osmolality of body fluids.

Diffusion. Diffusion is the movement of solute from an area of high concentration to an area of low concentration. The movement occurs in all directions throughout the solution or through a selectively permeable membrane. In the body there are only selectively permeable membranes; thus, diffusion occurs through the cell wall only when the membrane is permeable to a given solute.

Filtration. Filtration is the movement of solute and solvent by differences in hydrostatic pressure between the two solutions separated by a selectively permeable membrane. The solute and solvent pass from the compartment with the higher pressure into the compartment with the lower pressure. Regardless of the difference in pressures, only those particles to which the membrane is permeable will be able to pass through. In the body, filtration occurs at the aterioles to provide fluid and nutrients to the cells; at the venules to provide removal of cellular waste products, and in the kidneys, where the glomerular filtrate is formed.

Active Transport. Requires energy to move the solute against a concentration gradient. In active transport the substances are moved "uphill," or from an area of low concentration to an area of high concentration. The movement of glucose from the extracellular fluid to the intracellular fluid is an example of active transport. Insulin provides the energy to transport the glucose from the extracellular fluid to the intracellular fluid where there is actually more glucose present. Some other substances that move by active transport include sodium, potassium, calcium, and amino acids.

Hormone Control

Osmotic pressure and the volume of extracellular water are maintained by two hormones: antidiuretic hormone (ADH) and aldosterone. These hormones help maintain health by regulating the osmotic pressure and volume of extracellular water within normal limits.

Antidiuretic Hormone (ADH). ADH is manufactured by the hypothalamus and secreted by the anterior pituitary gland. ADH causes the distal tubules and the collecting ducts of the kidneys to be more permeable to water. With this increased permeability, more water is reabsorbed, the volume of urine decreases, and the urine becomes more concentrated.

ADH secretion is regulated by serum osmolality, emotional and physical stress, and blood volume. With an increase in serum osmolality, specialized neuronal cells in the hypothalamus (osmoreceptors), respond by shrinking, which then initiates more ADH secretion. With increased ADH secretion, the kidneys reabsorb more water, the body fluids approach a more normal osmolality, and the size of the neuronal cells returns to normal. As the neuronal cells return to a more normal size, ADH secretion is inhibited, and the cycle is complete.

The converse is also true. If the body fluids are dilute, water moves by osmosis from the extracellular fluid into the intracellular fluid. The neuronal cells then swell and ADH secretion is decreased; therefore, the kidneys reabsorb less water. As the body fluids approach a more normal osmolality, the neuronal cells return to a more normal size, and ADH secretion returns to normal. By responding to both increases and decreases in serum osmolality, ADH maintains a normal osmotic pressure in the body fluids.

With a decreased blood volume, pressure receptors in the left atrium stimulate increased ADH secretion. Increased ADH secretion causes increased renal reabsorption of water, thereby expanding blood volume. If the pressure in the left atrium is increased from too much blood volume, ADH secretion is inhibited. Inhibition of ADH secretion results in increased water loss through the kidneys, and the blood volume decreases.

Aldosterone. Aldosterone is a mineralcorticoid secreted by the adrenal cortex, which affects all segments of the renal tubules to reabsorb sodium and water and to excrete potassium. Aldosterone secretion is stimulated during volume depletion and inhibited during volume overload.

Aldosterone is regulated by the renin-angiotensin system. With hypovolemia there is a diminished pressure in the glomeruli of the kidneys. Next to the glomeruli are specialized cells that respond to changes in pressure of the glomeruli. With a decreased pressure, renin is released from the specialized cells and causes the formation of angiotensin I and II in the blood. Angiotensin II stimulates aldosterone secretion by the adrenal cortex, which causes increased reabsorption of sodium and water and increased potassium excretion. With the retention of sodium and water, blood volume increases, as does the pressure in the glomeruli, and aldosterone secretion is inhibited.

Physical stress has a transient, mild effect on aldosterone secretion and causes the kidneys to reabsorb sodium and water and to excrete potassium.

Assessment Modalities

Fluid and electrolyte assessment is based upon the client's history and clinical findings. Unfortunately, the same findings, such as lethargy, can be apparent in various syndromes, sometimes even in opposite

imbalances. Fluid and electrolyte imbalances often occur as a secondary syndrome from a disease or drug, so many of the signs and symptoms result from an underlying disorder. Assessing fluid and electrolyte balance is often a difficult challenge, since evidence may seem to be vague and contradictory. The clinical signs are determined through various measurements and observational skills, which include temperature, pulse, respirations, blood pressure, and weight.

Temperature. Body temperature is maintained by the hypothalamus in response to heat loss and heat production. Each increase of 1° increases the body's need for water by 15 percent. The pulse often is used to assess fluid volume and the effect of various electrolytes on the myocardium. Changes in respirations from fluid and electrolyte imbalances are related to effects of the nervous system, muscular system, or fluid volume. Blood pressure can also be used to assess fluid volume and the effects of various electrolytes on the heart and arterial walls (Table 20-10).

Weight. Weight is the best indicator of fluid gain or loss from the body, since it is much easier to measure accurately than intake and output. Relative weight gain accompanies retention of water while relative weight loss occurs with water loss. Five hundred milliliters of water weighs 500 milligrams (1 liter = 1 kilogram or 2.2 pounds). Therefore, if a person retains 500 milliliters—that is, intake is 500 milliliters greater than output—an accurate weight shows a weight gain of 500 milligrams (1 pound). The converse is also true. If output is 500 milliliters greater than intake, an accurate weight shows a loss of 500 milligrams (1 pound).

Although body weight gives an indication of total body water, the weight does not show fluids that are unavailable to the body by pooling in extravascular compartments ("third spacing"). For instance, in ascites there is fluid accumulation in the abdominal cavity. Although body weight increases, the amount of water available in the circulation is actually decreased; therefore, the patient has the signs and symptoms of volume deficit.

Additional measurements sometimes indicated are intake and output, serum and urine analysis, and venous pressure. Clinical observations include assessment of the skin, mucous membranes, and neuromuscular activity and behavior.

Intake and Output. A typical 24-hour fluid intake is approximately 1500 milliliters in a healthy adult in a temperate climate without any major physical exertion. In hot weather or during physical exertion the thirst mechanism is stimulated and more fluids are ingested.

Table 20-10.   Clinical Significance of Variations in Vital Signs

Finding	Associated Fluid and Electrolyte Disorders	Explanation for Finding
Pyrexia (fever)	Volume deficit Hypernatremia	Reduction in the amount of water ingestion and increased heat loss through the skin can cause a volume deficit, since with pyrexia, body metabolism is increased. Therefore, more water is lost through the skin and lungs.
Hypothermia	Hyponatremia	The reduced body metabolism that occurs with hyponatremia decreases body heat production.
Tachycardia	Magnesium deficit	A reduced serum magnesium causes hyperirritability of the heart muscle and stimulation of the CNS and ANS.
	Fever produced volume deficit	Cardiovascular response to increased metabolism occurs if circulating blood volume is also decreased.
	Sodium deficit Volume deficit	Cardiac response to decreased blood volume found in sodium deficit and extracellular fluid volume deficit.
Irregular, rapid heart rate	Potassium deficit	Direct effect of potassium on polarization and conduction of cardiac muscle. Also causes a broader T-wave, and many types of arrhythmias.
Irregular, slow heart rate	Calcium excess	Incomplete or complete AV block from excess calcium inhibiting cardiac depolarization.
	Potassium excess	Direct effect of potassium on polarization and conduction of cardiac muscle.
Cardiac standstill	Potassium excess	An increased serum potassium prevents transmission of the stimulus along the cardiac muscle. Before cardiac standstill occurs, the P-R interval increases, the T-wave is tall and peaked and progresses to an aberrant QRS, ventricular fibrillation, and then cardiac standstill.
	Calcium excess	An increased serum calcium inhibits cardiac depolarization.
	Magnesium excess	An increased serum magnesium inhibits cardiac depolarization.
Full, bounding pulse	Water and sodium excess	Cardiac response to an increased extracellular fluid volume or serum sodium excess.
Weak pulse	Volume deficit Sodium deficit	Cardiac response to a decreased extracellular fluid volume or serum sodium deficit.
Decreased respiratory rate and depth	Potassium deficit Potassium excess Magnesium excess	Imbalances produce a muscular weakness that progresses to paralysis of the diaphragm.
Increased respiratory rate and depth	Volume deficit with fever	Response to body's increased rate of metabolism that occurs with a fever.
Shortness of breath	Volume excess Sodium excess	Respiratory response to an overloaded circulatory system from volume excess or sodium excess.
Hypotension	Magnesium excess	Imbalance produces a muscular weakness, which depresses the force of ventricular contraction.
Orthostatic hypotension	Decreased vascular volume Sodium deficit	Decreased blood volume decreases amount of pressure exerted against arterial walls upon resuming upright position.
Hypertension	Magnesium deficit Volume excess Sodium excess Calcium excess	Imbalances produce a hyperirritability of muscles, including the heart, increased pressure against the arterial walls, and increased force of cardiac contraction.

In the absence of disease or hydration abnormalities, the amount of water added to the body is excreted from the body. Normally, if excretion of water is increased in one organ, the other organs compensate by not excreting as much water. For instance, in hot weather there is more perspiration, so water loss from the skin is increased, perhaps doubled. To compensate, urine output decreases, and the thirst mechanism is stimulated so that the water lost by perspiration is replenished.

Intake and output is a tool for assessing gains and losses of body fluids. The amounts and types of fluids gained and lost are reported. The content of specific body fluids varies considerably and this information aids in preventing or anticipating an imbalance (Table 20-11).

Intake and output measurements are indicated in any patient with a known or potential fluid and electrolyte imbalance; patients receiving intravenous therapy; patients with abnormal losses of body fluids such as nasogastric suctioning, fistulas, and drains, and patients whose fluid intake must be limited.

Urine volume varies considerably, although the average urine output in 24 hours is 1,500 milliliters (Table 20-12).

Urinalysis. In addition to urine volume, the specific gravity, pH, and composition of urine are measured in the assessment of fluid and electrolyte imbalances (Appendix 9).

One of the functions of the kidney is concentration or dilution of the urine in response to the needs of the body. If the body fluids are concentrated, the kidneys compensate through the hormonal control of ADH to reabsorb more water. The result is a more concentrated urine. If the body fluids are dilute, less ADH is secreted, and a dilute urine is excreted. The concentration of urine with normal renal function is approximately the same as the serum.

Urine concentration is measured by the laboratory as urine osmolality and has a range of 40 to 1,200 mOsm/1. The average urine osmolality is 310 mOsm/1, the same as the serum. Another way to measure urine concentration is the specific gravity. This is performed easily at the bedside, or outpatient facility, and measures the amount of dissolved solids in the urine by comparing the weight of the urine to the weight of an equal amount of distilled water. The

Table 20-11. Electrolyte Content of Selected Body Fluids (electrolytes in mEQ/L)

Fluid	*Volume*	*Na^+*	*K^+*	*Cl^-*	*HCO_3^-*
Gastric	40 ml./hr.	10-120	10-30	50-100	0-20
Bile	500-1,000 ml./24 hr.	130-150	4-6	90-110	30-60
Pancreas	1,000 ml./24 hr.	100-140	4-6	50-75	75-100
Small intestine	200 ml./24 hr.	70-120	3-7	65-125	30-40
Ileostomy					
Recent	1,000-4,000 ml./24 hr.	100-140	4-14	90-110	30-40
Old	100-500 ml./24 hr.	40-50	2-4	15-25	15-30
Feces	200 ml./24 hr.	5-10	0-2	5-10	5-10
Urine					
(mEq/24 hr.)	1,500 ml./24 hr.	10-200	15-200	170-250	0
Sweat	350 ml./24 hr.	30-70	2-4	30-70	0

Table 20-12. Clinical Significance of Urine Volume Variations

Finding	*Associated Fluid and Electrolyte Disorders*	*Explanation for Finding*
Decreased urine output Oliguria	Volume deficit, decreased fluid intake, diarrhea, vomiting, diaphoresis, hyperpnea	Normal renal compensatory mechanism associated with the disorders.
	Hypotension, shock, decreased cardiac output	Conditions decrease renal perfusion, which decreases the amount of glomerular filtrate formed.
	Renal failure	Diseased kidney unable to form normal amounts of urine.
Increased output Polyuria	Increased fluid intake, increased solute load in urine, diabetes, calcium excess, drugs, infection	Normal renal compensatory mechanism associated with the disorders.
	Decreased ADH, decreased aldosterone	Result of the direct effect of the decreased circulation of ADH and aldosterone.
	Renal insufficiency	In renal insufficiency the kidneys are unable to concentrate urine. A large volume of urine is needed to excrete the end products of metabolism.

specific gravity of distilled water is 1.000. The normal specific gravity of urine varies from 1.010 to 1.030. Specific gravity and urine osmolality change in the same direction.

Urine pH is measured with a nitrozine paper or dip stick and is therefore easy to perform at the beside or outpatient facility. Urine pH is the concentration of hydrogen ion in the urine and varies from 4.5 to 8.0 with an average of 6, depending on the acid-base status (Chapter 21). The kidneys have a major role in acid-base balance by reabsorbing base and excreting acid in various forms. Any condition that causes an acid-base imbalance, also causes a change in urine pH.

Venous Pressure. In the absence of cardiac disease, the venous pressure rises with an expanded blood volume. Venous pressure is measured by a catheter in the vena cava or right atrium (central venous pressure) or by noting the distention of the jugular veins (Chapter 11).

In fluid and electrolyte balance, the skin is dry, warm to the touch, and recoils immediately after being pinched (turgid). The mucous membranes are moist, with no drying or cracking. The client has the ability to control body movements and has no evidence of behavioral changes (Table 20-13).

Table 20-13. Clinical Observations in Fluid and Electrolyte Disorders

Finding	*Associated Fluid and Electrolyte Disorders*	*Explanation for Finding*
"Doughy" skin	Volume deficit	Skin feels thick and rubbery with a normal turgor.
Loss of skin turgor	Hyponatremia	After pinching the skin of the inner forearm, it remains folded for more than 30 seconds. Poor skin turgor is seen also in the elderly and emaciated but is not related to a low sodium.
Excessively dry and flushed skin	Volume excess	Sweating is decreased as a compensatory response to conserve body water.
Finger printing	Volume excess	A form of edema seen by the examiner by pressing or rolling a finger over a bony prominence, and this produces an imprint of the finger on the skin.
Pitting edema	Hypernatremia in congestive heart failure, cirrhosis, nephrotic syndrome, and Cushing's syndrome	Skin remains indented and blanched after pressing on it: 1+, edema barely detectable; 2+, indentation less than 5 mm.; 3+, indentation less than 10 mm. (1 cm.); 4+, indentation greater than 10 mm. (1 cm.).
Dry, fissured tongue and mucous membranes	Water deficit	Parched, dry tongue and mucous membranes of the mouth sometimes making phonation difficult. It is best detected by checking the mucous membranes where the gum and cheek meet. In moderate to severe situations the tongue has deep, longitudinal cracks.
Dry, fissured tongue	Mouth breather O_2 by mask	Parched, dry tongue with longitudinal cracking, but the mucous membranes at the junction of the gums and cheeks are moist.
Weakness	Potassium excess	Vague muscle weakness beginning in the legs and progressing to the torso and arms is an early symptom. Hyperpolarization of the cell membrane blocks the transmission of the stimulus along the muscle fiber.
	Potassium deficit	Hypopolarization of the cell membrane blocks the transmission of the stimulus along the muscle fiber.
	Water deficit	Water loss causes functional changes in the CNS. Also, severe water loss can cause subdural effusions or intracranial hemorrhages.
	Water excess	Gross muscle weakness occurs possibly from excessive water in the cells of the CNS.
	Calcium excess	Excess ionized calcium decreases neuromuscular transmission and may cause decreased muscle tone.
Paralysis	Potassium excess	Hyperpolarization of the cell membrane blocks the transmission of the stimulus along the muscle fiber. The respiratory muscles are affected last, and the muscles supplied by the cranial nerves are usually not affected.
	Potassium deficit	Hyperpolarization of the cell membrane blocks the transmission of the stimulus along the muscle fiber.

Table 20-13 *(continued)*

Finding	Associated Fluid and Electrolyte Disorders	Explanation for Finding
Spasms	Calcium deficit	A low ionized calcium increases neruromuscular transmission and causes neuromuscular irritability.
Paresthesias	Potassium excess	An increased potassium stimulates the pain receptors.
	Calcium deficit Magnesium deficit	Neuromuscular irritability from a deficit in calcium and magnesium.
Tremors	Water deficit	Desiccation of the cells causes neuromuscular irritability.
Isolated twitching	Water excess	The exact mechanism is unknown, but it is possibly from excessive amounts of water in the cells of the CNS.
Fasciculation	Magnesium deficit	Causes increased neruromuscular transmission and, therefore, neuromuscular irritability.
Cramps	Magnesium deficit Calcium deficit	Causes increased neuromuscular irritability.
	Potassium deficit	Occurs when potassium falls below 2.5 mEq/L. Hypopolarization of the cell membrane blocks the transmission of the stimulus along the muscle fiber.
+ Chvostek sign	Hypocalcemia	Tapping the facial nerve where it emerges from the parotid gland in front of the ear produces a contraction of the facial muscles on the side being tapped.
+ Trousseau sign	Hypocalcemia	Inflating a blood pressure cuff above the systolic pressure or by applying a tourniquet on the forearm produces carpal spasm within 3 minutes.
Apathy	Water excess	Excessive water in the cells causes apathy.
	Potassium deficit	Neuromuscular system is depressed from the hypopolarization of the cell membrane; this blocks the transmission of the stimulus along the muscle fiber.
	Sodium deficit	A deficit of extracellular sodium changes the osmotic equilibrium of the body and water shifts into the cells. This then causes a decreased circulating blood volume with associated signs and symptoms.
Lethargy	Water deficit	Decreased circulating blood volume and functional changes in the CNS produce a lethargic state.
	Potassium deficit	Decreased serum potassium depresses the neuromuscular system.
	Sodium deficit	Decreased serum sodium decreases circulating blood volume and causes functional changes in the CNS.
	Calcium deficit Magnesium excess	The electrolyte abnormalities depress the central nervous system.
Confusion	Water excess	Excessive water in the cells of the CNS possibly produces confusion.
	Sodium deficit	Decreased serum sodium decreases circulating blood volume and causes functional changes in the CNS.
	Calcium excess	Serum calcium excess produces a disturbance in neuronal transmission and functional changes in the CNS.
	Magnesium deficit	CNS depression occurs since there is a block or delay in neuromuscular transmission.

Life Cycle Variations

Childhood

The child's body weight is composed mainly of water. This amount varies from as high as 90 percent in premature infants to as low as 60 percent by the age of two (Table 20-14). As the infant becomes older, the body accumulates more fat and, therefore, the percentage of water decreases.

The amount of water needed to maintain balance depends upon the metabolic rate and water excreted by the kidneys, skin, lungs, and gastrointestinal tract. Although an infant consumes more water per unit of body weight than an adult, it is directly related to these factors.

Both infants and adults need 100 milliliters of water for every 100 calories metabolized. Since the infant's metabolic rate is two to three times greater than an adult's, the requirement for water is two to three times more per unit of weight than the adult. Therefore, as the infant grows, the metabolic rate and need for water decrease. By the age of 13, the adult requirement for water is reached (Table 20-15).

Another factor that affects the infant's water requirements is the solute load of the kidneys. Since the metabolic rate is higher in infants, there are more metabolic waste products for excretion and the urine pH is slightly more acidic (ranges from 5 to 5.5). In addition to excreting large volumes of water to rid the body of metabolic waste products, the infant has immature renal and hormonal systems. The kidneys are unable to efficiently concentrate the urine and the hormonal controls by aldosterone and ADH are unstable. The infant's urine osmolality can rise up to only 700-800 mOsm/L.

Infants also lose more water through the skin since their body surface area is proportionately larger than that of the adult. A premature infant has five times as much body surface area per unit of weight as an adult; a full-term newborn, three times as much.

The respiratory rate of infants is normally much faster than that of adults, so proportionately more water is lost through the lungs. Fecal losses of water in infants is relatively small.

The infant exchanges approximately half of his extracellular fluid each day. The water is lost mainly through the skin by evaporation and through the kidneys in urine and is replaced by the water in milk, fruits, and vegetables.

Table 20.14. Approximate Amount of Water in Body at Various Ages

Age	% Water
Premature infant	90
Newborn	75
1 year	70
2 years-adult	60

Table 20-15. Approximate Daily Requirement for Water

Age	Ml/Kg	Oz/lb
0-1*	150	$2\text{-}\frac{1}{4}$
1-3	125	2
4-6	100	$1\frac{1}{2}$
7-12	75	1.0+
13-adult	50	$\frac{3}{4}$

*First weeks lower; first 6 months relatively higher than last 6 months

Source: Adapted from V. Vaughan and R. McKay, editors, *Nelson Textbooks of Pediatrics*. Philadelphia. W. B. Saunders, 1975, p. 148.

Serum electrolytes vary little throughout the life span, although the daily requirements vary according to the needs of the body. During times of accelerated bone growth such as prepubescence and pubescence, greater quantities of calcium, magnesium, and phosphorous are needed. Chloride, potassium, and sodium needs remain relatively constant throughout the life span (Table 20-16).

Although infants have a higher percentage of body weight that is water, there is less of a water reserve

Table 20-16. Approximate Daily Requirements for Electrolytes

Electrolyte	Infants	Children	Adults
Calcium	0.4-0.6 gm	< 10yr. 0.7-1.9 gm > 10yr. 1.2-1.4 gm Amounts depend on vitamin D and sunlight	.65 gm
Chloride	0.5 gm	0.5 gm	3 gm
Magnesium	40-70 gm	1-3yr. 100-150 gm 3-12yr. 200-300 gm 12-18yr. 350-400 gm	20-40 mEq
Phosphorous	0.2-0.5 gm	< 10 0.7-1.0 gm > 10 1.2-1.4 gm	
Potassium	1-2 gm or 1.5 mEq/kg		80-200 mEq
Sodium	2.0 mEq/kg		50-85 mEq (3.5 gm)

Source: Adapted from V. Vaughan and R. McKay, R., editors, *Nelson Textbooks of Pediatrics*, Philadelphia; W. B. Saunders, 1975, pp. 152, 153, 154.

since so much of the water is exchanged each day. Infants are much more vulnerable to fluid volume deficit and can survive only three to four days without water. The signs and symptoms of fluid and electrolyte imbalances are the same in children as in adults; the major differences are the speed of the onset of the imbalance and the necessity to correct the imbalance rapidly.

The assessment modalities utilized in fluid and electrolyte imbalances in children are the same as for adults, although there are some inherent difficulties. Unfortunately, the small child is unable to describe symptoms. Crying may be the only sign, but crying occurs for a variety of reasons besides thirst. The anterior fontanelle is utilized in assessing fluid balance. A depressed fontanelle is indicative of decreased extracellular fluid volume. Skin turgor in a small child or infant is best palpated on the abdomen, sternum, or medial aspects of the thigh.

Intake and output is a real challenge in infants. As with adults, the most accurate method to assess fluid gains and losses from day to day is through daily weights. Measuring urine output is almost impossible in infants and small children. There are various methods utilized for measuring output. The number of voidings can be added, but this gives no information as to the quantity of the urine. In addition, the diapers can be weighed to determine how much urine is in the wet diaper (1 liter = 1 kilogram, 500 milliliters = 1.1 pounds). Various pediatric urine collectors can be used. Unfortunately, none of these methods are very accurate, even with the most meticulous nursing care. In severe cases of extracellular fluid volume deficit, a small child can go up to 18 hours without voiding.

Adolescence

The assessment of fluid and electrolyte balance in adolescents is the same as that in adults. Often, it is during this age that the body functions physiologically at its optimum. However, adolescents are not immune to fluid and electrolyte imbalances. Imbalances generally occur from improper diet or sports-related activities.

This age group is generally very weight-conscious and often follows various fad or starvation diets. Although these diets cause the desired effect of weight loss, they often are nutritionally unsound. Many of the body electrolytes are maintained through food ingestion. Of main concern are inadequate intakes of potassium, calcium, and phosphorous. Sodium intake is rarely a problem since it is present in soft drinks, candy, and prepared foods, which most dieting adolescents consume.

Another factor in weight control is the improper and dangerous use of diuretics. Since 500 milliliters of water weighs 500 milligrams, an increased urine output causes a decreased body weight. Unfortunately, electrolytes are lost with the water, and severe fluid and electrolyte imbalances can occur. Since this weight loss represents only water loss, once the diuretics are stopped, the body's normal compensatory mechanisms function to replace the lost water.

Physical sports such as football, soccer, and tennis may cause severe volume deficit, especially if they are played in a hot and dry environment. Generally, water and electrolyte replacement occurs with oranges, and other fluids containing water and electrolytes. If copious amounts of water are consumed, hyponatremia may result.

Pregnancy

Pregnancy is a healthful state in which physiologic changes occur. The most striking change in pregnancy is the increase in fluid volume. At term the pregnant woman has approximately 8 liters of excess water. Approximately 3.5 liters are from the water in the fetus, placenta, and amnionic fluid. Another 3.5 liters are from the expanded blood volume and increase in the size of the breasts and uterus. An additional 1 liter is present as edema of the interstitium. The edema is a result of four factors: increased venous pressure, decreased serum proteins, increased capillary permeability, and sodium retention.

When the pregnant woman is erect or supine, the enlarged uterus causes excessive pressure on the inferior vena cava. This increase in venous pressure increases the rate of filtration through the normal capillaries and, therefore, produces edema from a plasma to interstitial fluid shift. Characteristically, if the pregnant woman lies on her side for an extended period of time—for instance, while sleeping—the edema disappears since the uterus no longer exerts pressure on the inferior vena cava. This explanation applies to the edema of the lower extremities, not to the generalized edema sometimes exhibited by pregnant women.

Another factor in water retention is a lowered plasma albumin. Albumin is a plasma protein that affects the colloidal osmotic pressure. Colloidal osmotic pressure is the pressure exerted by the concentration of plasma proteins. With a decrease in the amount of plasma proteins, the colloidal osmotic pressure decreases, and there is a shift of fluid from the plasma to the interstitium. The plasma is unable to "hold onto" as much water as before. This fluid shift causes generalized edema.

A third factor in water retention is the increased permeability of the capillaries to water and electrolytes. This causes a generalized body edema from the shift of fluid from the plasma to the interstitium. This fluid shift generally occurs in the last few weeks of pregnancy.

A somewhat controversial explanation for water retention in pregnancy is sodium retention. Sodium retention is related to hormonal changes, especially the increase in aldosterone. It is thought that more aldosterone is secreted in response to elevated progesterone levels. This sodium retention represents a normal process in pregnancy.

The edema in pregnant women is assessed primarily by weight gain and the degree of pitting edema. Although the amount of weight gain varies considerably among women, most gain approximately 2 to 4 pounds in the first trimester and 10 pounds in each of the remaining trimesters. A sudden weight gain, or a weight gain well over the average, needs to be evaluated in terms of water retention. Mild pitting edema in the legs is a normal variant in pregnancy, especially when it occurs at the end of the day and disappears after resting with the legs elevated. Moderate or severe pitting edema and a more generalized body edema can be pathological.

Serum electrolytes also change somewhat during pregnancy. Serum osmolality and sodium decrease by about 3 percent to 290 mOsm/L and 140 mEq/L, respectively. This is most likely a result of the loss of plasma proteins. Calcium and magnesium decrease slightly, especially if the mother's intake is not adequate to meet the demands of the fetus. A pregnant or lactating woman needs more than 1 gram of calcium each day. Calcium deficits frequently cause leg cramps.

Late Adulthood

With increasing age there is a progressive decrease in renal function, since the kidney is unable to replace or regenerate injured nephrons. Therefore, there are fewer nephrons remaining to maintain normal renal function. This degeneration is not a problem during health, since the remaining nephrons are able to compensate adequately to maintain the composition and volume of body fluids. However, during periods of disease or environmental stress, the aged kidneys respond at a much slower rate than the healthy kidneys of youth.

The normal serum electrolyte values do not change with advancing age, but the specific gravity and osmolality of the urine do. The kidneys lose some of their ability to respond to change; this is evidenced by a decrease in the ability to concentrate the urine. The maximum specific gravity decreases from 1.032 in youth, to 1.024 in the aged. The maximum urine osmolality decreases from 1,200 mOsm/L in youth to 750 mOsm/L in the aged.

Although hypokalemia is not a normal condition for elderly people, it is a common finding and is characterized by fatigue. The elderly experience hypokalemia for a variety of reasons; most commonly it results from use of laxatives and diuretics and from malnutrition.

Elderly people generally have less frequent bowel movements than younger people and often are preoccupied with their bowel habits. In the early 1900s a bowel movement every day was considered normal. It is common for elderly people to abuse laxatives so that they can maintain this bowel-movement-per-day pattern. Many laxatives cause a loss of potassium from the body.

Diuretics are prescribed for many elderly people in the treatment of hypertension and heart disease. A side effect of most diuretics is hypokalemia. To prevent hypokalemia, supplemental potassium is administered either through diet or medication.

In a healthy person, potassium balance is maintained through diet. The aged commonly suffer from malnutrition. Some factors that affect malnutrition in the elderly are impaired mobility, which causes more difficulty shopping for food; soaring food costs with a fixed income; and the challenge of cooking nutritious and economical meals when living alone.

Physiology

Acid–base balance results from the regulation of hydrogen ion concentration in the body fluids and is expressed by the symbol pH. A pH of 7 indicates neutrality; anything above 7 is alkaline and anything below 7 is acidotic. The normal serum pH is 7.35-7.45; therefore, the blood is slightly alkaline. In the blood, a pH of less than 7.35 indicates an acidotic state and a pH above 7.45 indicates an alkalotic state (Figure 21-1). (A further discussion regarding pH appears later in the chapter.) Slight alterations in hydrogen, hence pH, cause marked acceleration or depression of cellular reactions. Since these alterations may produce death, it is essential that the body provide various mechanisms for the maintenance of hydrogen concentration. To accomplish this, there are three lines of defense that function simultaneously: the buffer systems, the respiratory system, and the renal system.

Buffers

The first line of defense is the buffers. Buffers are substances that react within seconds to absorb or release hydrogen, thereby maintaining a relatively constant pH. Although the buffers are in all body fluids and react within seconds to a change in pH, they are unable to correct a derangement completely. A buffer weakens an acid or base, but it does not neutralize it. For example, during normal metabolism the body produces approximately 60 mEq of hydrogen each day. This hydrogen is buffered and then transported to the lungs or kidneys for excretion. The buffers do not rid the body of excess acid produced, but weaken its effect and maintain the pH of the body fluids relatively constant until the other systems complete the task of excreting the excess hydrogen produced.

The major buffer systems in the body fluids are the bicarbonate, phosphate, hemoglobin, and protein buffer systems.

The bicarbonate and phosphate buffer systems are composed of weak acids and their conjugate bases. If a strong acid is added to the body fluids, the acid reacts chemically with the weak base from the buffer system to produce a weak acid and a salt. If a strong base is added to the body fluids, the base reacts chemically with the weak acid from the buffer system to produce a weak base and water. In the bicarbonate buffer system, the two components are carbonic acid (H_2CO_3), and sodium bicarbonate ($NaHCO_3$). Carbonic acid and sodium bicarbonate are present in both intracellular and extracellular fluids. If hydrochloric

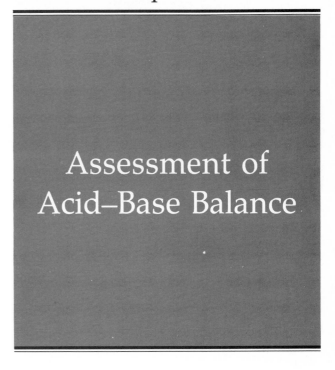

Chapter 21

Assessment of Acid–Base Balance

_____ Objectives _____

The examiner will be able to do the following:

1. Recognize signs and symptoms of acid-base imbalance
2. Recognize abnormalities in arterial blood gas values
3. Record the information obtained

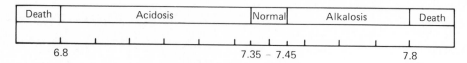

Figure 21-1. *Normal pH range.*

acid (HCl) is added to the body fluids, it reacts chemically with the sodium bicarbonate to form carbonic acid and sodium chloride (NaCl)—stated chemically:

$$HCl + NaHCO_3 \longrightarrow \quad H_2CO_3 + NaCl$$
(strong acid + base $\longrightarrow$ weak acid + salt)

A similar reaction occurs if a strong base is added to the body fluids. The strong base, sodium hydroxide (NaOH) reacts chemically with the carbonic acid to produce sodium bicarbonate and water—stated chemically:

$$NaOH + H_2CO_3 \longrightarrow \quad NaHCO_3 + H_2O$$
(strong base + buffer $\longrightarrow$ weak base + water)

The phosphate buffer system operates identically to the bicarbonate buffer system, except that it is most plentiful in the tubular fluid of the kidneys and in the intracellular fluid. The two components are monosodium dihydrogen phosphate (NaH_2PO_4) and disodium monohydrogen phosphate (Na_2HPO_4). If hydrochloric acid, is added to the body fluids, it reacts chemically with Na_2HPO_4 to form NaH_2PO_4 and NaCl—stated chemically:

$$HCl + Na_2HPO_4 \longrightarrow \quad NaH_2PO_4 + NaCl$$
(strong acid + buffer $\longrightarrow$ weak acid + salt)

Hemoglobin is a buffer since it functions as a weak acid or weak base by accepting or releasing some of the hydrogen dissociated from the carbonic acid in the serum. If the pH falls, hemoglobin absorbs hydrogen; if the pH rises, hemoglobin releases hydrogen.

Another buffer system in the body is the protein buffer system. It is the most plentiful buffer in the body and is found in the tissue cells and plasma. The body proteins are amino acids bound together by peptide linkages and function as weak acids or weak bases. Some of the amino acids have free acidic radicals and some have free basic radicals; in this way they can bind or release hydrogen in response to the body's pH. If an acid is introduced to the body, the proteins in the cell absorb hydrogen; if a base is introduced into the body, the proteins in the cell release hydrogen.

Respiratory System

The second line of defense is the respiratory system. The lungs help to maintain the pH of the blood by retaining or excreting volatile acids. A volatile acid is an acid that is excreted from the body as a gas. Carbonic acid is a volatile acid formed as a natural by-product from cellular metabolism. The oxidation of carbon in food produces carbon dioxide, CO_2, which diffuses into the vascular system. The carbon dioxide may be transported to the lungs, where it diffuses into the alveoli and is exhaled during pulmonary ventilation, or it reacts with water and forms carbonic acid ($CO_2 + H_2O \rightarrow H_2CO_3$). If it is necessary to remove acid from the body, the carbonic acid dissociates into carbon dioxide and water ($H_2CO_3 \rightarrow CO_2 + H_2O$), and the carbon dioxide diffuses into the alveoli and is exhaled during pulmonary ventilation (Figure 21-2).

The respiratory system not only removes acid produced by the body but responds to changes in hydrogen ion concentration, or pH, in one to three minutes.

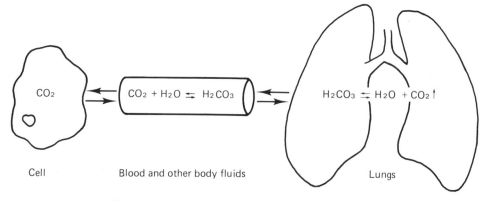

Figure 21-2. *Removal of acid by the respiratory system.*

The pH of the blood has a direct effect on the respiratory center in the medulla oblongata and a small indirect effect on the carotid body. If the pH falls the respiratory center is stimulated and hyperventilation occurs. With hyperventilation the rate of carbon dioxide excretion is increased, and, therefore, the amount of carbonic acid in the blood is reduced and the pH returns to normal. If the pH rises, the respiratory center is depressed and hypoventilation occurs. With hypoventilation, the rate of carbon dioxide excretion is reduced, and, therefore, the amount of carbonic acid in the blood is increased and the pH returns to normal (Figure 21-3).

This discussion is about normal acid-base balance and does not include disease states of the lungs or acid-base imbalance. If the change in pH is exogenous—that is, arising from outside of the body—the respiratory system is unable to return the pH completely to normal. As the pH approaches the normal range, the stimulus to the respiratory center in the medulla oblongata for hyperventilation or hypoventilation ceases. The lungs are approximately 50 to 75 percent effective in maintaining a normal pH if the change is from exogenous sources, but 100 percent effective if the variation results from normal carbon dioxide production from cellular metabolism.

Renal System

The third line of defense is the renal system. The kidneys produce the body's most powerful and most effective mechanism for maintaining a normal pH. The kidneys respond to a change in pH in approximately 12 to 24 hours and accomplish acid-base balance through hydrogen secretion, excretion of phosphoric acid and ammonium, and bicarbonate reabsorption.

Hydrogen ion secretion occurs throughout the tubules in exchange for sodium. During cellular metabolism, the tubular cells produce carbon dioxide, which reacts chemically with water and yields carbonic acid ($CO_2 + H_2O \rightarrow H_2CO_3$). The carbonic acid dissociates into hydrogen and bicarbonate ($H_2CO_3 \rightarrow H^+ + HCO_3^-$). The hydrogen is secreted into the tubular fluid while sodium is reabsorbed. The reabsorbed sodium combines with bicarbonate to pro-

duce sodium bicarbonate ($Na^+ + HCO_3^- \rightarrow NaHCO_3$) (Figure 21-4).

The pH of normal urine, and thus tubular fluid, is 6. The tubules can tolerate a pH as low as 4.5 without any damage. When the tubular fluid pH approaches 4.5, hydrogen secretion is inhibited.

To permit continued hydrogen secretion, the secreted hydrogen either reacts with the phosphate buffer system to produce phosphoric acid or combines with ammonia to produce ammonium ($H^+ + NH_3^= \rightarrow NH_4^-$).

The level of bicarbonate in the urine responds to the pH of the body fluids. In the presence of a low pH, most of the bicarbonate is reabsorbed. In the presence of a high pH, less bicarbonate is reabsorbed.

Assessment Modalities

Preparation

The first step in assessing acid-base balance is a computer analysis of the arterial blood gases. Arterial

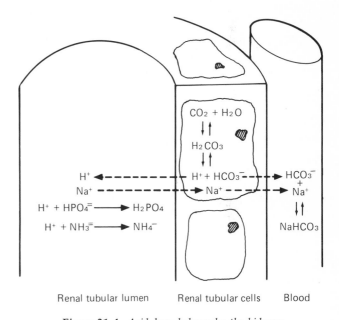

Figure 21-4. Acid–base balance by the kidneys.

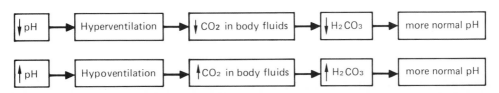

Figure 21-3. Respiratory response to changes in pH.

blood gas analysis is also performed to evaluate a patient's response to a change in respiratory treatment and to assess the progress of a patient with chronic lung disease. Arterial blood samples are obtained by direct arterial puncture or through an existing arterial line.

After the arterial blood sample is analyzed, the next step is interpretation of the results (Table 21-1). By progressing from simple to complex and treating the results as a simple mathematical problem, arterial blood gases are easily interpreted.

To assess acid-base balance, only three values from the arterial blood gases are needed: pH, P_aCO_2, and HCO_3^- (Table 21-1). The *pH* is the determination of the acid-to-base ratio in the body fluids. All the acid-base regulatory systems function to maintain a ratio of 1 part acid to 20 parts base (Figure 21-5). Since pH is an indication of hydrogen concentration and represents the negative logarithm of hydrogen, pH is inversely related to hydrogen concentration. That is, when the pH falls below 7.35, hydrogen ion concentration is up and acidosis is present. When the pH rises above 7.45, hydrogen ion concentration is down and alkalosis is present.

P_aco_2 is the partial pressure of CO_2 in the arterial blood. Partial pressure, or tension, is that portion of the total pressure that a gas exerts in a solution (Dalton's law), and is measured in millimeters of mercury (mm.Hg.). P_aCO_2 is the respiratory component and is an indicator of alveolar ventilation. If alveolar ventilation is poor as in hypoventilation, carbon dioxide is not exhaled. This in turn causes a rise in the P_aCO_2 above 42 mm.Hg. and more carbonic acid is formed in the body fluids. The converse is also true. If alveolar ventilation is accelerated, as in hyperventilation, the P_aCO_2 falls below 38 mm.Hg. and the carbonic acid levels fall. The P_aCO_2 is considered an indicator of the amount of acid in the body fluids from respiratory processes.

HCO_3^- is the metabolic component and is indicative of metabolic derangements. HCO_3^- levels are calculated from the pH and P_aCO_2. The HCO_3^- value is considered an indicator of the amount of base from metabolic processes in the body fluids. In metabolic imbalances an elevated HCO_3^- above 27 mEq/L is indicative of excess base in the body fluids and, hence, a metabolic alkalosis. Similarly, low HCO_3^- below 23 mEq/L is indicative of a base deficit in the body fluids and, hence, a metabolic acidosis. In respiratory imbalances the HCO_3^- level is indicative of the body's compensatory mechanisms.

In making an assessment, it is always better to have serial determinations so that the direction of the body's reactions are assessed. Given the following results, the arterial blood gases are analyzed as a simple mathematical problem:

pH 7.31
P_aCO_2 60 mm.Hg.
HCO_3^- 27 mEq/L.

Since the pH is low, it represents acidosis as the primary disorder. But the pH does not give any information regarding how the blood became acidotic. For that reason, the respiratory component, P_aCO_2, and the metabolic component, HCO_3^-, are assessed. Since P_aCO_2 is elevated, it is indicative of a respiratory acidosis. It is respiratory because the P_aCO_2 is the respiratory component, and acidosis, because a high P_aCO_2 in the blood reacts with water to form carbonic acid. Since HCO_3^- is within normal limits, it signifies that there is no metabolic imbalance. This information can be summarized as follows:

pH 7.31   low, primary acidosis
P_aCO_2 60 mm.Hg.   high, respiratory acidosis
HCO_3^- 27 mEq/L.   normal, metabolic component

After determining that the pH is acidotic, the respiratory and metabolic components are examined to see which one matches the pH. In this case, the pH shows an acidosis and the P_aCO_2 shows a respiratory acidosis. Therefore, the primary disorder is a respiratory acidosis. Since the HCO_3^- is normal, there is no metabolic compensation. Therefore, the inter-

Table 21-1. Arterial Blood Gas Samples

Symbol	Normal Value	Definition
pH	7.35 - 7.45	Negative logarithm of hydrogen ion concentration. Indicates relative acid-base balance or the primary imbalance
P_aCO_2	40 mm.Hg. ± 2	Partial pressure of CO_2, respiratory component, indicator for respiratory imbalance
HCO_3^-	25 mEq/L. ± 2	Concentration of bicarbonate ion, metabolic component, indicator for metabolic imbalances

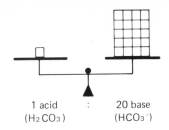

1 acid   :   20 base
(H_2CO_3)   (HCO_3^-)

Acidosis — pH less than 7.35

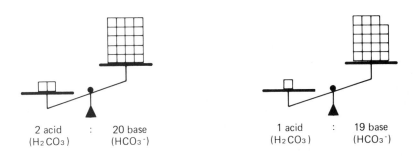

2 acid   :   20 base   1 acid   :   19 base
(H_2CO_3)   (HCO_3^-)   (H_2CO_3)   (HCO_3^-)

Alkalosis — pH greater than 7.45

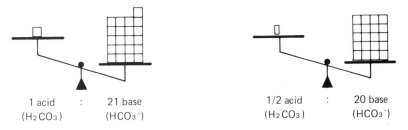

1 acid   :   21 base   1/2 acid   :   20 base
(H_2CO_3)   (HCO_3^-)   (H_2CO_3)   (HCO_3^-)

Figure 21-5. Ratio of acid to base.

pretation is an acute respiratory acidosis. With this formula in mind, the four primary acid-base imbalances with and without compensation are discussed.

Respiratory Acidosis

Respiratory acidosis occurs from problems of the respiratory component in acid-base balance. Anything that decreases or blocks alveolar ventilation interferes with the exhalation of carbon dioxide. This interference causes a rise in P_aCO_2, and therefore a rise in carbonic acid. With more carbonic acid in the serum, the normal ratio between acid and base is upset, and the pH falls to the acid side (Figure 21-5).

Regardless of the condition that causes respiratory acidosis, changes in mentation range from restlessness and confusion to CNS depression. This is a result of the high P_aCO_2, often called CO_2 narcosis, and from the change in pH and its effect on cellular activities. Although hypoventilation caused the respiratory acidosis, hyperventilation can occur in the late stages as a compensatory mechanism to rid the body of excess CO_2. Other signs and symptoms are a result of the underlying condition. If the acidotic state persists beyond 12 to 24 hours, the kidneys compensate by retaining more bicarbonate (HCO_3^-), and an elevated HCO_3^- appears in the arterial blood gases. The more chronic the respiratory acidosis is, the higher the HCO_3^- . (Table 21-2, 21-3).

Respiratory Alkalosis

Respiratory alkalosis also occurs from problems of the respiratory component in acid-base balance, but in respiratory alkalosis there is hyperventilation. In hyperventilation the respiratory rate and depth increase and excessive amounts of carbon dioxide are exhaled, which reduces the amount of carbonic acid in the body fluids. With less carbonic acid in the serum, the normal ratio between acid and base is upset, and the pH rises to the alkalotic side (Figure 21-5).

In respiratory alkalosis there are changes in sensorium from the effect of an altered pH on cellular activity. Also associated with the alkalotic state are paresthesias, muscle twitching, and a positive Chvostek's sign (Table 20-13). These result from a decrease in ionized calcium that occurs during an alkalotic state. If the alkalosis continues, tetany can occur.

With hyperventilation, dizziness and syncope frequently occur since the cerebral blood vessels constrict and the blood flow to the brain is impaired. Other signs and symptoms during respiratory alkalosis are those of the underlying condition (Tables 21-4 and 21-5).

Metabolic Acidosis

Metabolic acidosis occurs from an accumulation of acids or a loss of base in the body fluids. Anything that causes an excess production of acid, interferes with acid excretion, or causes a loss of bicarbonate causes a metabolic acidosis. In metabolic acidosis the acid-to-base ratio is upset, and the pH falls from either too much acid or too little base (Figure 21-5).

In metabolic acidosis there is usually hyperventilation as an attempt of the respiratory system to compensate for the acidotic state by exhaling carbon dioxide. This decreases the cabonic acid levels in the body fluids. Mentation degenerates from restlessness and confusion to CNS depression from the effect of the low pH on cellular metabolism. Other signs and symptoms are a result of the underlying condition (Tables 21-6, 21-7).

Table 21-2.   Respiratory Acidosis.

Finding	Possible Conditions	Description and Explanation
Acute, no renal compensation pH ↓ P_aCO_2 ↑ HCO_3^- normal	Pneumonia Pulmonary edema	Hypoventilation from accumulation of fluid in alveoli. Hyperventilation may occur in late stages to assist with the excretion of CO_2.
	Oversedation Head injuries	Hypoventilation from depressed respiratory center.
Chronic renal compensation pH ↓ P_aCO_2 ↑ HCO_3 ↑	Chronic obstructive pulmonary disease	Hypoventilation from poor pulmonary function, often associated with pursed lip breathing and use of accessory muscles.
	Gross obesity Neuromuscular weakness	Hypoventilation from inability of lungs to expand fully.

Table 21-3.   Chinical Example: Respiratory Acidosis

	Respiratory Acidosis without Renal Compensation	Respiratory Acidosis with Renal Compensation
pH	7.22 (acidosis)	7.32 (acidosis)
P_aCO_2	60 mm.Hg. (respiratory acidosis)	60 mm.Hg. (respiratory acidosis)
HCO_3^-	26 mEq./L. (normal)	31 mEq./L. (metabolic alkalosis)
Interpretation	Respiratory acidosis	Chronic respiratory acidosis or respiratory acidosis with partial renal compensation

Table 21-4. Respiratory Alkalosis

Finding	Possible Conditions	Explanation
Acute, no renal compensation pH ↑ P_aCO_2 ↓ HCO_3^- normal	Anxiety	Hyperventilation can occur as a physiologic component of the anxiety syndrome.
	Fever, pain	Hyperventilation can occur as a physiologic component.
	Salicylate poisoning	Large or toxic doses of acetylsalicylic acid (aspirin) stimulate the respiratory center and therefore cause hyperventilation.
Chronic, renal compensation pH ↑ P_aCO_2 ↓ HCO_3^- ↓	Pregnancy	The respiratory center is "reset" to a lower level of P_aCO_2 from the high levels of progesterone. Hyperventilation occurs to lower the P_aCO_2, which protects the fetus from high levels of CO_2, but little change occurs in the pH since the kidneys excrete more HCO_3^-. Also, the increased weight and pressure against the diaphragm cause the pregnant woman to hyperventilate.
	Pulmonary emboli	Respiratory rate is increased from the resultant pulmonary infarction and is out of proportion to the degree of fever and tachycardia.
	Improper mechanical ventilation	Increased respiratory rate or an increased tidal volume is produced regardless of the needs of the patient. The patient is unable to override the "settings" of the ventilator.
	Hypoxemia	Hyperventilation occurs as a compensatory mechanism to raise the P_aCO_2.
	Encephalitis	Hyperventilation occurs from the inflammation to the CNS and the accompanying high fever.

Table 21-5.   Clinical Example: Respiratory Alkalosis

	Respiratory Alkalosis without Renal Compensation	Respiratory Alkalosis with Renal Compensation
pH	7.6 (alkalosis)	7.56 (alkalosis)
P_aCO_2	25 mm.Hg (respiratory alkalosis)	25 mm.Hg (respiratory alkalosis)
HCO_3^-	22 mEq/L. (normal)	18 mEq/L. (metabolic acidosis)
Interpretation	Respiratory alkalosis	Chronic respiratory alkalosis or respiratory alkalosis with partial renal compensation

Table 21-6.   Metabolic Acidosis

Finding	Possible Conditions	Explanation
pH ↓ P_aCO_2 ↓ HCO_3^- ↓	Diabetic ketoacidosis, starvation	Metabolism of fats and proteins produce excessive amounts of hydrogen, which are inadequately excreted by the kidneys.
	Heart failure	Cellular anaerobic metabolism occurs from tissue hypoxia, which produces lactin and then lactic acidosis.
	Acidifying agents	Hydrogen ion concentration increases from overadministration of hydrogen-containing substances, e.g., ammonium, diamox, methyl alcohol.
	Renal failure	Inability of renal tubules to reabsorb bicarbonate.
	Diuretics	Excessive renal loss of bicarbonate.
	Severe diarrhea Ileostomy	Loss of bicarbonate from body fluids since it is plentiful in the lower GI tract.

Table 21-7. Clinical Example: Metabolic Acidosis

	Metabolic Acidosis without Compensation	Metabolic Acidosis with Compensation
pH	7.25 (acidosis)	7.30 (acidosis)
P_aCO_2	38 mm.Hg (normal)	32 mm.Hg (respiratory alkalosis)
HCO_3^-	13 mEq/L. (metabolic acidosis)	13 mEq./L (metabolic acidosis)
Interpretation	Metabolic acidosis	Metabolic acidosis with partial respiratory compensation

Metabolic Alkalosis

Metabolic alkalosis occurs from the ingestion or administration of bicarbonate or from the loss of acids. In metabolic alkalosis the acid-to-base ratio is upset from too much base or too little acid, and the pH rises (Figure 21-5).

The physical signs associated with metabolic alkalosis are rather vague and nonspecific. Hypoventilation occurs as a compensatory mechanism to raise carbonic acid levels. The main clinical features—paresthesias, muscular twitching, and a positive Chvostek's sign—result from a decrease in ionized cal-

cium during an alkalotic state. If the alkalosis continues, tetany can occur (Tables 21-8, 21-9).

Life Cycle Variations

Childhood

The maintenance of acid-base balance in children is identical to that of adults. The buffers, respiratory system, and renal system respond in the same ways as previously discussed in both acid-base balance and imbalance. The laboratory data in infants are slightly

Table 21-8. Metabolic Alkalosis

Finding	Possible Conditions	Explanation
pH ↑ P_aCO_2 ↑ HCO_3^- ↑	Overzealous use of antacids Overtreatment of metabolic acidosis with IV sodium bicarbonate	Body fluids are overloaded with base (HCO_3^-), which the kidneys are unable to excrete effectively.
	Severe vomiting Gastric suctioning	Loss of excessive amounts of acid (HCl) from body fluids.
	Ethacrynic acid Furosemide Thiazides	No bicarbonate is lost in the urine, but large volumes of extracellular fluid are excreted; therefore, the bicarbonate is dissolved in a decreased amount of fluid. This is sometimes referred to as contraction alkalosis. The action of these diuretics also causes an increased hydrogen ion presence in the urine. The result of volume contraction and increased urinary excretion of hydrogen produces a mild metabolic alkalosis.
	Hyperaldosteronism Cushing's disease Corticosteroid therapy	Metabolic alkalosis as a result of sodium reabsorption in the distal tubule while potassium and hydrogen are secreted.

Table 21-9. Clinical Example: Metabolic Alkalosis

	Metabolic Alkalosis without Compensation	Metabolic Alkalosis with Compensation
pH	7.55 (alkalosis)	7.50 (alkalosis)
P_aCO_2	40 mm.Hg (normal)	50 mm.Hg (respiratory acidosis)
HCO_3^-	40 mEq/L. (metabolic alkalosis)	40 mEq/L (metabolic alkalosis)
Interpretation	Metabolic alkalosis	Metabolic alkalosis with partial respiratory compensation

different from adults, but adult values are reached by adolesence (Table 21-10).

Table 21-10. Pediatric Normal Values

	Infancy	Adolescence
pH	7.37	7.4
P_aCO_2	35	40
HCO_3^-	19	24

Obtaining arterial blood is a problem in children. The umbilical cord is used in neonates, and an ear lobe or heel stick is performed in infants and children.

Pregnancy

During pregnancy it is normal for a mild, chronic respiratory alkalosis to exist from hyperventilation. The respiratory center is "reset" by high levels of progesterone to a lower level of P_aCO_2 in order to protect the fetus from high levels of carbon dioxide. Hyperventilation also occurs from the increased weight and pressure against the diaphragm. Both these conditions lower the P_aCO_2, and the HCO_3^- falls from 25 to approximately 22 mEq/1. to compensate effectively for the respiratory changes. Because of the renal compensation, there is little change in the pH of body fluids.

Late Adulthood

With aging there is no direct change in acid-base balance. If no disease state is present, the arterial blood gases are identical to younger people. Renal function is depressed with aging, but the kidneys retain the ability to maintain acid-base balance in the absence of disease. However, the kidneys are slower to react to changes in pH as seen by the decreased ability of the kidney to acidify urine. Although there are pulmonary changes with aging, they do not affect carbon dioxide diffusion or the P_aCO_2.

Health is a state of physical, psychosocial, and socioeconomic well-being. It exists in varying degrees on a continuum from optimal functioning to cessation of functioning (death). Individuals can exhibit different levels of functioning in the three aspects of healthful living although most frequently one aspect is influenced in some degree by the others. Health assessment consists of four steps: data gathering, analysis of data, formulation of a plan, and evaluation of the plan. The range and depth of each step of the assessment process are influenced by examiner, client, and situational variables. Some examiner variables include baseline of knowledge ("he can't find something he doesn't know exists or doesn't look for"), clinical experience, skill at performing examination techniques, role in the health care agency, ability to establish rapport, and feelings toward the client as contributor in the assessment process. Some of the client variables include attitude toward health, attitude toward the examiner, purpose for seeking assessment, trust in the examiner, risk factors, knowledge of health, and willingness to discuss and intervene in health. Some situational variables include the setting and time allotted for assessment.

Data gathering involves the collection of subjective and objective data. The subjective data are told by the client and are called the history; the objective data are observed by the examiner and include the physical examination, laboratory tests, X-ray, and other specialized diagnostic techniques, for example ECG, EEG, and cystoscopy.

The analysis of data has various models: nursing model (formulation of client needs), Weed model (statement of the problem), and medical model (differential diagnosis). Whichever model is used, at this stage the examiner reviews the collected data and summarizes the client's level of health. Based on this analysis a plan is formulated with three goals: diagnostic, therapeutic, and educational.

Diagnostic goals indicate what further assessment modalities are indicated to confirm a suspicion. For example, one or several laboratory tests may be necessary. Therapeutic goals provide some kind of relief to the client. This could be in the form of periodic counseling sessions, medication, or application of heat or cold to a body part. Educational goals instruct the client in a better understanding of health and his role in maintaining or regaining it. This includes providing positive reinforcement for healthful practices and behavior.

The final step is evaluation of the plan. At some later point, the client and examiner meet to assess how the client's health has changed as a result of the plan.

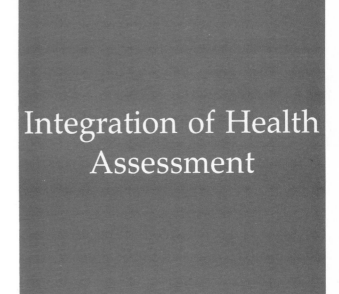

Chapter 22

Integration of Health Assessment

Objectives

The examiner will be able to do the following:

1. Understand clinical applications of health assessment skills in a variety of nursing settings
2. Internalize an organized method of performing a comprehensive physical examination for adult, neonatal, child, and pregnant clients
3. Perform and record a comprehensive physical examination

There is a continuum of health assessment skills among professional roles. For example, the public health nurse assesses all three aspects of the client's health: physical, psychosocial, and socioeconomic. In contrast a recovery room nurse concentrates on assessment of the client's physiologic responses to surgery. The prime concerns are maintenance of vital functions and proper functioning of surgical drains, dressings, and appliances. Although psychosocial and socioeconomic factors may be considered, physiologic factors are primary.

This text presents many methods of data collection, methods that are useful in a variety of settings and circumstances and some that are especially important for certain life cycle stages. There is great variety in the settings where health assessment occurs (Table 22-1). Some settings provide more opportunities for the examiner to perform certain aspects of health assessment. However, in any setting the more assessment skills the examiner utilizes, the more fruitful the interaction with an individual client can be.

Circumstances altering the depth and range of assessment include the client's reason for seeking care and the time, equipment and finances available. Some clients request a comprehensive health assessment at first contact, while others request ongoing periodic assessment in their interest for preventive care. Still others require help with resolution of an acute crisis.

Time can be a major factor influencing health assessment. Although possessing a multitude of health assessment skills, the charge nurse on a medical-surgical ward might have to rely on initial daily assessment of key aspects of each patient during bedside rounds and reports of changes from other staff members. Even if time were not a factor, it would not be practical to perform a comprehensive health assessment on each patient on each shift.

Equipment is also a determining factor in assessment. For example, screening for glaucoma would not be complete if a tonometer were not available; a coronary care unit nurse would be unable to detect arrhythmias without monitors.

Finances influence the extent of assessment. For example, in a setting where a Dopler is considered too expensive a purchase, fetal heart tones are inaudible until about the twentieth week in contrast to auscultation at the ninth to the tenth week where Doplers are used. Obstetric nurses are unable to observe early signs of fetal distress without fetal monitoring devices. Of course, the best-equipped setting can ensure assessment only as good as the people using it.

This chapter presents tables with suggestions for comprehensive health assessment for the "routine checkup" during several life cycle stages: adulthood, infancy, childhood, and pregnancy. These suggestions are for periodic evaluation of "healthy" clients. Healthy is in quotation marks because two of the purposes and outcomes of health assessment are illness screening and identification of disease.

There is considerable controversy about the efficacy of periodic health assessment and what techniques should be included if it is performed (Table 22-2). Proponents of periodic health assessment view it as a process more complex and many-faceted than searching for disease. They view it as providing subjective values such as positive feedback for healthful living practices, an opportunity for clients to increase their knowledge of health practices, and an opportunity to obtain counseling for psychosocial problems. Opponents of health assessment believe that there is a low yield in identifying health problems in comparison with the amount of time and money expended during routine checkups of well persons.

The material in this text is organized mainly by systems, with the exception of the head and neck. However, in conducting the physical examination, the examiner proceeds regionally in order to facilitate client comfort, avoid client fatigue, and use time efficiently. The examiner uses all the necessary techniques for a given region or body part before proceeding to the next region. This minimizes client changes of position, which is particularly important for debilitated people. For example, when assessing the chest, the examiner performs the lung and heart assessment, the assessment of the skin of the chest and back, and the breast and axillary examination. The recording or write-up is done systemically.

It is not only important to be able to assess clients and patients; it is essential that the examiner be able to record this information. Because more items are assessed than recorded, some items are included only if abnormal findings are present. For example, in the eye examination the condition of the eyelids, eyebrows, and eyelashes is not recorded unless abnormalities are present. When present, abnormalities are described in detail including the following characteristics: location, size, appearance, texture, tenderness, radiation, and mobility.

Ideally the health professional obtains the health history while the client is fully clothed, prior to the physical examination. The client and examiner face each other at eye level. During the examination, however, the professional frequently becomes aware of an omission from the history; this information is obtained during the physical examination. For example, a client relates that he has never had surgery, but the examiner notes an abdominal scar during inspection of the abdomen.

Table 22-1. Differences in Data Gathering Related to Professional Setting

Professional Setting	Strengths	Weaknesses
Home visit (public health nurse)	Opportunity to evaluate home environment, interrelationships between household members, coping mechanisms, safety, environmental risk factors, how household handles stress.	Lack of equipment precludes certain types of assessment, for example, tonometry, biochemical tests, and measurements such as weight.
Health office in industrial plant (occupational nurse)	Opportunity to evaluate interrelationships among co-workers and occupational risk factors. Access to job performance evaluations. Employees see health professional on a regular basis and may feel more comfortable to discuss problems.	Amount of equipment available varies. Large industry often has fully equipped examination room and means for obtaining biochemical tests.
Rehabilitation center (rehabilitation nurse)	Opportunity to evaluate response to disability.	Assessment tends to focus on disability and rehabilitation. Seemingly unrelated problems may be missed unless actively sought; for example, response of significant others to disability of client.
Summer camp (camp nurse)	Opportunity to evaluate children at play with peers and how they approach new activities.	Lack of time to perform comprehensive health assessment.
School (school nurse)	Opportunity to assess achievement of developmental goals, children at play, how children relate to peers and teachers, how they approach learning new skills, and how they handle responsibility. Children can seek health care independently of parents.	Lack of time to perform comprehensive health assessment.
Psychiatric setting (psychiatric nurse specialist)	High degree of interviewing skills and ability to assess psychosocial status of clients.	Frequently may not be able to observe client interact with significant others, must rely on client's perceptions and reports, usually able to assess physiologic well-being as it relates to psychologic health, but unable to assess other aspects of physiologic health, such as performance of health screening.
Primary care clinic (family nurse practitioner)	Possesses ability to perform comprehensive health assessment including physiologic, psychologic, social, and nutritional status.	Clients who are unfamiliar with role are sometimes reluctant to be seen by nurse practitioner. Frequently other health professionals do not accept the nurse practitioner.
Perinatal setting (perinatal nurse)	Frequently can assess client's response to pregnancy and her particular methods of coping and the partner's role in pregnancy.	Usually able to assess only one or several aspects of perinatal course, for example, prenatal care, labor and delivery, or postpartum course.
Operating room (nurse anesthetist)	High level of skill in assessment of vital functions (temperature, pulse, respirations, blood pressure, fluid and electrolyte balance, and acid-base balance).	Aside from initial interview and follow up interview must necessarily focus on assessment of vital functions only. Insufficient time to perform other assessment skills.
Office (office nurse)	Most assessment equipment is available.	Although office may be well equipped, nurse usually is too busy to utilize equipment other than what traditional roles dictate, for example, taking of vital signs and anthropometric measurements. Frequently clients see nurse as physician's assistant and are reluctant to discuss openly or to have the nurse perform assessment skills.
Client's bedside (primary nurse)	Maximal time available for thorough assessment of client's physical, psychological, and social status as well as coping mechanisms of significant others.	When seeing a client on a prolonged and frequent basis, subtle changes are sometimes missed.
Clinical preceptorship (nursing instructor)	Assessment enriched by information gained by students who frequently have intensive involvement with client.	Assessment of individual clients is limited by students' abilities and the instructors' capacity for expanding the students' abilities.

Table 22-2. Recommendations for Health Assessment of Adults

Assessment Modalities	18-20 Yrs. Of Age	20-40 Yrs. Of Age	Over 40 Yrs. Of Age	Over 50 Yrs. Of age
Comprehensive health history and examination (Tables 22-3 and 22-4)	Usually obtained for military health assessment, precollege, or pre-employment health assessment	Every 3 years	Annually	Annually
Self-breast examination	Monthly	Monthly	Monthly	Monthly
Self-head and neck examination	Semi-annually	Semi-annually	Semi-annually	Semi-annually
Self-testicular examination	Monthly	Monthly	Monthly	Monthly
Urine dipstick, hematocrit/ hemoglobin	Usually obtained with comprehensive health examination	Every 3 years	Annually	Annually
Tuberculosis tine test	Usually obtained with comprehensive health history	Annually for health professionals; otherwise every 3 years	Annually for health professionals; otherwise every 3 years	Annually for professionals; otherwise every 3 years
VDRL (and rubella immunity test in females)	Usually obtained with premarital health examination and initiation of obstetric care	Usually obtained with premarital health examination and initiation of obstetric care		
Pap smear	American Cancer Society recommendation: Sexually active females—every 3 years after 2 normal tests one year apart American College of Obstetricians and Gynecologists recommendation: Annually	Every 3 years after 2 initial normal tests 1 year apart	Annually	Annually
Mammogram		Women between the ages of 35 and 40—1 baseline mammogram; if breast mass is palpable or with family history (mother or sister with breast cancer)—annually	Annually	Annually
Stool specimen for occult blood (guiaic or hemoccult)		Every three years	Annually	Annually
Chest X-ray			Biannually	Biannually
Proctosigmoidoscopy			2 baseline studies 1 year apart; with a change in bowel habits or with family history of bowel carcinoma—annually	Every 3-5 years after 2 initial normal examinations 1 year apart

Table 22-2 (continued)

Assessment Modalities	18-20 Yrs. of Age	20-40 Yrs. of Age	Over 40 Yrs. of Age	Over 50 Yrs. of Age
ECG			Males—every 2 years	Males and females every 2 years
Tonometry		With signs or symptoms of increased intra-ocular pressure or family history of glaucoma—annually	Annually	Annually
Dental Examination	Annually	Annually	Annually	Annually

The comprehensive health history is ideally obtained when the health professional first meets the client (Table 22-3.) Subsequent visits with clients who have provided a comprehensive health history contain the following information:

1. Statement about the general state of health since last interview

2. Statement about what brought the client to the health professional this time

Table 22-3. Components of the Comprehensive Health History

Identifying data
  Name, address and telephone number of client and contact, birthdate, sex, race, religion, marital status and number of children, Social Security number, occupation, birthplace, referral source, informant and reliability, and date of interview

Chief complaint or reason for presenting for health care

Present illness or present state of health
  Introduction
    Description of client
    Usual health
  Chronological investigation of symptoms
    Course of symptomatology: onset, manner, duration, incidence, remissions, and exacerbations
    Clarification: location; quantity; quality; setting; aggravating, alleviating, and associated factors
  Pertinent negatives
  Relevant family history and psychosocial and socioeconomic data
  Assessment of disability
  Medications

Past history
  Childhood diseases
  Serious injuries, accidents, and disabilities
  Hospitalizations
  Surgical procedures
  Transfusions
  Major illnesses
  Allergies: food, drug, and environmental
  Immunizations
  Military service
  Foreign travel

Family history
  Health of relatives
  Cause of death of deceased family members
  Presence in family of conditions with familial tendencies

Psychosocial history
  Personal life: state of well-being, general level of satisfaction with significant others, developmental history with occupational and educational factors

Socioeconomic history.
  Cultural considerations: Members of household, role and position in household, position in extended family
  Environmental factors: Description of neighborhood, pattern of moving, description of home, occupational health risks
  Economic profile: existence of health insurance, effect of health on finances, effect of finances on health
  Activities of daily living: example of a normal day, sleep and activity patterns, identification of unhealthy habits (smoking, alcohol use, and illicit drug use), hobbies and recreational interests
  Health practices: orientation to and philosophy of health care, hygiene facilities, sanitation and refrigeration, safety precautions, source of health care, emergency readiness

Nutritional history—diet history *

Review of systems

* The examiner may determine that a more extensive nutritional assessment is indicated when the following risk factors and conditions are identified during history taking or weight and height measurements: reliance on fad diets, overweight, underweight, multiple food allergies or intolerances, alcoholism, diabetes mellitus, hospitalization, inability to obtain or prepare food, prolonged NPO status, and major surgery. This can include a food diary, biochemical measurements such as fasting blood sugar, two-hour postprandial blood sugar, white blood cell count, hematocrit, hemoglobin, serum protein and albumin, cholesterol and triglycerides, skinfold thickness measurements, creatinine height index, and immune system response.

3. Follow-up statement about any problems identified at previous interviews

4. Identification of stress-producing factors: death of spouse, death of a family member, divorce, financial difficulties, change in occupation, change in makeup of household

5. Complete review of systems and family history

6. Statement about feelings toward role and developmental tasks; for example, how does the client feel about the new role as parent

Tables 22-4, 22-5, 22-6, and 22-8 present outlines for the examination of the adult, neonate, child, and pregnant woman. Table 22-7 presents recommendations for health assessment of children. Hospitalized or debilitated clients require many additional assessment techniques to provide information regarding response to and progression of illness and return to the healthy state. Examples of these are assessment of incisional wounds, stomas, and stumps following amputation and progress in rehabilitative programs. Discussion of these conditions, however, is beyond the scope of this text.

Table 22-4. Outline for Examination of the Adult (Items in brackets are assessed but not usually recorded unless abnormal)

Body Region	Client Position	Examiner Position	Techniques	Where Recorded
Overall body	Sitting on examination table, wearing examination gown	Standing facing client	Inspection of client's apparent age, sex, race, body build, stature, symmetry, posture, hygiene, skin condition, apparent state of health and motor activity. Observation of speech, and presence of any odors of breath or body.	General survey
Vital signs	As preceding	As preceding	Temperature. Pulses (carotid, radial, brachial, femoral, popliteal, posterior tibial, and dorsalis pedis).	General survey Cardiovascular
			Rate of radial pulse. Respiratory rate. Blood pressure, both arms.	General survey General survey General survey
	Standing	As preceding	Blood pressure, both arms	General survey
Overall body	Walking to scale	As preceding	Inspection of gait	Neurologic General survey
			Height and weight measurements	
Eyes	Standing 6 m. (20 ft.) from Snellen eye chart	6 m. (20 ft.) from client, beside Snellen eye chart	Visual acuity (if chart is not available, reading newspaper print or Snellen chart on a small card can be done with head examination).	Eye and neurologic (cranial nerve II)
Nutritional status	Sitting on table	As preceding	Triceps skinfold thickness (done if client's height and weight seem disproportionate).	Nutritional assessment
Head	As preceding	As preceding	Inspection and palpation of head includes skull, (scalp), face (temporomandibular joints), and sinuses.	Head

Table 22-4. Outline for Examination of the Adult (*continued*)

Body Region	Client Position	Examiner Position	Techniques	Where Recorded
Eyes	As preceding	Standing or sitting, facing client at eye level	Inspection (eyebrows, eyes, eyelids, cornea, slcera, iris, lens, conjunctiva).	Eyes
			Inspection of alignment of eyes (alternate cover test or corneal light reflex).	Eyes
			Visual field testing.	Eyes and neurologic (cranial nerve II)
			Extraocular movement testing.	Eyes and neurologic (cranial nerves II, IV, VI)
			Pupillary response testing.	Eyes and neurologic (cranial nerves, II, III)
			Ophthalmoscopy.	Eyes and neurologic (cranial nerve II)
			Corneal reflex testing.	Eyes and neurologic (cranial nerve V)
Ears	As preceding	Standing	(Inspection of pinnae).	Ears
			Otoscopy.	Ears
			Measurement of auditory acuity.	Ears and neurologic (cranial nerve VIII)
			Weber, Rinne, Schwaback.	Ears and neurologic (cranial nerve VII)
Nose	As preceding	Standing	(Inspection)	Nose
			(Checking of patency of each nostril).	Nose
			Using nasal speculum inspection of internal nose, mucosa (turbinates), septum.	Nose
			Testing for olfaction.	Neurologic (cranial nerve I)
Mouth and pharynx	As preceding	Standing	Inspection of (lips,) mucosa, tongue, teeth, gingivae (floor of the mouth, palates), tonsils and pharynx.	Mouth and pharynx
			Testing of glossopharyngeal ("ah") and vagus nerves ("gag")	Mouth and pharynx and neurologic (cranial nerves IX, X)
			Testing of hypoglossal nerve.	Mouth and pharynx and neurologic (cranial nerve XII)
			Testing of taste.	Neurologic (cranial nerve VII)
Face and neck	As preceding	Standing	Completion of cranial nerve examination: Testing of trigeminal nerve (jaw clenching, lateral jaw movements, and light touch).	Neurologic (cranial nerve V)

Table 22-4. Outline for Examination of the Adult (*continued*)

Body Region	Client Position	Examiner Position	Techniques	Where Recorded
			Testing of facial nerve (raising of eyebrows, showing teeth, puffing out cheeks, keeping eyes closed against resistance.	Neurologic (cranial nerve VII)
			Testing of spinal accessory nerve (raising of shoulder against pressure, turning head against pressure).	Neurologic (cranial nerve XII)
Neck	As preceding	Standing	Inspection of neck, including jugular vein.	Neck and cardiovascular
			Testing of range of motion.	Musculoskeletal
			Palpation of lymph nodes.	Hematologic
			Palpation of thyroid.	Neck
			Palpation of trachea.	Neck
			Discussion of self-examination of head and neck.	
Upper extremities	As preceding	Standing	Inspection of skin and nails.	Skin
			Inspection of muscle mass.	Musculosketetal
			Testing of deep tendon reflexes (DTRs).	Neurologic Musculosketetal
			Testing of muscle strength and range of motion.	
			Testing of coordination, sensation, vibration, position sense, and rapid alternating movements.	Neurologic
Chest	As preceding	Standing behind client	Inspection of skin.	Skin
			Inspection of back.	Musculoskeletal
			Palpation over spine.	Musculoskeletal
			Percussion over costovertebral angles (CVAs).	Abdomen
			Observation of respiratory pattern, rate, and rhythm.	Lungs
			Percussion of lungs and determination of degree of descent of the diaphragm.	Lungs
		Standing behind and in front of the client	Auscultation of lungs for breath sounds.	
			Palpation for chest expansion and (fremmitus).	
Breasts	As preceding	Standing in front of the client	Inspection of breasts with client's arms at the sides, overhead, and with hands pressed together and with client leaning forward.	Breasts
			Palpation of breasts.	Breasts
			Palpation of axillae.	Hematologic

Table 22-4. Outline for Examination of the Adult (*continued*)

Body Region	Client Positon	Examiner Position	Techniques	Where Recorded
Heart	As preceding	As preceding	Inspection of precordium.	Cardiovascular
			Palpation of precordium.	Cardiovascular
			Auscultation of precordium.	Cardiovascular
Breasts	Supine	Standing at right side of client	Inspection and palpation of breasts and nipples.	Breasts
			Discussion of monthly breast self-examination.	
Chest	As preceding	As preceding	Inspection of precordium.	Cardiovascular
			Palpation of precordium.	Cardiovascular
			Auscultation of precordium.	Cardiovascular
			Blood pressure in both arms.	Cardiovascular
			Inspection of jugular venous pulses.	Cardiovascular
Abdomen	Supine	As preceding	Inspection of abdomen.	Abdomen
			Auscultation of abdomen.	Abdomen
			Percussion of liver.	Abdomen
			Percussion of spleen.	Hematologic
			Palpation of liver.	Abdomen
			Palpation of spleen.	Hematologic
			Palpation of inguinal and femoral nodes.	Hematologic
Male genitalia	Supine	As preceding	Inspection of penis and scrotum.	Male genitalia
			Palpation of scrotum.	Male genitalia
			Discussion of monthly testicular self-examination.	
Lower extremities	Sitting	As preceding	Inspection of skin and hair.	Skin
			Inspection of muscle mass and skeletal proportions.	Musculoskeletal
			Palpation of temperature.	Cardiovascular
			Testing of range of motion.	Musculoskeletal
			Testing of strength, sensation, position sense, vibration, deep tendon reflexes (DTRs), and Babinski reflex.	Neurologic
			Testing of cerebellar function (heel to calf).	Neurologic
Female genitalia	Lithotomy	Sitting	Inspection of external genitalia.	Female genitalia
			Palpation of external genitalia.	Female genitalia
			Speculum examination.	Female genitalia
			Collection of cytologic specimen (Pap smear).	Female genitalia

Table 22-4. Outline for Examination of the Adult (*continued*)

Body Region	Client Position	Examiner Position	Techniques	Where Recorded
Female genitalia	As preceding	As preceding	Collection of smears and cultures if necessary.	Female genitalia
Female genitalia	As preceding	Standing	Bimanual vaginal palpation.	Female genitalia
			Rectovaginal examination.	Female genitalia
Back	Standing	Standing behind client	Inspection of spine.	Musculoskeletal
Back	Bending over	Standing beside client	Inspection of spine.	Musculoskeletal
Back	Bending laterally and twisting	As preceding	Testing of range of motion.	Musculoskeletal
Neurologic	Standing	As preceding	Performance of Romberg test.	Neurologic
Rectal (male client)	Leaning over table	Standing behind client	Inspection of anus. Palpation of rectum and prostate.	Male genitalia Male genitalia

Since the neonate is small and is positioned by an adult throughout the examination, the order of performing techniques is not critical with a few exceptions:

1. Auscultation is performed whenever the infant is quiet; therefore, this is frequently the first modality completed. Once the baby begins to cry, it is often difficult to auscultate the heart and lungs.

2. Inspection of the mouth and pharynx is reserved until the end because this is particularly uncomfortable to children.

Observation is most complete when it includes various stages of activity—quietude to crying. It includes the parent's response to the infant's activity as well.

The history includes the course of pregnancy, labor, and delivery; feelings toward the baby; and statements about how the parents are coping with the presence of the new baby, how the baby's presence has affected relationships with others, that is, the baby's father, relatives, friends, and babysitter.

The nutritional history is of particular importance during early childhood (Chapter 4).

Table 22-5. Outline for examination of the Neonate

Region	Client Position	Examiner Position	Techniques	Where Recorded
Interplay between parent and baby	Occurs throughout examination in all positions	Standing	Observation of how the parent holds the baby, talks to the baby, and picks up baby's cues	General Survey
General appearance	Supine on table Prone on table Held by parent	Standing in front of client	Inspection of appearance, including maturity, state of well-being, response to parent's attempts to calm, respiratory pattern, skin color and characteristics, character of sleep, resting posture	General survey Psychosocial Psychosocial Lungs Skin Neurologic Neurologic
Chest	Supine Prone	Standing beside client	Inspection of thorax Auscultation of breath sounds Palpation of precordium Auscultation over precordium	Skin Neurologic Lungs Cardiovascular

Table 22-5. Outline for Examination of the Neonate (*continued*)

Region	Client Position	Examiner Position	Techniques	Where Recorded
Pulses	Supine	As preceding	Comparison of femoral and brachial pulses	Cardiovascular
Extremities	Supine	As preceding	Inspection of extremities for symmetry and form	Musculoskeletal
			Performance of check for hip dislocation	Musculoskeletal
			Muscle tone checks Recoil of extremities, heel-to-ear test, pull to sitting position (neck extensors and neck flexors), hold in standing position (Body extensors)	Musculosketetal
Abdomen	Supine	As preceding	Inspection of abdomen and umbilical cord	Abdomen
			Palpation of abdomen	Abdomen
External genitalia	Supine	As preceding	Inspection and palpation of the external genitalia	Genitalia
Anus and rectum	Supine	As preceding	Inspection	Anus and rectum
			Check for patency with fifth finger or soft catheter if meconium has not been passed	Anus and rectum
Reflexes	Supine	As preceding	Sucking, rooting, grasp (fingers and toes), Moro, tonic neck, and Babinski	Neurologic
	Prone	As preceding	Spontaneous crawling	Neurologic
	Held in standing position	As preceding	Placing and stepping	Neurologic
Head	Supine	As preceding	Inspection of size, shape, and symmetry of head	Head
			Inspection of fontanelles and sutures	Head
			Palpation of fontanelles and sutures	Head
			Measurement of fontanelles and head circumference	General survey
Face	Supine	As preceding	Inspection of face	Head
Neck	Supine	As preceding	Inspection of neck	Neck
Eyes	Supine	As preceding	Inspection of eye accessory structures (lids, lacrimal ducts, brows, lashes)	Eyes
			Inspection of eyes with ophthalmoscope including red reflex	Eyes
Nose	Supine	As preceding	Inspection of nose	Nose
			Inspection of nose and respiratory pattern while each naris is occluded	Nose

Table 22-5. Outline for Examination of the Neonate *(continued)*

Region	Client Position	Examiner Position	Techniques	Where Recorded
Ears	Supine or held on parent's lap	As preceding	Inspection of external ears	Ears
			Inspection of tympanic membrane with otoscope	Ears
			Screening for hearing acuity by clapping hands or ringing a bell	Ears
Mouth and pharynx	Supine	As preceding	Inspection of mouth and pharynx	Mouth and pharynx
			Gag reflex	Neurologic system
Measurements	Supine on scale	Standing in front of client	Weight	General Survey
			Length	General survey
			Measurement of temperature, pulse, respirations, and blood pressure	General survey

The examination of the child from infancy to four years of age is often best performed with the child held on an adult's lap (Table 22-6). The format for assessing older children is the same as for adults with the addition of some screening tests listed in Table 22-7 and the omission of the vaginal and rectal examinations.

Table 22-6. Outline For the Pediatric Lap Examination

Region	Client Position	Examiner Position	Techniques	Where Recorded
Measurements	Up to age 2—lying on table After age 2— standing on floor scale	Standing beside client	Height and weight	Measurement
Vital signs	Up to age 3—lying on examining table or on parent's lap	As preceding	Rectal temperature	Vital signs
	After age 3—sitting on parent's lap	As preceding	Oral temperature	Vital signs
	Sitting on parent's lap	As preceding	Pulse, respiration, and blood pressure	Vital signs
General survey	Walking across room	Standing across from client	Inspection of gait	Neurologic
			Feet position	Musculoskeletal
			Motor coordination	Neurologic
			Balance	Neurologic
			Symmetry of body	Musculoskeletal
Thorax	Sitting on parent's lap	Sitting, facing client	Inspection of thorax and precordium	Cardiovascular
			Auscultation of precordium	Cardiovascular
			Auscultation of lungs	Lungs
Head	As preceding	As preceding	Inspection and palpation	Head
Joints	As preceding	As preceding	Inspection of joint mobility	Musculoskeletal
Extremities	As preceding	As preceding	Inspection of color	Skin
			Inspection of symmetry and range of motion	Musculoskeletal
Lymph nodes	As preceding	As preceding	Palpation of inguinal, axillary, and cervical lymph nodes	Hematologic

Table 22-6. Outline for the Pediatric Lap Examination (*continued*)

Region	Client Position	Examiner Position	Techniques	Where Recorded
Genitalia and anus	As preceding	As preceding	Inspection of genitalia Palpation of external genitalia Inspection of anus	Genitalia Genitalia Anus
Back	Sitting on parent's lap, facing parent	As preceding	Inspection of back Auscultation of lungs	Musculoskeletal Lungs
Eyes	Sitting on parent's lap, facing examiner	Sitting facing client	Inspection of eyes Alternate cover test Testing of extraocular movements Testing of visual fields Ophthalmoscopy Visual acuity testing. For infants the examiner notes whether child focuses on the examiner and follows her movements. For preverbal toddlers the examiner asks the child to point to various pictures of objects, for example, "show me the ball, where's the dog?" Verbal children— Snellen picture or E chart.	Eyes Eyes Eyes Eyes Eyes Eyes
Ears	Sitting on lap, facing examiner, with head and arms restrained by parent or lying supine on table with head and arms restrained by parent	Sitting or standing, facing the client	Inspection of external ear Otoscopy Pneumonoscopy Hearing behavior— Response to bell or hand clap Watch tick or whisper test Hearing acuity tested by audiometry every year beginning at age 3	Ear Ear Ear Ear
Abdomen	Supine on table	Standing, facing client	Inspection of abdomen Palpation of abdomen	Abdomen Abdomen
Mouth and pharynx	Sitting on lap with head and arms restrained by parent or lying supine on the table with head and arms restrained by parent	Standing, facing client	Inspection of mouth and pharynx Gag reflex	Mouth and pharynx Neurologic system

Table 22-7. Recommendations for Health Assessment of Children

History		NB	1 mo	2 mo	4 mo	6 mo	9 mo	12 mo	18 mo	2 yr	4 yr	6 yr	9 yr	12 yr	15 yr
	Approximate Age														
Comprehensive		+													
Health History		+	+	+	+	+	+	+	+	+	+	+	+	+	+
Eating		+	+	+	+	+	+	+	+	+	+	+	+	+	+
Sleeping		+	+	+	+	+	+	+	+	+	+	+	+	+	+
Elimination		+	+	+	+	+	+	+	+	+	+				
Crying		+	+	+	+	+									
Behavior		+	+	+	+	+	+	+	+	+	+	+	+	+	+
Vocalizes				+											
Smiles				+											
Happiness				+	+	+	+	+	+	+	+	+	+	+	+
Parent/child interaction		+	+	+	+	+	+	+	+	+	+	+	+	+	+
Current living situation			+	+	+	+	+	+	+	+	+	+	+	+	+
Holds head up					+										
Laughs					+										
Grasps rattle					+										
Eyes follow object for 180°					+										
Rolls over					+	+									
Reaches for object						+									
Feeds self cracker							+								
Sits alone						+									
Stands								+							
Says "da da" or "ma ma"								+							
Walks, holding on to furniture								+							
Plays pat-a-cake								+							
Walks well									+	+					
Indicates wants										+					
Language									+	+	+				
Drinks from cup well									+						
Peer reaction										+	+	+	+	+	+
Toilet training										+					
Brushes teeth										+					
Pedals tricycle										+	+				
Tantrums										+	+				
Sex education										+	+	+			
Plays with other children										+	+	+	+		
Preschool											+				
School												+			
Safety		+	+	+	+	+	+	+	+	+	+	+	+	+	+
Responsibility in household										+	+	+	+	+	+
Discipline										+	+	+	+	+	+
Obedience										+	+	+	+	+	+
Interests and activities outside home										+	+	+	+	+	+
Perception of self											+	+	+	+	+
School success											+	+	+	+	+
Competitive athletics												+	+	+	+
Sexual behavior												+	+	+	+
Drug, alcohol, tobacco use														+	+

Table 22-7. Recommendations For Health Assessment of Children (continued)

Physical Examination	NB	1 mo	2 mo	4 mo	6 mo	9 mo	12 mo	18 mo	2 yr	4 yr	6 yr	9 yr	12 yr	15 yr
Height	+	+	+	+	+	+	+	+	+	+	+	+	+	+
Weight	+	+	+	+	+	+	+	+	+	+	+	+	+	+
Head circumference	+	+	+	+	+	+	+	+						
Temperature	+	+	+	+	+	+	+	+	+	+	+	+	+	+
Pulse	+	+	+	+	+	+	+	+	+	+	+	+	+	+
Respiratory rate	+	+	+	+	+	+	+	+	+	+	+	+	+	+
Blood pressure		+							+	+	+	+	+	+
Parent-child interaction	+	+	+	+	+	+	+	+	+	+	+	+	+	+
Thorax	+	+	+	+	+	+	+	+	+	+	+	+	+	+
Lungs	+	+	+	+	+	+	+	+	+	+	+	+	+	+
Heart	+	+	+	+	+	+	+	+	+	+	+	+	+	+
Breasts	+	+	+	+	+	+	+	+	+	+	+	+	+	+
Back and Extremities	+	+	+	+	+	+	+	+	+	+	+	+	+	+
Skin	+	+	+	+	+	+	+	+	+	+	+	+	+	+
Neurologic	+	+	+	+	+	+	+	+	+	+	+	+	+	+
Head and neck	+	+	+	+	+	+	+	+	+	+	+	+	+	+
Genitalia	+	+	+	+	+	+	+	+	+	+	+	+	+	+
Eyes	+	+	+	+	+	+	+	+	+	+	+	+	+	+
Ears	+	+	+	+	+	+	+	+	+	+	+	+	+	+
Nose	+	+	+	+	+	+	+	+	+	+	+	+	+	+
Throat	+	+	+	+	+	+	+	+	+	+	+	+	+	+
Abdomen	+	+	+	+	+	+	+	+	+	+	+	+	+	+
Lymph nodes	+	+	+	+	+	+	+	+	+	+	+	+	+	+
Screening tests														
Vision	+	+	+	+	+	+	+	+	+	+	+	+	+	+
Hearing acuity	+	+	+	+	+	+	+	+	+	+	+	+	+	
Tuberculosis							+		+	+	+	+	+	+
Hemoglobin S and C Traits													+	+
Sickle cell disease	+													
PKU, galactosemia, and hypothyroidism	+													
Bactiuria (girls only)										+	+	+	+	+
Anemia	+					+							+	
Strabismus			+	+	+	+	+	+	+	+				
Hip dislocation	+					+								
Scoliosis												+	+	+

Adapted from Abraham Rudolph, ed., *Pediatrics*, 16th Ed. New York: Appleton-Century-Crofts, 1977.

Example of a Normal Recording

General Survey. Forty-year-old black male who appears his stated age and is of normal weight and athletic build. He is well-groomed, alert, interested, and cooperative; responds appropriately.

Height. 180 cm.   Weight: 82 kg.

V.S. T = 37.0° centigrade (orally)

P = 72/min.; regular

R = 16/min.; regular

BP = 122/84/78 (left arm, sitting)

Skin. Uniform dark brown color, warm, dry, and turgid. Hair: early frontal alopecia and thinning. Nails: Nail beds pink, well-manicured.

Head and neck. Normocephalic; trachea midline; thyroid isthmus palpable, soft and small, lobes not palpable.

Eyes. Visual acuity—OD 20/20, OS 20/40, OU 20/40 with glasses (Snellen eye chart)

OD 20/40, OS 20/100, OU 20/60 without glasses (Snellen eye chart)

Conjunctivae clear. Sclerae clear. PERRLA. Visual fields normal by confrontation. Extraocular muscles intact.

Fundi: Discs well-delineated; no arteriovenous nicking, arteriolar narrowing, hemorrhages, or exudates.

Table 22-8.   Recommendations For Health Assessment during Pregnancy

Initial Visit	Monthly until 8th month Bimonthly during 8th month Weekly during 9th month	Screening tests

Comprehensive history and examination
Pregnancy test
CBC
Blood type and Rh factor
VDRL
Rubella titre
Urinalysis
	History questions:
	  Nausea, vomiting, dizziness, edema
	  headaches
	  constipation
	  pain
	  hemorrhoids, varicose veins
	  bleeding
	Urine dipstick for glucose and protein
	Blood pressure
	Weight
	Palpation of height of fundus
	Auscultation of fetal heart tones (starting between ninth and twelfth week with dopler and twentieth week with fetuscope)
		Fasting blood sugar, 2-hour postprandial blood sugar if family history of diabetes mellitus or previous delivery of large baby (over 9 lbs.)
		Sonogram if uterine fundus is not at expected level, dates are confused, previous Caesarian section, bleeding occurs, or prior to amniocentesis
		Amniocentesis with history of or predisposition to birth defects (maternal age over 35), indication for induction of labor (for example, diabetes mellitus) to determine fetal lung maturity

Ears. Canals—soft cerumen easily removed by irrigation prior to examination. Tympanic membranes—translucent, pearly gray with light reflex and other landmarks visible.

Hearing acuity: Whispered voice heard at 2 feet bilaterally.

Weber: No lateralization.

Rinne: AC > BC bilaterally.

Mouth and Pharynx: Mucosa—pink; teeth—32 present, and in good repair; gingiva—pink, firm, nontender; tonsils—absent.

Nose. Mucosa—pink; septum midline; sinuses: nontender

Lungs. Breath sounds—vesicular with no adventitious sounds; fremitus—equal bilaterally; lung fields resonant to percussion.

Cardiovascular. Heart—point of maximum impulse at fifth intercostal space in the left midclavicular line; no heaves, lifts, or thrills; apical pulse = 80/min.; S-1 loudest at apex; S-2 loudest at base; physiologic splitting of S-2 (A-2 louder than P-2); no murmurs.

BP.

	Left arm	Right arm
Sitting	122/84/76	122/80/76
Supine	124/80/72	122/80/70
Standing	120/80/72	120/80/70

Arterial Pulses:

	Left	Right
Temporal	+3	+3
Carotid	+3	+3 (no bruits)
Brachial	+3	+3
Radial	+3	+3
Femoral	+3	+3
Popliteal	+3	+3
Posterior tibial	+3	+3
Dorsal pedal	+3	+3

Venous pulses and pressures:
Jugular venous pressure = 1 cm. at 45°; a wave > v wave

Breasts: Symmetrical; no masses, tenderness, or nipple discharge.

Abdomen: Scaphoid, supple, nontender, and without masses; liver, kidneys, and spleen not palpable; liver span = 10 cm. in right midclavicular line; bowel sounds present; abdomen tympanitic to percussion.

Rectum: Mucosa—smooth, nontender, and without masses; prostate—rubbery firm, and smooth; brown feces negative for occult blood.

Genitalia: Penis uncircumcized, foreskin easily retractable; scrotum nontender and without masses or hernia.

Musculoskeletal: Extremities symmetrical; posture—erect; gait and stance normal; full ROM; no swelling, tenderness, redness, crepitation, or deformities of back, joints, muscles, or bones.

Mental Status: Cheerful, cooperative, and calm; fully alert and oriented to time, place, person, and situation; memory—intact; mood—stable; affect—appropriate; thought content—appropriate; thought processes—coherent.

Neurologic—cranial nerves:

I—identifies 3 of 3 odors accurately.

II, III, IV, VI—see eye examination.

V—sensation to light touch, pin prick, hot and cold, and vibration present and equal bilaterally; corneal reflexes present and equal; jaw symmetrical, muscles of mastication strong.

VII—wrinkles forehead bilaterally, raises eyebrows; smiles and frowns symmetrically; opens eyes against resistance, taste sensations present bilaterally.

VIII—see ear examination.

IX, X—soft palate moves symmetrically, moves on side stroked; uvula moves in midline; gag reflex present; swallows easily, voice clear, without hoarseness; taste sensations present bilaterally.

VII—tongue symmetrical in midline; protrudes with good force against resistance; speech clear and crisp.

Cerebellar Function: Gait smooth and coordinated. Finger to nose and heel to skin movements coordinated bilaterally. Dresses without difficulty. Romberg negative.

Motor System: Strength in upper and lower extremities equal bilaterally. Makes a fist, grasps, extends, and flexes joints against resistance. Full ROM. Rises to standing easily; stands on toes and heels.

Sensory System: Sensation present to light touch, pin prick, hot and cold, and vibration; equal bilaterally on trunk and extremities. Two point and position sense intact. No extinction phenomenon.

Hematologic: No lymphadenopathy or hepatosplenomegaly.

Appendix 1.   Metric-Fahrenheit Equivalents
              for Temperature

C	F
36.00	96.6
36.50	97.7
37.00	98.6
37.50	99.5
38.00	100.4
38.50	101.3
39.00	102.2
39.50	103.1
40.00	104.9
40.50	104.9
41.00	105.8

Appendix 2.   Chronologic Variations in Pulse Rate

Age	Pulse Rate/Minute
Newborn	110–150
14 months	100–140
2 years	90–110
4 years	80–120
6 years	80–100
8 years	76–90
10 years	70–110
Adult	60–100

Appendix 3.   Chronologic Variations in Respiratory Rate

Age	Respirations/Minute
Neonate	30–50
2 years	20–30
10 years	14–22
Adolescent	12–20
Adult	12–20

Appendix 4.   Normal Ranges of Arterial Blood Pressure in
              Children

Ages	Mean Systolic ± 2 S.D.	Mean Diastolic ± 2 S.D.
Newborn	80 ± 16	46 ± 16
6–12 months	89 ± 29	60 ± 10
1 year	96 ± 30	66 ± 25
2 years	99 ± 25	64 ± 25
3 years	100 ± 25	67 ± 23
4 years	99 ± 20	65 ± 20
5–6 years	94 ± 14	55 ± 9
6–7 years	100 ± 15	56 ± 8
8–9 years	105 ± 16	57 ± 9
9–10 years	107 ± 16	57 ± 9
10–11 years	111 ± 17	58 ± 10
11–12 years	113 ± 18	59 ± 10
12–13 years	115 ± 19	59 ± 10
13–14 years	117 ± 19	60 ± 10

R. J. Haggerty, M. W. Maroney, and A. S. Nadas, "Essential hypertension in infancy and childhood," *A.M.A.J. Dis. Child*, 92:536, 1956. Copyright 1956, American Medical Association.

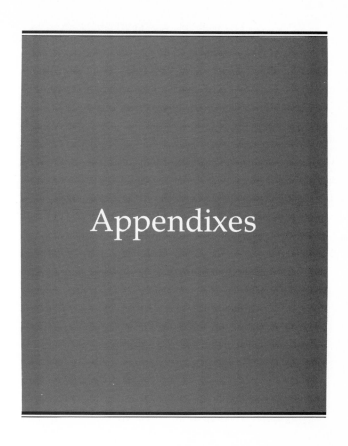

Appendixes

Appendix 5. Height and Weight Standards for Adult Females

			Women (in indoor clothing)*					
			Small Frame		Medium Frame		Large Frame	
Feet	Inches	Centimeters	Pounds	Kilograms	Pounds	Kilograms	Pounds	Kilograms
4	8	142.2	92–98	41.7–44.4	96–107	43.5–48.5	104–119	47.2–54.0
4	9	144.8	94–101	42.6–45.8	98–110	44.4–49.9	106–122	48.1–55.3
4	10	147.3	96–104	43.5–47.2	101–113	45.8–51.3	109–125	49.4–56.7
4	11	149.9	99–107	44.9–48.5	104–116	47.2–52.6	112–128	50.8–58.1
5	0	152.4	102–110	46.3–49.9	107–119	48.5–54.0	115–131	52.2–59.4
5	1	154.9	105–113	47.6–51.3	110–122	49.9–55.3	118–134	53.5–60.8
5	2	157.5	108–116	49.0–52.6	113–126	51.3–57.2	121–138	54.9–62.6
5	3	160.0	111–119	50.3–54.0	116–130	52.6–59.0	125–142	56.7–64.4
5	4	162.6	114–123	51.7–55.8	120–135	54.4–61.2	129–146	58.5–66.2
5	5	165.1	118–127	53.5–57.6	124–139	56.2–63.0	133–150	60.3–68.0
5	6	167.6	122–131	55.3–59.4	128–143	58.1–64.9	137–154	62.1–69.9
5	7	170.2	126–135	57.2–61.2	132–147	59.9–66.7	141–158	64.0–71.7
5	8	172.7	130–140	59.0–63.5	136–151	61.7–68.5	145–163	65.8–73.9
5	9	175.3	134–144	60.8–65.3	140–155	63.5–70.3	149–168	67.6–76.2
5	10	177.8	138–148	62.6–67.1	144–159	65.3–72.1	153–173	69.4–78.5

*Allow 2-4 pounds for women.
These tables correct the 1959 Metropolitan Standards to height without shoe heels.

Appendix 6. Height and Weight Standards for Adult Males

			Men (in indoor clothing)*					
			Small frame		Medium frame		Large frame	
Feet	Inches	Centimeters	Pounds	Kilograms	Pounds	Kilograms	Pounds	Kilograms
5	1	154.9	112–120	50.8–54.4	118–129	53.5–58.5	126–141	57.2–64.0
5	2	157.5	115–123	52.2–55.8	121–133	54.9–60.3	129–144	58.5–65.3
5	3	160.0	118–126	53.5–57.2	124–136	56.2–61.7	132–148	59.9–67.1
5	4	162.6	121–129	54.9–58.5	127–139	57.6–63.0	135–152	61.2–68.9
5	5	165.1	124–133	56.2–60.3	130–143	59.0–64.9	138–156	62.6–70.8
5	6	167.6	128–137	58.1–62.1	134–147	60.8–66.7	142–161	64.4–73.0
5	7	170.2	132–141	59.9–64.0	138–152	62.6–68.9	147–166	66.7–75.3
5	8	172.7	136–145	61.7–65.8	142–156	64.4–70.8	151–170	68.5–77.1
5	9	175.3	140–150	63.5–68.0	146–160	66.2–72.5	155–174	70.3–78.9
5	10	177.8	144–154	65.3–69.9	150–165	68.0–74.8	159–179	72.1–81.2
5	11	180.3	148–158	67.1–71.7	154–170	69.9–77.1	164–184	74.4–83.5
6	0	182.9	152–162	68.9–73.4	158–175	71.7–79.4	168–189	76.2–85.7
6	1	185.4	156–167	70.8–75.7	162–180	73.4–81.6	173–194	78.5–88.0
6	2	188.0	160–171	72.5–77.6	167–185	75.7–83.9	178–199	80.7–90.3
6	3	190.5	164–175	74.4–79.4	172–190	78.0–86.2	182–204	82.6–92.5

*Allow 5-7 pounds for men.
These tables correct the 1959 Metropolitan Standards to height without shoe heels.

Appendix 7. Physical Growth

Age	Boys 5th	Boys 10th	Boys 25th	Boys 50th	Boys 75th	Boys 90th	Boys 95th		Girls 5th	Girls 10th	Girls 25th	Girls 50th	Girls 75th	Girls 90th	Girls 95th
AT BIRTH	**46.4**	**47.5**	**49.0**	**50.5**	**51.8**	**53.5**	**54.4**	**Length-cm.**	**45.4**	**46.5**	**48.2**	**49.9**	**51.0**	**52.0**	**52.9**
	18¼	18¾	19¼	20	20½	21	21½	Length-in.	17¾	18¼	19	19¾	20	20½	20¾
	2.54	**2.78**	**3.00**	**3.27**	**3.64**	**3.82**	**4.15**	**Weight-kg.**	**2.36**	**2.58**	**2.93**	**3.23**	**3.52**	**3.64**	**3.81**
	5½	6¼	6½	7¼	8	8½	9¼	Weight-lb.	5¼	5¾	6½	7	7¾	8	8½
	32.6	**33.0**	**33.9**	**34.8**	**35.6**	**36.6**	**37.2**	**Head C-cm.**	**32.1**	**32.9**	**33.5**	**34.3**	**34.8**	**35.5**	**35.9**
	12¾	13	13¼	13¾	14	14½	14¾	Head C-in	12¾	13	13¼	13½	13¾	14	14¼
3 MONTHS	**56.7**	**57.7**	**59.4**	**61.1**	**63.0**	**64.5**	**65.4**	**Length-cm.**	**55.4**	**56.2**	**57.8**	**59.5**	**61.2**	**62.7**	**63.4**
	22¼	22¾	23½	24	24¾	25½	25¾	Length-in.	21¾	22¼	22¾	23½	24	24¾	25
	4.43	**4.78**	**5.32**	**5.98**	**6.56**	**7.14**	**7.37**	**Weight-kg.**	**4.18**	**4.47**	**4.88**	**5.40**	**5.90**	**6.39**	**6.74**
	9¾	10½	11¾	13¼	14½	15¾	16¼	Weight-lb.	9¼	9¾	10¾	12	13	14	14¾
	38.4	**38.9**	**39.7**	**40.6**	**41.7**	**42.5**	**43.1**	**Head C-cm.**	**37.3**	**37.8**	**38.7**	**39.5**	**40.4**	**41.2**	**41.7**
	15	15¼	15¾	16	16½	16¾	17	Head C-in.	14¾	15	15¼	15½	16	16¼	16½
6 MONTHS	**63.4**	**64.4**	**66.1**	**67.8**	**69.7**	**71.3**	**72.3**	**Length-cm.**	**61.8**	**62.6**	**64.2**	**65.9**	**67.8**	**69.4**	**70.2**
	25	25¼	26	26¾	27½	28	28½	Length-in.	24½	24¾	25¼	26	26¾	27¼	27¾
	6.20	**6.61**	**7.20**	**7.85**	**8.49**	**9.10**	**9.46**	**Weight-kg.**	**5.79**	**6.12**	**6.60**	**7.21**	**7.83**	**8.38**	**8.73**
	13¾	14½	15¾	17¼	18¾	20	20¾	Weight-lb.	12¾	13½	14½	16	17¼	18½	19¼
	41.5	**42.0**	**42.8**	**43.8**	**44.7**	**45.6**	**46.2**	**Head C-cm.**	**40.3**	**40.9**	**41.6**	**42.4**	**43.3**	**44.1**	**44.6**
	16¼	16½	16¾	17¼	17½	18	18¼	Head C-in.	15¾	16	16½	16¾	17	17¼	17½
12 MONTHS	**71.7**	**72.8**	**74.3**	**76.1**	**77.7**	**79.8**	**81.2**	**Length-cm.**	**69.8**	**70.8**	**72.4**	**74.3**	**76.3**	**78.0**	**79.1**
	28¼	28¾	29¼	30	30½	31½	32	Length-in.	27½	27¾	28½	29¼	30	30¾	31¼
	8.43	**8.84**	**9.49**	**10.15**	**10.91**	**11.54**	**11.99**	**Weight-kg.**	**7.84**	**8.19**	**8.81**	**9.53**	**10.23**	**10.87**	**11.24**
	18½	19½	21	22½	24	25½	26½	Weight-lb.	17¼	18	19½	21	22½	24	24¾
	44.8	**45.3**	**46.1**	**47.0**	**47.9**	**48.8**	**49.3**	**Head C-cm.**	**43.5**	**44.1**	**44.8**	**45.6**	**46.4**	**47.2**	**47.6**
	17¾	17¾	18¼	18½	18¾	19¼	19½	Head C-in.	17¼	17¼	17¾	18	18¼	18½	18¾
18 MONTHS	**77.5**	**78.7**	**80.5**	**82.4**	**84.3**	**86.6**	**88.1**	**Length-cm.**	**76.0**	**77.2**	**78.8**	**80.9**	**83.0**	**85.0**	**86.1**
	30½	31	31¾	32½	33¼	34	34¾	Length-in.	30	30½	31	31¾	32¾	33½	34
	9.59	**9.92**	**10.67**	**11.47**	**12.31**	**13.05**	**13.44**	**Weight-kg.**	**8.92**	**9.30**	**10.04**	**10.82**	**11.55**	**12.30**	**12.76**
	21¼	21¾	23½	25¼	27¼	28¾	29½	Weight-lb.	19¾	20½	22¼	23¾	25½	27	28¼
	46.3	**46.7**	**47.4**	**48.4**	**49.3**	**50.1**	**50.6**	**Head C-cm.**	**45.0**	**45.6**	**46.3**	**47.1**	**47.9**	**48.6**	**49.1**
	18¼	18½	18¾	19	19½	19¾	20	Head C-in.	17¾	18	18¼	18½	18¾	19¼	19¼

Appendix 7. Physical Growth (*continued*)

Age	Measurement	Boys 5th	Boys 10th	Boys 25th	Boys 50th	Boys 75th	Boys 90th	Boys 95th	Girls 5th	Girls 10th	Girls 25th	Girls 50th	Girls 75th	Girls 90th	Girls 95th
24 MONTHS	**Length-cm.**	82.3	83.5	85.6	87.6	89.9	92.2	93.8	81.3	82.5	84.2	86.5	88.7	90.8	92.0
	Length-in.	32½	32¾	33¾	34½	35½	36¼	37	32	32½	33¼	34	35	35¾	36¼
	Weight-kg.	10.54	10.85	11.65	12.59	13.44	14.29	14.70	9.87	10.26	11.10	11.90	12.74	13.57	14.08
	Weight-lb.	23¼	24	25¾	27¾	29¾	31½	32½	21¾	22½	24½	26¼	28	30	31
	Head C-cm.	47.3	47.7	48.3	49.2	50.2	51.0	51.4	46.1	46.5	47.3	48.1	48.8	49.6	50.1
	Head C-in.	18½	18¾	19	19¼	19¾	20	20¼	18¼	18¼	18½	19	19¼	19½	19¾
36 MONTHS	**Length-cm.**	91.2	92.4	94.2	96.5	98.9	101.4	103.1	90.0	91.0	93.1	95.6	98.1	100.0	101.5
	Length-in.	36	36½	37	38	39	40	40½	35½	35¾	36¾	37¾	38½	39¼	40
	Weight-kg.	12.26	12.69	13.58	14.69	15.59	16.66	17.28	11.60	12.07	12.99	13.93	15.03	15.97	16.54
	Weight-lb.	27	28	30	32¼	34¼	36¾	38	25½	26½	28¾	30¾	33¼	35¼	36½
	Head C-cm.	48.6	49	49.7	50.5	51.5	52.3	52.8	47.6	47.9	48.5	49.3	50.0	50.8	51.4
	Head C-in.	19¼	19¼	19½	20	20¼	20½	20¾	18¾	18¾	19	19½	19¾	20	20¼
4 YEARS	**Stature-cm.**	95.8	97.3	100.0	102.9	105.7	108.2	109.9	95.0	96.4	98.8	101.6	104.3	106.6	108.3
	Stature-in.	37¾	38¼	39¼	40½	41½	42½	43¼	37½	38	39	40	41	42	42¾
	Weight-kg.	13.64	14.24	15.39	16.69	17.99	19.32	20.27	13.11	13.84	14.80	15.96	17.56	18.93	19.91
	Weight-lbs.	30	31½	34	36¾	39¾	42½	44¾	29	30½	32¾	35¼	38¾	41¾	44
5 YEARS	**Stature-cm.**	102.0	103.7	106.5	109.9	112.8	115.4	117.0	101.1	102.7	105.4	108.4	111.4	113.8	115.6
	Stature-in.	40¼	40¾	42	43¼	44½	45½	46	39¾	40½	41½	42¾	43¾	44¾	45½
	Weight-kg.	15.27	15.96	17.22	18.67	20.14	21.70	23.09	14.55	15.26	16.29	17.66	19.39	21.23	22.62
	Weight-lbs.	33¾	35¼	38	41¼	44½	47¾	51	32	33¾	36	39	42¾	46¾	49¾
6 YEARS	**Stature-cm.**	107.7	109.6	112.5	116.1	119.2	121.9	123.5	106.6	108.4	111.3	114.6	118.1	120.8	122.7
	Stature-in.	42½	43¼	44¼	45¾	47	48	48½	42	42¾	43¾	45	46½	47½	48¼
	Weight-kg.	16.93	17.72	19.07	20.69	22.40	24.31	26.34	16.05	16.72	17.86	19.52	21.44	23.89	25.75
	Weight-lbs.	37¼	39	42	45½	49½	53½	58	35½	36¾	39¼	43	47¼	52¾	56¾
8 YEARS	**Stature-cm.**	118.1	120.2	123.2	127.0	130.5	133.6	135.7	116.9	118.7	122.2	126.4	130.6	134.2	136.2
	Stature-in.	46½	47¼	48½	50	51½	52½	53½	46	46¾	48	49¾	51½	52¾	53½
	Weight-kg.	20.40	21.39	23.09	25.30	27.91	31.06	34.51	19.62	20.45	22.26	24.84	27.88	32.04	34.71
	Weight-lbs.	45	47¼	51	55¾	61½	68½	76	43¼	45	49	54¾	61½	70¾	76½
10 YEARS	**Stature-cm.**	127.7	130.1	133.4	137.5	141.6	145.5	148.1	127.5	129.5	133.6	138.3	142.9	147.2	149.5
	Stature-in.	50¼	51¼	52½	54¼	55¾	57¼	58¼	50¼	51	52½	54½	56¼	58	58¾
	Weight-kg.	24.33	25.52	28.07	31.44	35.61	40.80	45.27	24.36	25.76	28.71	32.55	37.53	43.70	47.17
	Weight-lbs.	53¾	56¼	62	69¼	78½	90	99¾	53¾	56¾	63¼	71¾	82¾	96¼	104

National Center for Health Statistics, Health Resources Administration, D.H.E.W., Hyattsville, Md. Data from Fels Research Institute, Yellow Springs, Ohio; smoothed by least squares-cubic-spline technique. Conversion of metric data to inches and pounds by Ross Laboratories.

Appendix 7. Physical Growth (*continued*)

Age	Percentiles, Boys								Percentiles, Girls						
	5th	10th	25th	50th	75th	90th	95th		5th	10th	25th	50th	75th	90th	95th
12 YEARS	**137.6**	**140.3**	**144.4**	**149.7**	**154.6**	**159.4**	**162.3**	**Stature-cm.**	**139.8**	**142.3**	**147.0**	**151.5**	**155.8**	**160.0**	**162.7**
	54¼	55¼	56¾	59	60¾	62¾	64	Stature-in.	55	56	57¾	59¾	61¼	63	64
	29.85	**31.46**	**35.09**	**39.78**	**45.77**	**52.73**	**58.09**	**Weight-kg.**	**30.52**	**32.53**	**36.52**	**41.53**	**48.07**	**55.99**	**60.81**
	65¾	69¼	77¼	87¾	101	116¼	128	Weight-lbs.	67¼	71¾	80½	91½	106	123½	134
14 YEARS	**148.8**	**151.8**	**156.9**	**163.1**	**168.5**	**173.8**	**176.7**	**Stature-cm.**	**148.7**	**151.5**	**155.9**	**160.4**	**164.6**	**168.7**	**171.3**
	58½	59¾	61¾	64¼	66¼	68½	69½	Stature-cm.	58½	59¾	61½	63¼	64¾	66½	67½
	38.22	**40.64**	**45.21**	**50.77**	**58.31**	**65.57**	**72.13**	**Weight-kg.**	**37.76**	**40.11**	**44.54**	**50.28**	**57.09**	**66.04**	**73.08**
	84¼	89½	99¾	112	128½	144½	159	Weight-lbs.	83¼	88½	98¼	110¾	125¾	145½	161
16 YEARS	**161.1**	**163.9**	**168.7**	**173.5**	**178.1**	**182.4**	**185.4**	**Stature-cm.**	**151.6**	**154.1**	**157.8**	**162.4**	**166.9**	**171.1**	**173.3**
	63½	64½	66½	68¼	70	71¾	73	Stature-in.	59¾	60¾	62¼	64	65¾	67¼	68¼
	47.74	**51.16**	**56.16**	**62.10**	**70.26**	**77.97**	**85.62**	**Weight-kg.**	**43.41**	**45.78**	**50.09**	**55.89**	**62.29**	**71.68**	**80.99**
	105¼	112¾	123¾	137	155	172	188¾	Weight-lbs.	95¾	101	110½	123¼	137¼	158	178½
18 YEARS	**165.7**	**168.7**	**172.3**	**176.8**	**181.2**	**185.3**	**187.6**	**Stature-cm.**	**153.6**	**156.0**	**159.6**	**163.7**	**167.6**	**171.0**	**173.6**
	65¼	66½	67¾	69½	71¼	73	73¾	Stature-in.	60½	61½	62¾	64½	66	67¼	68¼
	53.97	**57.89**	**62.61**	**68.88**	**76.04**	**88.41**	**95.76**	**Weight-kg.**	**45.26**	**47.47**	**51.39**	**56.62**	**62.78**	**72.25**	**82.47**
	119	127¼	138	151¾	167¾	195	211	Weight-lbs.	99¾	104¾	113¼	124¾	138½	159¼	181¾

National Center for Health Statistics, Health Resources Administration, D.H.E.W., Hyattsville, Maryland 20782. Data from N.C.H.S. National Health Surveys, smoothed by least-square-cubic-spline technique. Conversion of metric data to inches and pounds by Ross Laboratories.

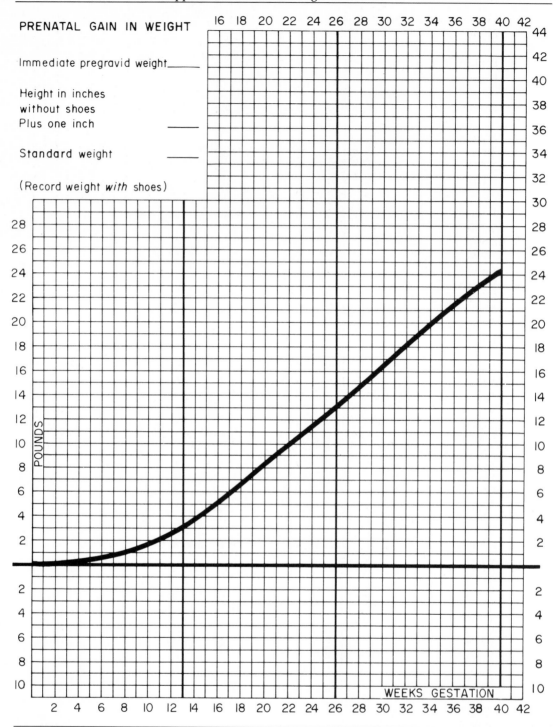

PRENATAL GAIN IN WEIGHT

Immediate pregravid weight_____

Height in inches
without shoes
Plus one inch   _____

Standard weight   _____

(Record weight *with* shoes)

POUNDS

WEEKS GESTATION

Reprinted with permission from *Clinical Obstetrics*, 1953, J. B. Lippincott and Co.

Test	Normal Value	

Complete Blood Count

Erythrocyte count	Male: $4.6\text{-}6.2 \times 10^6$/ul	
	Female: $4.25\text{-}5.4 \text{ s } 10^6$/ul	
Leukocyte count	4,500-11,000/ul	
Hemoglobin	Male: 13.5-18.0 gm/dl	
	Female: 12.0-16.0 gm/dl	
Hematocrit	Male: 40-54%	
	Female: 38-47%	

Erythrocyte indices

MCV	82-98 cu. microns (fl)	
MCH	27-31 pg	
MCHC	32-36%	
Platelet count	150,000-400,000/ul	

White blood cell differential	Mean percent	Range of absolute counts
Segmented neutrophils	56%	1,800-7000/ul
Bands	3%	0-700/ul
Eosinophils	0-3%	0-450/ul
Basophils	0-1%	0-200/ul
Lymphocytes	34%	1,000-4,800/ul
Monocytes	4%	0-800/ul

Coagulation Tests

Pro Time	10-13 seconds
PTT	28-40 seconds
Bleeding Time	Less than 9 minutes

Serum Chemistry

Sodium	135-145 mmol/1
Potassium	3.5-5.0 mmol/1
Calcium	4.5-5.5 mg/dl
Magnesium	1.5-2.5 mEq/L
Chloride	95-105 mmol/1
Bicarbonate	23-28 mmol/1
Phosphate	2-4 mg/dl
Glucose (fasting)	61-110 mg/dl
Triglyceride	23-158 mg/dl
Cholesterol	114-262 mg/dl
Protein	6-8 g/dl
Albumin	3.4-4.9 g/dl

Urinalysis

Macroscopic:	
specific gravity	1.003-1.030
pH	4.6-8.0
Protein	negative
Glucose	negative
Ketones	negative
Bilirubin	negative
Occult Blood	negative
Urobilinogen	negative
Microscopic:	
RBC/HPF	males-neg. females 0-2
WBC/HPF	negative
Epithelial cell/LPF	negative
Bacterial/HPF	negative
Casts/LPF	negative
Crystals/LPF	negative

NEONATAL PERIOD (FIRST 4 WEEKS)

Prone: Lies in flexed attitude; turns head from side to side; head sags on ventral suspension

Supine: Generally flexed and a little stiff

Visual: May fixate face of light in line of vision, "doll's eye" movement of eyes on turning of the body

Reflex: Moro response active; stepping and placing reflexes; grasp reflex active

AT 4 WEEKS

Prone: Legs more extended; holds chin up; turns head; head lifted momentarily to plane of body on ventral suspension

Supine: Tonic neck posture predominates; supple and relaxed; head lags on pull to sitting position

Visual: Watches person; follows moving object a few degrees

AT 8 WEEKS

Prone: Raises head slightly farther; head sustained in plane of body on ventral suspension

Supine: Tonic neck posture predominates; head lags on pull to sitting position

Visual: Follows moving object 180 degrees

Social: Smiles on social contact; listens to voice and coos

AT 12 WEEKS

Prone: Lifts head and chest, arms extended; head above plane of body on ventral suspension

Supine: Tonic neck posture predominates; reaches toward and misses objects; waves at toy

Sitting: Head lag partially compensated on pull to sitting position; early head control with bobbing motion; back rounded

Reflex: Typical Moro response has not persisted; makes defense movements or selective withdrawal reactions

Social: Sustained social contact; listens to music; says "aah, ngah"

AT 16 WEEKS

Prone: Lifts head and chest, head in approximately vertical axis; legs extended

Supine: Symmetrical posture predominates, hands in midline; reaches and grasps objects and brings them to mouth

Sitting: No head lag on pull to sitting position; head steady, held forward; enjoys sitting with full truncal support

Standing: When held erect, pushes with feet

Adaptive: Sees pellet, but makes no move to it

Social: Laughs out loud; may show displeasure if social contact is broken; excited at sight of food

AT 28 WEEKS

Prone: Rolls over; may pivot

Supine: Lifts head; rolls over; squirming movements

Sitting: Sits briefly, with support of pelvis; leans forward on hands; back rounded

Standing: May support most of weight; bounces actively

Adaptive: Reaches out for and grasps large object; transfers objects from hand to hand; grasp uses radial palm; rakes at pellet

Language: Polysyllabic vowel sounds formed

Social: Prefers mother; babbles; enjoys mirror; responds to changes in emotional content of social contact

AT 40 WEEKS

Sitting: Sits up alone and indefinitely without support, back straight

Standing: Pulls to standing position

Motor: Creeps or crawls

Adaptive: Grasps objects with thumb and forefinger; pokes at things with forefinger; picks up pellet with assisted pincer movement; uncovers hidden toy; attempts to retrieve dropped object; releases object grasped by other person

Language: Repetitive consonant sounds (mama, dada)

Social: Responds to sound of name; plays peek-a-boo or pat-a-cake; waves bye-bye

AT 52 WEEKS

Motor: Walks with one hand held; "cruises" or walks holding on to furniture

Adaptive: Picks up pellet with unassisted pincer movement of forefinger and thumb; releases object to other person on request or gesture

Language: 2 "words" besides mama, dada

Social: Plays simple ball game; makes postural adjustment to dressing

V. Vaughan and R. J. McKay, editors, *Nelson Textbook of Pediatrics*, 10th ed., W. B. Saunders Co., Philadelphia, 1975, p. 49.

15 MONTHS

Motor: Walks alone; crawls up stairs

Adaptive: Makes tower of 2 cubes; makes a line with crayon; inserts pellet in bottle

Language: Jargon; follows simple commands; may name a familiar object (ball)

Social: Indicates some desires or needs by pointing

18 MONTHS

Motor: Runs stiffly; sits on small chair; walks up stairs with one hand held; explores drawers and waste baskets

Adaptive: Piles 3 cubes; imitates scribbling; imitates vertical stroke; dumps pellet from bottle

Language: 10 words (average); names pictures

Social: Feeds self; seeks help when in trouble; may complain when wet or soiled

24 MONTHS

Motor: Runs well; walks up and down stairs, one step at a time; opens doors; climbs on furniture

Adaptive: Tower of 6 cubes; circular scribbling; imitates horizontal stroke; folds paper once imitatively

Language: Puts 3 words together (pronoun, verb, object)

Social: Handles spoon well; often tells immediate experiences; helps to undress; listens to stories with pictures

30 MONTHS

Motor: Jumps

Adaptive: Tower of 8 cubes; makes vertical and horizontal strokes, but generally will not join them to make a cross; imitates circular stroke, forming closed figure

Language: Refers to self by pronoun "I"; knows full name

Social: Helps put things away

36 MONTHS

Motor: Goes up stairs alternating feet; rides tricycle; stands momentarily on one foot

Adaptive: Tower of 9 cubes; imitates construction of "bridge" of 3 cubes; copies a circle; imitates a cross

Language: Knows age and sex; counts 3 objects correctly; repeats 3 numbers or a sentence of 6 syllables

Social: Plays simple games (in "parallel" with other children); helps in dressing (unbuttons clothing and puts on shoes); washes hands

48 MONTHS

Motor: Hops on one foot; throws ball overhand; uses scissors to cut out pictures; climbs well

Adaptive: Copies bridge from model; imitates construction of "gate" of 5 cubes; copies cross and square; draws a man with 2 to 4 parts besides head; names longer of 2 lines

Language: Counts 4 pennies accurately; tells a story

Social: Plays with several children with beginning of social interaction and role-playing; goes to toilet alone

60 MONTHS

Motor: Skips

Adaptive: Draws triangle from copy; names heavier of 2 weights

Language: Names 4 colors; repeats sentence of 10 syllables; counts 10 pennies correctly

Social: Dresses and undresses; asks questions about meaning of words; domestic role-playing

After 5 years the Stanford-Binet, Wechsler-Bellevue, and other scales offer the most precise estimates of developmental level. In order to have their greatest value, they should be administered only by an experienced and qualified person.

V. Vaughan and R. J. McKay, editors. *Nelson Textbook of Pediatrics.* 10th ed. Philadelphia; W. B. Saunders Co., 1975, p. 50.

Health Assessment—General

Bates, Barbara. *A Guide to Physical Examination.* 2nd ed., Philadelphia: Lippincott, 1979.

Bennett, A. E., ed. *Communication between Doctors and Patients.* Oxford, England: Oxford University Press, 1976.

Berger, K., and Fields, W. *Pocket Guide to Health Assessment.* Reston, Virginia: Reston Publishing Co., 1980.

Bernstein, L., and Dana, R. *Interviewing: A Guide for Health Professionals.* 2d ed., New York: Appleton-Century-Crofts, 1974.

Bird, B. *Talking with Patients.* 2d ed., Philadelphia: J. B. Lippincott, 1973.

Buckingham, W. B. *A Primer of Clinical Diagnosis.* 2nd ed. New York: Harper and Row, 1979.

Burns, K., and Johnson, P. *Health Assessment in Clinical Practice.* Englewood Cliffs, New Jersey: Prentice-Hall, 1979.

Burnside, J. W. *Adam's Physical Diagnosis, An Introduction to Clinical Medicine.* Baltimore: Williams and Williams, 1974.

DeGowin, E. L., and DeGowin, R. L. *Bedside Diagnostic Examination.* 3d ed. New York: Macmillan, 1976.

Delp, M., and Manning, R. *Major's Physical Diagnosis.* 8th ed. Philadelphia: W. B. Saunders Co., 1976.

Diekelmann, N. *Primary Health Care of the Well Adult.* New York: McGraw-Hill, 1977.

Engel, G. L., and Morgan, W. L. *Interviewing the Patient.* Philadelphia: W. B. Saunders Co., 1973.

Fowkes, W. C., and Hunn, V. K. *Clinical Assessment for the Nurse Practitioner.* St. Louis: C. V. Mosby, 1973.

Gillies, D., and Alyn, S. *Patient Assessment and Management by the Nurse Practitioner.* Philadelphia: W. B. Saunders Co., 1976.

Harlem, O. K. *Communication in Medicine.* New York: S. Karger, 1977.

Hochstein, E., and Rubin, Albert L. *Physical Diagnosis.* New York: McGraw-Hill, 1964

Judge, R., and Zuidema, G. *Methods of Clinical Examination: A Physiologic Approach.* 3d ed. Boston: Little, Brown and Company, 1974

Macleod, J., et al. *Introduction to Clinical Examination.* 2d ed. Edinburgh: Churchill Livingstone, 1977.

Malasanos, L.; Borkauska, V.; Moso, M; and Stoltenberg, Allen, K. *Health Assessment.* St. Louis: C. V. Mosby, 1977.

Morgan, W. L., and Engel, George L. *The Clincial Approach to the Patient.* Philadelphia: W. B. Saunders Co., 1969.

Parkins, R. A., and G. D., Pegrum. *The Basis of Clinical Diagnosis.* New York: Arco, 1975.

Prior, J. A., and Silberstein, J. S. *Physical Diagnosis, The History and Examination of the Patient.* 5th ed. St. Louis: C. V. Mosby, 1977.

Raus, E. E., and Raus, M. M. *Manual of History Taking, Physical Examination and Record Keeping.* Philadelphia: J. B. Lippincott, 1974.

Sauvé, M. J., and Pecherer, A. *Concepts and Skills in Physical Assessment.* Philadelphia: W. B. Saunders Co., 1977.

Sherman, J., and Fields, S. *Guide to Patient Evaluation.* 2d ed. Flushing, New York: Medical Examination Publishing Company, Inc., 1976.

Wiener, S. L., and Nathanson, M. "Frequent Errors in Doing a Physical," *Medical Times* 105, no. 12 (December 1977): 79-82.

Yarnall, S. R., and Wakefield, J. S. 2nd ed. *Acquisition of the History Data Base.* Seattle: Medical Computer Services Association, 1972.

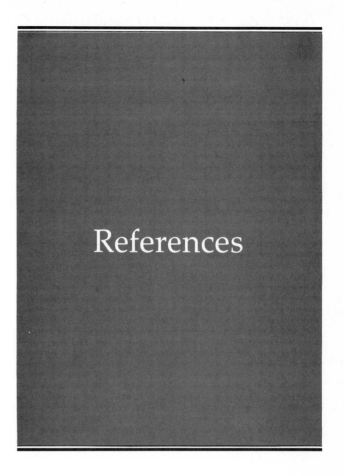

References

Clinical Nursing and Medicine—General

Beeson, P. B., and McDermott, W. *Cecil Textbook of Medicine.* 15th ed. Philadelphia: W. B. Saunders Co, 1979.

Beland, Irene. *Clinical Nursing.* 3d ed. New York: Macmillan, 1975.

Brunner, L., and Suddarth, D. *Textbook of Medical-Surgical Nursing.* 3d ed. Philadelphia: J. B. Lippincott Company, 1975.

Collins, R. Douglas. *Illustrated Manual of Laboratory Diagnosis.* 2nd ed. Philadelphia: J. B. Lippincott Company, 1975.

Hudak, C. M., et al. *Clinical Protocols: A Guide for Nurses and Physicians.* Philadelphia: J. B. Lippincott Company, 1976.

Komaroff, A. L., and Winickoff, R. N. *Common Acute Illnesses.* Boston: Little, Brown and Company, 1977.

MacBryde, C. M., and Blacklow, R. S. *Signs and Symptoms.* 5h ed. Philadelphia: J. B. Lippincott Company, 1970.

Williams, W. J. et al. *Hematology.* 2d ed. New York: McGraw-Hill, 1972.

Wylie, W. D., and Churchill-Davidson, H. C. *A Practice of Anesthesia.* 3d ed. Chicago, Illinois: Year Book Medical Publishers, Inc., 1979.

Anatomy and Physiology— General

Anthony, C. P., and Thibodeau, G. A. *Textbook of Anatomy and Physiology.* 10th ed. St. Louis: C. V. Mosby Co., 1979.

Gray, H. *Anatomy of the Human Body.* 29th ed. Philadelphia: Lea Febinger, 1973.

Guyton, A. C. *Textbook of Medical Physiology.* Philadelphia: W. B. Saunders Co., 1976.

Guyton, A. C. *Basic Human Physiology: Normal Function and Mechanisms of Disease.* 2d ed. Philadelphia: W. B. Saunders Co., 1977.

Pansky, B. *Dynamic Anatomy and Physiology.* New York: Macmillan, 1975.

Sutterley, D., and Donnelly, Gloria. *Perspectives in Human Development.* Philadelphia: J. B. Lippincott Company, 1973.

Late Adulthood— General

Andrew, W. *The Anatomy of Aging in Man and Animals.* New York: Grune and Stratton, 1971.

Brocklehurst, J. *Textbook of Geriatric Medicine and Gerontology.* London: Churchill Livingstone, 1978.

Caird, F., and Judge, T. G. *Assessment of the Elderly Patient.* New York: Pitman Publishing Corporation, 1979.

Carnevali, D. L. and Patrick, M. *Nursing Management for the Elderly.* Philadelphia: J. B. Lippincott, 1979.

Goldman, R., and Rackstein, M. *The Physiology and Pathology of Human Aging.* New York: Academic Press, 1975.

Kart, C.; Metress, E.; and Metress, J. *Aging and Health: Biologic and Social Perspectives.* Menlo Park, California: Addison-Wesley Publishing Co., 1978.

Kiem, Robert J. "How Aging Affects the Ear." *Geriatrics* 32, no. 6: 97.

Kimmel, Douglas C. *Adulthood and Aging.* New York: John Wiley and Sons, 1974.

Rossman, I. "Human Aging Changes." in *Nursing and the Aged,* edited by Irene Mortenson Burnside. New York: McGraw-Hill, 1976.

Rossman, I. Ph.D., M.D., *Clinical Geriatrics.* Philadelphia: J. B. Lippincott Company, 1971.

Saxon, S. V. and Etten, M. J. *Physical Change and Aging.* New York: Tiresias Press, 1978.

Steinberg, F., ed. *Cowdry's Care of the Geriatric Patient.* St. Louis: C. V. Mosby, 1976.

Pediatrics—General

Alexander, Mary M., Brown, Marie S. *Pediatric History Taking and Physical Diagnosis for Nurses.* New York: McGraw-Hill, 1979.

Barness, L. *Manual of Pediatric Physical Diagnosis.* 4th ed. Chicago: Year Book Medical Publishers, Inc., 1972.

Davis, J., and Dobbing, J. *Scientific Foundations of Pediatrics.* Philadelphia: W. B. Saunders Co., 1974.

Dower, John C. "Assessment and Care of the Child." in *Pediatrics,* edited by Abraham Rudolph. 16th ed. New York: Appleton-Century Crofts, 1977.

Kempe, C. H.; Silver, H. K.; and O'Brien, D. *Current Pediatric Diagnosis and Treatment.* Los Altos: Lange, 1976.

Lowrey, G. H. *Growth and Development of Children.* 6th ed. Chicago: Year Book Medical Publishers, 1973.

Nelson, W. E., M.D., sr. ed. *Textbook of Pediatrics.* 11th ed. Philadelphia: W. B. Saunders Co., 1979.

Obstetrics

Broadribb, V., and Corliss, C. *Maternal-Child Nursing.* Philadelphia: J. B. Lippincott Company, 1973.

Kreutner, A. Karen and Hollingsworth, Dorothy R., eds. *Adolescent Obstetrics and Gynecology.* Chicago: Year Book Medical Publishers, 1978.

Macdonald, R. *Scientific Basis of Obstetrics and Gynecology.* 2d ed. New York: Churchill Livingston, 1978.

McLennan, Charles E., Sandberg, Eugene C. *Synopsis of Obstetrics.* 9th ed. St. Louis: C. V. Mosby, 1974.

Pritchard, Jack A., and MacDonald, Paul C. *Williams Obstetrics.* 15th ed. New York: Appleton-Century-Crofts, 1976.

Romney, Seymore L., et al. *Gynecology and Obstetrics, the Health Care of Women.* New York: McGraw-Hill, 1975.

Psychosocial

American Psychiatric Association, *DSM-III (Diagnostic and Statistical Manual of Mental Disorders).* 3d ed. Washington, D. C., 1980.

Freedman, A. et al. *Modern Synopsis of Comprehensive Textbook of Psychiatry.* Baltimore: The Williams and Wilkins Co., 1976.

Freud, A. *The Writings of Anna Freud. Vol. IV, Normality and Pathology in Childhood: Assessments of Development.* New York: International University Press Inc, 1975.

Levinson, D.; Darrow, C.; Klein, E.; Levinson, M.; and McKeeb, B. *Seasons of a Man's Life.* New York: Alfred A. Knopf, 1978.

Mahler, M. *Psychological Birth of the Human Infant.* New York: Basic Books, Inc., 1975.

Rosenbaum, C. *Psychiatric Treatment: Crisis/Clinic/Consultation.* New York: McGraw-Hill, 1975.

Nutrition

Grant, Anne. *Nutritional Assessment Guide.* P. O. Box 25057 Northgate Station, Seattle, Washington 98125, 1979.

Warner, Susan C. *Nutrition Assessment Manual.* Ames, Iowa: University of Iowa Hospitals and Clinics, 1977

Skin

Fitzpatrick, T. B., et al. *Dermatology in General Medicine.* New York: McGraw-Hill, 1979.

Harmon, V. M., and Steele, S. M. *Nursing Care of the Skin: A Developmental Approach.* New York: Appleton-Century-Crofts, 1975.

Moschella, S., et al. *Dermatology.* Vol. 1. Philadelphia: W. B. Saunders, 1975.

Sutton, R. L., and Waisman, M. *The Practitioners' Dermatology.* New York: Dunn-Donnelley, 1975.

Head and Neck

DeWeese, D., and Saunders, W. *Textbook of Otolaryngology.* 5h ed. Saint Louis: C. V. Mosby, 1977.

Fried, L. A. *Anatomy of the Head, Neck, Face, and Jaws.* Philadelphia: Lea and Febiger, 1976.

Glass, R. T., et al. "Teaching Self-Examination of the Head and Neck: Another Aspect of Preventive Dentistry." *Journal of the American Dental Association* 90 (June 1975): 1265–1268.

Harley, R. D., ed. *Pediatric Ophthalmology.* Philadelphia: W. B. Saunders, 1975.

Havener, W. H., et al. *Nursing Care in Eye, Ear, Nose, and Throat Disorders.* Saint Louis: C. V. Mosby, 1974.

Jackson, C. R. S. *The Eye in General Practice.* Baltimore: Williams and Wilkins, 1975.

Kerr, D. A. et al. *Oral Diagnosis.* 5th ed. St. Louis: C. V. Mosby, 1978.

Newell, F. W., and Ernest, J. T. *Ophthalmology, Principles and Concepts.* 4th ed. St. Louis: C. V. Mosby, 1978.

Vaughan, D.; Asbury, T.; and Cook, R. *General Ophthalmology.* 8th ed. Los Altos, Ca.: Lange, 1977.

Lungs

Burton, G.; Gee, G.; and Hodgkin, J., ed. *Respiratory Care: A Guide to Clinical Practice.* Philadelphia: J. B. Lippincott Company, 1977.

Forgacs, P. *Lung Sounds.* New York: Macmillan, 1978.

Murray, J. *The Normal Lung.* Philadelphia: W. B. Saunders Co., 1976.

Romanes, G. J., ed. *Manual of Practical Anatomy: Thorax and Abdomen. Vol. 2.* New York: Oxford University Press, 1977.

Sacknea, M., ed. *Diagnostic Techniques in Pulmonary Disease, Part I.* New York: Marcel Dekker, Inc., 1980.

Shapiro, B.; Harrison, R.; and Trout, C. *Clinical Application of Respiratory Care.* Chicago: Year Book Medical Publishers, Inc., 1979.

Heart

Duben, D. *Rapid Interpretation of EKGs.* Tampa, Florida: Cover Pub. Co., 1974.

Hurst, J. W.; and Logue, R. B. *The Heart, Arteries and Veins.* 4th ed. New York: McGraw-Hill, 1978.

Littman, D., "Stethoscopes and Auscultation." *American Journal of Nursing,* July 1972: 1238.

Marriott, Henry. *Practical Electrocardiography.* Baltimore: Williams and Wilkins Co., 1977.

Moser R. H., ed. "Standards for Cardiopulmonary Resuscitation (CPR) and Emergency Cardiac Care (ECC)." *Journal of the American Medical Association* (supplement) 227, no. 7: 838.

Breasts

Gallager, H. S., et al. *The Breast.* St. Louis: C. V. Mosby, 1978.

Hagensen, C. D. *Diseases of the Breast.* Philadelphia: W. B. Saunders Co., 1971.

Leis, H. P. *Diagnosis and Treatment of Breast Lesions.* Flushing: Medical Examination Publishing Co., 1970.

Genitalia

Harrison, J. H., et al. *Campbell's Urology.* 4th ed. Philadelphia: W. B. Saunders Co., 1978.

Hellinga, G. *Clinical Andrology.* London: William Heinemann Medical Books Ltd., 1976.

Martin, L., "Impotence in Diabetes: An Overview." *Psychosomatics* 22, no. 4 (April 1981): 318

Masters, W., and Johnson, V. *Human Sexual Response.* Boston: Little, Brown and Co., 1966.

Murray, Barbara, and Wilcox, Linda. "Testicular Self-Examination." *American Journal of Nursing* (December 1978): 2074.

Watts, R. "Dimensions of Sexual Health." *American Journal of Nursing* (September 1979): 1568

Woods, N., and Mandetta, A. "Human Sexual Response Patterns." *Nursing Clinics of North America* 10, no. 13 (September 1975): 529.

Musculoskeletal

Daniels, L., and Worthingham, C. *Muscle Testing Techniques of Manual Examination.* 3d ed. Philadelphia: W. B. Saunders Co. 1972.

Hoppenfeld, S. *Physical Examination of the Spine and Extremities.* New York: Appleton-Century-Crofts, 1976.

Shanck, A. H. "Musculoskeletal Problems in Aging." In *Nursing and the Aged,* edited by Irene Mortenson Burnside. New York: McGraw-Hill, 1976.

Neurologic

Burnside, Irene M. "The Special Senses and Sensory Deprivation." In *Nursing and the Aged* edited by Irene Mortenson Burnside. New York: McGraw-Hill, 1976.

Clark, R. G. *Essentials of Clinical Neuroanatomy and Neurophysiology.* 5th ed. Philadelphia: F. A. Davis Company, 1975.

DeJong, R. N., et al. *Essentials of the Neurological Examination.* Philadelphia: Smith Kline Corporation, 1978.

Gardner, E. *Fundamentals of Neurology.* 6h ed. Philadelphia: W. B. Saunders Co., 1975.

Gribbin, K. "Cognitive Processes in Aging." In *Nursing and the Aged* edited by Irene Mortenson Burnside. New York: McGraw-Hill, 1976.

"Patient Assessment: Neurological Examination, Part I." *American Journal of Nursing* 75, no. 9 (September 1975): 1–24.

"Patient Assessment: Neurological Examination, Part II." *American Journal of Nursing* 75, no. 11 (November 1975): 1–24.

"Patient Assessment: Neurological Examination, Part III." *American Journal of Nursing* 76, no. 4 (April 1976): 1–25.

Fluid, Electrolyte, and Acid-Base Balance

Andreoli, T. et al, ed. *Disturbances in Body Fluid Osmolality.* Bethesda, Maryland: American Physiological Society, 1977.

Carroll, H., and Man, O. L. *Water, Electrolytes, and Acid-Base Metabolism.* Philadelphia: J. B. Lippincott, 1978.

Davenport, H. *The ABC of Acid-Base Chemistry.* 6th ed. Chicago: University of Chicago Press, 1974.

Goldberger, E. *A Primer of Water, Electrolytes, and Acid-Base Syndromes.* 5th ed. Philadelphia: Lea and Febiger, 1975.

Keyes, J. "Basic Mechanisms Involved in Acid-Base Homeostasis." *Heart and Lung* 5, no. 2 (March-April 1976): 239.

Keyes, J. "Blood Gas Analysis and the Assessment of Acid-Base Status," *Heart and Lung* 5, no. 2 (March-April 1976): 247.

Metheny, N., and Snively, W. *Nurses' Handbook of Fluid Balance.* 3d ed. Philadelphia: J. B. Lippincott Company, 1979.

Rooth, G. *Introduction to Acid-Base and Electrolyte Balance.* New York: Barnes and Noble, 1969.

Schwartz, A., and Lyons, H. *Acid-Base and Electrolyte Balance.* New York: Grune and Stratton, 1977.

Tuller, M. *Acid-Base Homeostasis and Its Disorders.* Flushing, New York: Medical Examination Publishing Co., 1971.

Weil, W., and Bailie, M. *Fluid and Electrolyte Metabolism in Infants and Children: A Unified Approach.* New York: Grune and Stratton, 1977.

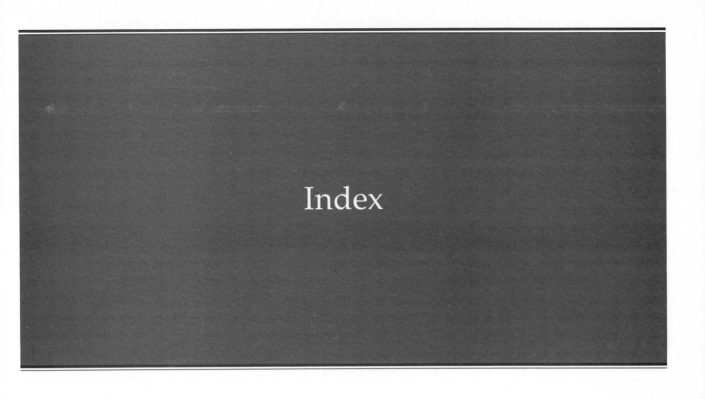

Index